MRCS
Core Modules
Essential Revision Notes

second edition

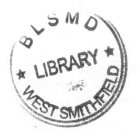
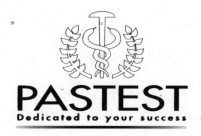

PASTEST
Dedicated to your success

MRCS
Core Modules
Essential Revision Notes

second edition

edited by

Sam Andrews MA MS FRCS (Gen)

Consultant General and Vascular Surgeon
Department of General and Vascular Surgery
Maidstone and Tunbridge Wells NHS Trust
Maidstone Hospital
Maidstone
Kent

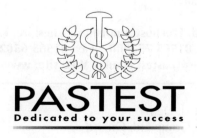

PASTEST
Dedicated to your success

© 2002 PasTest Ltd

Egerton Court
Parkgate Estate
Knutsford
Cheshire WA16 8DX
Telephone: 01565 752000

First published 1999
Reprinted 2001
Second edition 2002
Reprinted 2003

ISBN: 1 901198 71 5

A catalogue record for this book is available from the British Library.

The information contained within this book was obtained by the authors from reliable sources. However, while every effort has been made to ensure its accuracy, no responsibility for loss, damage or injury occasioned to any person acting or refraining from action as a result of information contained herein can be accepted by the publisher or the authors.

PasTest Revision Books and Intensive Courses

PasTest has been established in the field of postgraduate medical education since 1972, providing revision books and intensive study courses for doctors preparing for their professional examinations. Books and courses are available for the following specialties:

MRCS, MRCP Part 1 and Part 2, MRCPCH Part 1 and Part 2, MRCOG, DRCOG, MRCGP, MRCPsych, DCH, FRCA and PLAB.

For further details contact:

PasTest Ltd, Freepost, Knutsford, Cheshire, WA16 7BR
Tel: 01565 752000   Fax: 01565 650264
Email: enquiries@pastest.co.uk   Web site: www.pastest.co.uk

Typeset by Saxon Graphics Ltd, Derby
Printed and Bound by Alden Group Ltd, Oxford

Contents

Acknowledgements

All my co-authors for their help and contributions to this manuscript.
Kirsten Baxter and Cathy Dickens of PasTest, for their help on the Editorial side.
Lou Brimson and Phoebe Cooper for secretarial assistance.
Astrid, Bryony and Daisy for their forbearance.

Sam Andrews

Contributors

SECOND EDITION

Sam Andrews MA MS FRCS (Gen)
Consultant General and Vascular Surgeon, Department of General and Vascular Surgery, Maidstone and Tunbridge Wells NHS Trust, Maidstone Hospital, Maidstone, Kent
Peri-operative Management 1, Intensive Care and Neoplasia

James Brown MRCS
Specialist Registrar in Surgery, South East Thames Surgical Rotation
Neoplasia

Alistair R K Challiner FRCA FIMC.RCSEd DCH
Consultant Anaesthetist and Director Intensive Care Unit, Department of Anaesthetics, Maidstone Hospital, Maidstone, Kent
Intensive Care and Peri-operative Management 1

Nicholas D Maynard BA Hons (OXON) MS FRCS (Gen)
Consultant Upper Gastrointestinal Surgeon, Department of Upper Gastrointestinal Surgery, John Radcliffe Hospital, Headington, Oxford
Peri-operative Management 2

Gillian M Sadler MBBS MRCP FRCR
Consultant Clinical Oncologist, Kent Oncology Centre, Maidstone Hospital, Maidstone, Kent
Neoplasia

Hank Schneider FRCS (Gen. Surg)
Consultant General Surgeon, Department of Surgery, The James Paget Hospital, Great Yarmouth, Norfolk
Trauma

FIRST EDITION

Editors

Jeremy J Elkabir MBBS FRCS (Eng) FRCS (Urol) FEBU
Consultant Urologist, Northwick Park and St. Marks Hospital, London

Abbas Khadra MBChB AFRCS
Honorary Research Fellow, University College Medical School, London

Contributors

Ishtiaq Ahmed BSc (Hons) MRCS
Senior House Officer, General Surgery, St James University Hospital, Leeds
Perioperative Management 2

Sudipta Banerjee MBChB MRCS
Senior House Officer, Manchester Royal Infirmary, Manchester
Neoplasia

Ardeshir Bayat BSc (Hons) MBBS MRCS AFRCS
Senior House Officer, Plastic and Reconstructive Surgery Unit, Withington Hospital, Manchester
Neoplasia

William Cross BMed Sci BMBS MRCS
Senior House Officer, General Surgery, Royal Infirmary Hospital, Huddersfield
Perioperative Management 2

Daniel Fletcher MB ChB
Senior House Officer, General Surgery, Chesterfield and North Derbyshire Royal Hospital, Chesterfield
Intensive Care

Rachel Harling Bmed Sci BMBS
Senior House Officer, General Surgery, Southmead Hospital, Bristol
Trauma

Charles Imber BSc (Hons) FRCS MB BChir
Surgical Specialist Registrar, St Mary's Hospital, London
Perioperative Management 1

Paul Latimer MB ChB
Senior House Officer, Trauma and Orthopaedics, Frenchay Hospital, Bristol
Trauma

Oliver Priest MB ChB
Senior House Officer, Cardiothoracic Unit, St. Thomas' Hospital, London
Perioperative Management 1

Ghufran Syed BSc BM AFRCS (Edin)
Specialist Registrar in Accident & Emergency, Accident & Emergency Department, Kings College Hospital, London
Intensive Care

Introduction

It is now seven years since the new MRCS examination replaced the "old style" FRCS, and after some difficulties during the change over, the new system of surgical examinations is up and running well. The current system involves an entry to higher surgical training examination – the MRCS (or AFRCS) Diploma – of which the four Royal Colleges of Surgery each have their own examinations; and an exit examination – the Intercollegiate Fellowship Examination in Surgery.

Trainees in all surgical disciplines are expected to pass the common entry examination, whilst each discipline has its own Intercollegiate exit exam, e.g. General Surgery, Orthopaedic Surgery, Cardiothoracic surgery etc.

The four surgical Royal Colleges (Royal College of Surgeons of England, Royal College of Surgeons of Edinburgh, Royal College of Physicians and Surgeons of Glasgow and Royal College of Surgeons of Ireland) all have their own entry examination for surgical training. They are all very similar, interchangeable, and all allow qualification for the Intercollegiate exit examinations after the appropriate number of years of higher surgical training.

This book is designed as a revision guide for all the entry examinations, (MRCS, AFRCS) to higher surgical training. It is based loosely on the syllabus of the core modules of the MRCS of the English college. However, it is equally suitable as a revision aid for the examinations of the Edinburgh, Glasgow and Irish Colleges.

The aim of this book is not to cover all aspects of the syllabus for these examinations in detail, but rather to act as a guide to revision, to be used in combination with the more detailed texts such as the STEP course of the English College and the many other "heavy" texts on the market.

The style is designed to highlight "bullet" learning points and lists as a guide to the Multiple choice sections of the exams. However, aspects of critical care and tumour biology have been covered in more detail, to clarify these areas which are often considered the more difficult aspects of the examination.

This second edition has been revised and expanded to bring some of the clinical details up to date. Much of the basic science has been left unchanged from the first edition, although the text has been simplified, clinical examples added where appropriate, and a number of new tables and figures inserted.

We hope that you find this book useful in your revision and wish you well for your forth-coming examinations.

Sam Andrews
Nick Maynard
Hank Schneider
Alistair Challiner

Format of the Examination

The Royal College of Surgeons of England

The MRCS Diploma consists of:

- The multiple-choice question section
- The viva section
- The clinical section

The multiple-choice question (MCQ) section

- The MCQ section consists of two papers each of 2½ hours duration. The first will be based upon the core modules of the syllabus and the second on the system modules.
- Candidates may enter one or both papers on any occasion.
- Each paper will stand alone, candidates being awarded either a 'pass' or a 'fail'.
- Candidates may resit each of the MCQ papers as often as they wish.
- There is full reciprocity of recognition of a 'pass' in the MCQ section between all surgical colleges.

The viva section

- Candidates must have been awarded a 'pass' in both MCQ papers and completed 22 months of clinical surgical training before entering the viva section.
- The viva section consists of three vivas lasting 1 hour in total and comprising:
  - applied surgical anatomy with operative surgery
  - applied physiology and critical care
  - clinical pathology with principles of surgery
  Each viva lasts 20 minutes and consists of two 10-minute oral examinations.
- Communication skills.

The clinical section

- Candidates must have been awarded a 'pass' in both the MCQ and viva sections before entering this section of the examination.
- It lasts approximately 50 minutes and is based upon five bays of 'short cases' derived from all surgical specialties and relevant to the whole syllabus. It is likely that these bays will comprise of:
  - Superficial lesions (lumps and bumps)
  - Musculoskeletal and neurological cases
  - Circulatory and lymphatic cases
  - The trunk and abdomen

The format for the AFRCS offered by the Royal College of Surgeons in Edinburgh is almost identical to the MRCS, and consists of two multiple choice exams – Principles of Surgery in General and Systematic Surgery. Both papers can be taken at any time during the two years of basic surgical training.

The Royal College of Surgeons in Glasgow contain four 1-hour MCQ question papers covering: Anatomy, Physiology, Pathology and Clinical Surgery. These papers can be taken after a minimum of 9 months of basic surgical training. The MCQ papers are all held on the same day.

The Royal College of Surgeons in Ireland has three parts. There are four 1-hour papers, each containing 20 questions on: Surgical Anatomy, Surgical Physiology, Applied pathology, microbiology, immunology and Clinical surgery.

There is full reciprocity of recognition of a 'pass' in the whole MCQ section between all three UK Royal Surgical Colleges and the Royal College of Surgeons of Ireland.

Exam Technique

In the MCQ paper you **must** read the question carefully. Many wrong answers are given through misreading even though candidates know the answers. If you think an answer is true, but are not entirely sure, mark it as true. Additionally, you almost certainly will be correct more than 50% of the time, so you will score more marks overall than if you do not answer.

As far as Vivas go, start with single, common answers and build up slowly. Have your own system for answering a question. For example, when asked about the presentation of a tumour – All tumours present with – with features of the primary lesion, features of secondary spread and/or general effects of malignancy.

Both Viva and MCQ practice is very important and if you practice enough of them you will encounter questions in the examination that you have previously thought about.

Chapter 1

Peri-operative Management 1

CONTENTS

Peri-operative Management 1

1. PRE-OPERATIVE CARE

1.1 Assessment of fitness for anaesthesia and surgery

Prior to consideration of surgical intervention, it is necessary to prepare the patient as fully as possible. The extent of pre-operative preparation will depend on the:

- Situation: emergency: life-threatening condition requiring immediate action, (e.g. ruptured aneurysm, penetrating trauma)
  - urgent: surgery required within a few hours (e.g. appendicitis, wound debridement)
  - elective: (e.g. hip replacement, varicose vein surgery)
- Nature of the surgery, for example minor operations under local require less preparation than major abdominal operations
- Location: A&E, endoscopy, minor theatre, main theatre
- Facilities available

The rationale for pre-operative preparation is to

- Anticipate difficulties
- Make advanced preparation and organize facilities, equipment and expertise
- Enhance patient safety and minimize chance of errors
- Alleviate any relevant fear/anxiety perceived by patient

Assessment of fitness for surgery and anaesthesia includes:

- History
- Examination
- Special investigations
- Informed consent
- Marking the site/side of operation

- Thromboembolic prophylaxis
- Antibiotic prophylaxis

Assessment in advance of hospital admission, by pre-admission clerking appointment is growing in popularity, driven by the need for more efficient hospital bed occupancy. Protocols for adequate investigation should be available and an early anaesthetic opinion obtained for patients with significant co-existent morbidity.

Surgical history

History of presenting complaint

- This dictates the urgency for surgery and can influence anaesthetic management
- Systemic effects of the presenting pathology (e.g. bowel cancer – anaemia)

Past medical history

Many diseases have a direct effect on anaesthetic treatment and outcome, especially those of the cardiovascular and respiratory systems.

Anaesthetic history (and previous anaesthetic records): History of adverse effects to previous anaesthetic agents, post-operative pain, etc.

Family history: e.g. malignant hyperthermia, pseudocholinesterase deficiency, porphyria can influence safety.

Drug history

- Interaction with anaesthesia (e.g. MAOI – reaction with opioids causing possible coma)
- Problems related to sudden withdrawal (e.g. steroids)
- Allergy and acute anaphylaxis

Social history: smoking is related to an adverse peri-operative outcome.

Short-term: nicotine increases myocardial oxygen demand but paradoxically carbon monoxide reduces oxygen delivery by binding to haemoglobin (reversible if stopped prior to 12 hours pre-surgery).
Long-term: reduces immune function, reduced clearance of secretions and chronic airway disease (cessation needs to be >6–8 weeks to have an improvement) also related to ischaemic heart disease.

Examination

This should include a full physical examination. Don't rely on the examination of others – surgical signs may change and others may miss important pathologies.

- Examination of the surgical pathology, confirm the site, side etc.
- General examination – anaemia, jaundice etc.
- Cardiac examination – pulse, BP, JVP, heart sounds

- Respiratory examination – RR, trachea, percussion, auscultation, accessory muscles
- Abdominal examination – tenderness, scars, organomegaly
- CNS
- Musculoskeletal } as required
- Peripheral vasculature

1.2 Pre-operative investigations

Blood tests

Full blood count (FBC) provides:

- Haemoglobin concentration (12–16 g/dl in male, 11–14 g/dl in female)
- White cell count (5–10 × 10^9/l)
- Platelet count (150–450 × 10^9/l)

Also may reveal details of red cell morphology (e.g. macrocytosis in alcoholism, microcytosis in iron deficiency anaemia) and white cell differential (e.g. lymphopenia, neutrophilia).

When to perform an FBC:

- All emergency pre-operative cases especially abdominal conditions, trauma, sepsis
- All elective pre-operative cases over 60 years
- All elective pre-operative cases in adult females
- If surgery is likely to result in significant blood loss
- Suspicion of blood loss, anaemia, haemopoietic disease, sepsis, cardiorespiratory disease, coagulation problems

Urea and electrolytes (U & Es)

Provide: Sodium   (133–144 mmol/l)
          Potassium   (3.3–4.8 mmol/l)
          Urea   (2.5–6.5 mmol/l)
          Creatinine (55–150 μmol/l)

When to perform U&Es:

- All pre-operative cases over 65
- Positive result from urinalysis (e.g. ketonuria)
- All patients with cardiopulmonary disease, or taking diuretics, steroids or drugs active on the cardiovascular system
- All patients with a history of renal/liver disease or an abnormal nutritional state
- All patients with a history of diarrhoea/vomiting or other metabolic/endocrine disease
- All patients on an intravenous infusion for more than 24 hours

The incidence of an unexpected abnormality in apparently fit patients under 40 years of age is <1% but increases with age and ASA grading (American Society of Anaesthesiologists).

Amylase

Normal range varies with different reference laboratories.

Perform in all adult emergency admissions with abdominal pain, prior to consideration of surgery.

Random Blood Glucose (RBG)

Normal range 3–7 mmol/l
When to perform an RBG:

- Emergency admissions with abdominal pain, especially if suspecting pancreatitis
- Pre-operative elective cases with diabetes mellitus, malnutrition or obesity
- All elective pre-operative cases over 60 years
- When glycosuria or ketonuria are present on urinanalysis

Clotting

Prothrombin time (11–13 sec) measures the functional components of the extrinsic pathway prolonged with warfarin therapy, liver disease and disseminated intravascular coagulation (DIC).

Activated partial thromboplastin time (<35 sec) measures the functional components of the intrinsic pathway and is prolonged in haemophilia A and B, heparin therapy and DIC.

Bleeding time (<10 min) prolonged with platelet dysfunction and thrombocytopenia.

Sickle Cell Test

All patients of Afro-Caribbean origin.

Liver Function Tests

All patients with upper abdominal pain, jaundice, known hepatic dysfunction or history of alcohol abuse.

Group and Save/Crossmatch

When to perform a Group and Save:

- Emergency pre-operative cases likely to result in significant operative blood loss, especially trauma, acute abdomen, vascular cases
- Suspicion of blood loss, anaemia, haemopoietic disease, coagulation defects
- Procedures on pregnant females

For quantity of blood required in elective surgical operations refer to blood transfusion, Chapter 2.

Chest X-Ray (CXR)

When to perform a pre-operative CXR:

- All elective pre-operative cases over 60 years
- All cases of cervical, thoracic or abdominal trauma
- Acute respiratory symptoms or signs
- Previous cardiorespiratory disease and no recent CXR
- Thoracic surgery
- Patients with malignancy
- Suspicion of perforated intra-abdominal viscus
- Recent history of tuberculosis
- Recent immigrants from areas with a high prevalence of tuberculosis
- Thyroid enlargement

Urinanalysis

When to perform pre-operative urinanalysis:

- All emergency cases with abdominal or pelvic pain
- All elective cases with diabetes mellitus
- All pre-operative cases with thoracic, abdominal or pelvic trauma

A mid stream urine (MSU) specimen should be considered prior to genitourinary operations and in pre-operative patients with abdominal or loin pain.

Urine Pregnancy Test should be performed in all women of childbearing age with abdominal symptoms, or who require X-rays.

Electrocardiography (ECG)

A 12 lead ECG is capable of detecting acute or long-standing pathological conditions affecting the heart, particularly changes in rhythm, myocardial perfusion or prior infarction.

NB. The resting ECG is not a sensitive test for coronary heart disease, being normal in up to 50%. An exercise test is preferred.

When to perform a 12 lead ECG:

- Patients over 60, with hypertension/other vascular disease
- Patients undergoing cardiothoracic surgery, taking cardiotoxic drugs/with an irregular pulse
- Any suspicion of hitherto undiagnosed cardiac disease

Specific pre-operative investigations for patients with associated medical conditions are covered in section 2.

1.3 Thromboembolic prophylaxis

Venous thrombosis or deep vein thrombosis (DVT) is common in surgical patients. It can cause pulmonary embolism, which carries a high mortality and therefore should be prevented. It may also cause a post-phlebitic limb with ulceration many years later. This subject is covered in more detail in Chapter 2.

Incidence of DVT after common surgical procedures	
Type of operation	**Incidence (%)**
• Knee surgery	75
• Hip fracture surgery	60
• Elective hip surgery	50–55
• Retropubic prostatectomy	40
• General abdominal surgery	30–35
• Gynaecological surgery	25–30
• Neurosurgery	20–30
• Transurethral resection of prostate	10
• Inguinal hernia repair	10

Risk factors for venous thromboembolism

- Age
- Obesity
- Immobility (e.g. cardiac illness, stroke, infection)
- Malignancy
- Trauma, post-surgical
- Pregnancy, puerperium
- Past history of thromboembolism
- Oral contraceptives, hormone replacement treatment
- Thrombophilic patients (deficiency of ATIII, protein C, protein S, lupus anticoagulant positive, resistance to activated protein C)
- Dehydration

Prophylaxis: the highest risk of thromboembolism occurs at and immediately after surgery. Measures are therefore required to prevent venous thromboembolism in the peri-operative period:

Graded Elastic Compression stockings: should be well fitting, and applied pre surgery, and left on until mobile, except in cases of peripheral vascular ischaemia, e.g. patients for femoro-crural bypass.

Intermittent pneumatic calf compression: various devices available.

Electrical calf muscle stimulation

Post-operative leg elevation and early ambulation

Heparin prophylaxis: traditional unfractionated heparin, given 5000 units subcutaneously 2–4 hours before surgery and continued twice daily until mobile. This has been largely superceded by low molecular weight heparin (LMWH). Various regimes are available. Advantages of LMWH are less propensity to bleeding, longer half-life, requiring only once daily administration and a lower incidence of heparin induced thrombocytopenia and heparin induced osteoporosis. Heparin prophylaxis should be discontinued 24 hours prior to administration or withdrawal of epidural anaesthesia, to prevent bleeding into the epidural space.

Other agents affecting blood coagulability: anti-platelet agents, e.g. aspirin, dipyridamole, dextran have been tried. Although they do reduce platelet activity, none are widely used for DVT prophylaxis. Oral anticoagulants, e.g. warfarin are not used for surgical DVT prophylaxis due to the unacceptably high risk of haemorrhage.

1.4 Consent

Patients have a right to information about their condition and the treatment options available to them. Informed consent should be sought prior to investigation, treatment, screening or research.

Informed consent should include

- Details of the diagnosis and prognosis, and the prognosis if the condition is left untreated
- Options for management of the condition, including the option not to treat
- A detailed explanation of the proposed procedure(s), including subsidiary treatment such as pain relief
- What the patient may experience during or after the procedure, including common and serious side-effects
- For each option explanation of risks and benefits
- The name of the doctor(s) who will have responsibility for treatment
- A reminder that patients may change their minds and/or seek further opinions
- An opportunity for patients and relatives to ask questions

The amount of information given to a patient will vary with factors such as the nature of the condition, the complexity of the treatment and the patient's wishes and understanding. Generally speaking it is necessary to warn patients of complications with >1% incidence.

Ideally the clinician performing the treatment should obtain consent. If this is not possible consent should be obtained by a suitably qualified person with sufficient knowledge of the proposed investigation, treatment and risks. Informed consent can be verbal, or written, although it is always better to have a written record that consent has been obtained. Patient advice leaflets and visual aides are a useful adjunct to obtaining consent.

Special considerations

Emergencies

In an emergency where consent cannot be obtained, medical treatment should be limited to what is immediately necessary to save life or to avoid significant deterioration, until full informed consent can be obtained.

Diminished or fluctuating capacity

Where patients have difficulty retaining information, or are only intermittently competent to make a decision, it may be necessary to provide assistance in the decision(s). This should be carefully documented. If patients lack capacity to decide, provided they comply, you may initiate investigation or treatment judged to be in their best interest.

Children

- At age 16 a young person can be treated as an adult
- Age under 16, depends on ability to understand
- When too young to understand requires parental consent

1.5 Criteria for consideration of day care surgery

Definition: *A patient admitted for investigation or operation on a planned non-resident basis, but who nonetheless requires facilities for recovery.*

May be performed under general, regional or local anaesthesia.

Advantages

- A firm date and time for operation with less risk of cancellation
- Minimum time away from home (especially in paediatric surgery)
- Greater efficiency of operating list scheduling
- Release of inpatient beds
- Cost effectiveness

Disadvantages

- Requirement of adequate aftercare at home
- Restriction of surgery and anaesthesia to experienced staff
- Requirement for inpatient admission or readmission in cases of unexpected, complications, inadequate analgesia etc.

Patients should have full verbal and printed instructions including

- A brief description of the surgical problem
- An outline of the nature of the surgery to be undertaken
- Pre-operative instructions
- Post-operative instructions, as well as details about the nature of possible complications, what to do about them, and when and who to contact for advice
- Advice on when to return to work and other activities
- Instructions about any appropriate appointments for follow-up or suture removal

Contraindications to day surgery

Medical

- Unfit (not ASA class I or II)
- Obese – body mass index >35
- Specific problems (e.g. recurrent hernias)
- Extent of pathology (e.g. large scrotal hernia)
- Operation longer than 1 hour
- Psychologically unsuitable
- Concept of day surgery unacceptable to patient

Social

- Lives over 1 hour drive from the unit
- No competent relative or friend to accompany or drive patient home after surgery and/or look after the patient at home for the first 24–48 hours post-operatively
- At home, no access to a lift (for an upper floor flat), telephone or indoor toilet and bathroom

Some common procedures suitable for day care surgery

General Surgery

- OGD
- Colonoscopy
- Hernia repair – inguinal, femoral, umbilical, para-umbilical and epigastric
- Varicose vein surgery
- Excision of breast lumps
- Anal stretch
- Pilonidal sinus

Urological Surgery

- Circumcision
- Cystoscopy ± biopsy
- Hydrocoele surgery
- Excision of epididymal cyst
- Reversal of vasectomy

ENT Surgery

- Myringotomy and insertion of grommets
- Direct laryngoscopy and pharyngoscopy
- Submucous resection
- Submucosal diathermy of turbinates

Orthopaedic Surgery

- Carpal tunnel release
- Release of trigger finger
- Dupuytren's contracture surgery
- Arthroscopy
- Amputation of finger or toe
- Ingrowing toenails

cont...

continued...

Paediatric Surgery
- Circumcision
- Inguinal herniotomy
- Hydrocoele surgery

- Repair umbilical hernia
- Orchidopexy

Ophthalmic Surgery
- Cataract surgery

- Correction of squint

Plastic Surgery
- Correction of 'bat' ears
- Blepharoplasty
- Breast augmentation

- Insertion of tissue expanders
- Nipple and areola reconstruction

Gynaecological Surgery
- D & C
- Termination of pregnancy

- Laparoscopy
- Laparoscopic sterilization

Other considerations
Day surgery should ideally be performed in dedicated day-case units, controlling their own waiting lists, scheduling etc. They should ideally be on the ground floor, with their own entrance, wards, theatres, staff etc. Patient satisfaction, adequacy of post operative analgesia, complications and admission rates should be regularly audited.

2. MANAGEMENT OF ASSOCIATED MEDICAL CONDITIONS

2.1 Respiratory disease

Chronic obstructive pulmonary disease and asthma

Chronic obstructive pulmonary disease (COPD) is pathologically distinct, but frequently co-exists with bronchospasm. It may be difficult to determine the importance of each condition in an individual. Generalized air flow obstruction is the dominant feature of both diseases.

History and examination

- Patient exercise tolerance (e.g. walking distance on flat)
- Recent deterioration resulting in hospital admission
- Previous admission to ITU for ventilation
- Need for home oxygen/present medical therapy (i.e. need for steroids)
- Whether currently smoking, or when stopped
- Changes on examination consistent with chronic lung disease/focal infective exacerbations etc.

Investigation

Assess baseline levels with lung function tests, for example:

- FEV_1/FVC ratio, if <50% the risk of post-op respiratory failure is increased
- Arterial blood gases confirming carbon dioxide retention in pure chronic bronchitis
- Sputum cultures and sensitivity in the presence of a productive cough
- Chest X-ray

Management

- Pre-operative salbutamol (nebulizers)
- Any reversible component must be treated (e.g. infective exacerbations)
- Consider regional anaesthesia for body surface/lower extremity surgery
- Intra-operatively nitrous oxide can rupture bullae leading to a tension pneumothorax, use opioids in doses that are not associated with pronounced respiratory depression
- Humidification of inspired gases
- Post-op: advice regarding smoking; chest physiotherapy; continuous positive airway pressure (CPAP) administration in an HDU setting; adequate pain relief allowing deep breathing and early mobilization; nurse in an upright position in bed, monitoring oxygen saturation.

Hypoxia in the peri-operative setting is most commonly due to inadequate ventilation or respiratory depression with opiates rather than loss of hypoxic drive due to prolonged high concentration oxygen therapy. However, the latter should always be borne in mind when dealing with a patient with chronic respiratory disease.

Tuberculosis (TB)

Many patients have evidence of old TB disease or previous anti TB surgery on CXR. This is not usually a problem, but the resulting lung change and reduced respiratory capacity may need consideration.

Active TB should be considered in recent immigrants from areas where TB is endemic, immunosuppressed and HIV patients. They may require a pre-operative CXR, sputum culture, Mantoux testing (if they haven't had previous BCG) and treatment if appropriate.

2.2 Cardiovascular conditions and hypertension

Ischaemic heart disease

Pre-operatively

Known risk factors must be identified in the history (e.g. smoking, hypertension, hyperlipidaemia, diabetes, including a positive family history). A careful examination of the heart and lungs must be performed.

New York Heart Association (NYHA) classification

- **Grade 1**
  No limitation on ordinary physical activity

- **Grade 2**
  Slight limitation on physical activity; ordinary activity results in palpitations, dyspnoea or angina

- **Grade 3**
  Marked limitation of physical activity; less than ordinary activity results in palpitations, dyspnoea or angina

- **Grade 4**
  Inability to carry out any physical activity without discomfort; symptoms may be present at rest

Recent myocardial infarction dramatically increases the risk of re-infarction in the peri-operative period, i.e. 80% in the first 3 weeks, 25–40% in the first 3 months and 10–15% from 3–6 months. After 6 months the risk drops to 5% and is normally the minimum time period that is an acceptable risk for an elective procedure. Obviously the risk must be balanced against any potential benefit of a surgical procedure.

Investigation of all patients with previous cardiac disease includes an ECG, CXR and monitoring of FBC (correction of anaemia if present) and electrolytes if not performed recently. An anaesthetist/cardiologist may well require more sensitive tests of cardiac function in a patient with ongoing symptoms, such as an exercise ECG or an echocardiogram with left ventricular ejection fraction measurement. The most detailed information can be obtained by a coronary angiogram, if possible therapeutic intervention is being considered for severe disease.

Intra-operatively

- Keep the patient well oxygenated
- Avoid changes in heart rate
- Avoid falls in blood pressure, especially diastolic
- Avoid fluid overload
- Good surgical technique resulting in as short an operating time as can safely be performed with the minimal amount of blood loss. Such 'high-risk' patients should be operated on by a more experienced surgeon.

Hypertension

If the diastolic blood pressure is >110 mmHg then elective procedures should be discussed with the anaesthetist and possibly postponed until better control can be achieved. (Always be aware of patient anxiety about being in hospital or the forthcoming surgery, i.e. 'white coat hypertension', and if necessary take three separate BP readings, separated by a period of at least an hour.)

Newly diagnosed hypertension must be assessed for possible reversible aetiological factors (e.g. renal disease, endocrine disease, pregnancy, oral contraceptive pill and coarctation of the aorta).

Chronic (longstanding) hypertension puts the patient at increased risk of cardiovascular disease, cerebrovascular events and renal impairment. These conditions need to be excluded or optimized if possible prior to an elective surgical procedure. Left ventricular hypertrophy (whether clinically, radiologically or electrocardiographically detected) is directly related to myocardial ischaemia. Poorly controlled hypertension in the immediate pre-operative period predisposes the patient to peri-operative cardiac morbidity and must be avoided.

Post-operative hypertension is common and most often due to pain.

2.3 Diabetes mellitus

Reasons for good glycaemic control

- Prevention of ketosis and acidaemia
- Prevention of electrolyte abnormalities and volume depletion secondary to osmotic diuresis
- Impaired wound strength and wound healing when plasma glucose concentration >11 mmol/l
- Hyperglycaemia interferes with leucocyte chemotaxis, opsonization and phagocytosis and thus leads to an impaired immune response
- Avoidance of hypoglycaemia in an anaesthetized patient

Pre-operative precautions

- Full pre-operative history and examination – diabetes is associated with increased risk of ischaemic heart disease, hypertension, peripheral vascular disease (PVD), autonomic and peripheral neuropathy, renal failure, impaired vision.
- Check urea and electrolytes
- Urinalysis for proteinuria
- ECG
- Confirm adequate glycaemic control (see below)

Peri-operative precautions

- Place first on operating list (reduces period of starvation and risk of hypoglycaemia)
- Protect pressure areas (especially with PVD and neuropathy)

NIDDM: optimize control pre-operatively and continue normal oral hypoglycaemic control until the morning of surgery (except chlorpropamide which may need to be reduced or stopped 48 hours in advance). Post-operatively monitor BM regularly and institute a sliding scale of intravenous insulin if the patient is unable to tolerate oral diet immediately. Restart the patient back on their normal oral hypoglycaemic regimen as soon as enteral diet is recommenced.

IDDM: achieve good pre-operative control and admit the patient the night before surgery. Monitor the patient's BM from admission, and commence the patient on a sliding scale of insulin on the morning of surgery. Restart insulin once the patient is eating and drinking normally and observe closely for sepsis. Only discharge the patient once their control is within recognized limits as their insulin requirements may well increase transiently after a stressful stimulus such as surgery.

2.4 Renal failure

Classification of renal failure

- **Pre-renal**
  e.g. haemorrhage (blood)
  burns (plasma)
  vomiting (crystalloid)
- **Renal**
  e.g. diabetes
  glomerulonephritis
- **Post-renal**
  e.g. retroperitoneal fibrosis (medially deviated ureters)
  benign prostatic hyperplasia (with chronic retention)
  pelvic malignancies

Fluid and electrolyte balance may be deranged and drug/metabolite excretion disturbed. Severe uraemia can directly affect the cardiovascular, pulmonary, haematological, immunological and central nervous systems.

Complications encountered may include:

- Fluid overload, oedema
- Hypoalbuminaemia (nephrotic syndrome)
- Electrolyte abnormalities – hyperkalaemia, hyponatraemia
- Metabolic acidosis

Management of established renal failure:

- Dialysis prior to surgery with regular monitoring of fluid/electrolyte balance
- Reduce doses of drugs excreted by kidney

NB. When establishing IV access in a patient with severe end-stage renal failure avoid potential arteriovenous fistula sites (e.g. cephalic vein).

2.5 Jaundice

Fluid balance

Hypoalbuminaemia and fluid overload are common in jaundiced patients and lead to pulmonary/peripheral oedema as well as ascites. There may be sodium retention and hypokalaemia due to secondary hyperaldosteronism which may be further complicated by the use of spironolactone or other diuretics.

Acid-base balance

A combined metabolic and respiratory alkalosis may occur. This will cause the oxygen dissociation curve to shift to the left and decrease oxygen delivery to the tissues.

Clotting

Due to a decrease in vitamin K absorption in cholestatic jaundice there is reduced synthesis of factors II, VII, IX and X and there may also be a thrombocytopenia if there is portal hypertension (due to hypersplenism).

Hepatorenal syndrome

Renal failure may be precipitated by hypovolaemia.

Drug metabolism

Many drugs, including anaesthetic agents, undergo metabolism by the liver and may therefore have a prolonged duration of action.

Other complications

Hypoglycaemia may occur due to depleted glycogen stores.

Wound failure and infection increased in the jaundiced patient.

Risk of infectivity to surgeon and hospital personnel if infective hepatitis. Patients require hepatitis screen if considered high-risk.

Child's classification of the severity of chronic liver disease

	A	B	C
Bilirubin	<35	35–50	>50
Albumin	>35	30–35	<30
Ascites	None	Mild–moderate	Severe
Encephalopathy	None	Mild	Advanced
Nutrition*	Good	Moderate	Poor
Risk of surgery	Good	Fair	Poor

*Pugh's modification replaces nutrition with prothrombin time

Management of a jaundiced patient

- If possible relieve jaundice prior to surgery (e.g. an endoscopically performed sphincterotomy to drain common bile duct stones)
- Keep the patient well hydrated in an attempt to avoid hepato-renal syndrome
- Check the prothrombin time and administer vitamin K 10 mg IV daily (maximum effect after 3 doses) or fresh frozen plasma within 2 hours of a surgical procedure
- In the presence of biliary obstruction/anticipated manipulation of the biliary tree administer prophylactic antibiotics to avoid cholangitis

2.6 Malnutrition and obesity

Malnutrition

Many patients, especially those with chronic disorders, malignancy and dementia may be suffering from malnutrition. Surgery may induce anorexia and temporary intestinal failure, exacerbating the problem. The post-operative catabolic state and the stress (inhibition of the normal ketotic response) can cause muscle metabolism and weaken the patient.

Malnutrition predisposes to:

- Delayed wound healing
- Delayed maturation of collagen
- Predisposition to respiratory problems

Assessment of malnourished patients

History

- Duration of illness
- Weight loss
- Reduced appetite
- Risk factors e.g. alcohol, malignancy

Examination

- Sunken eyes
- Loose skin
- Reduced tissue turgor
- Apathy
- Weight loss

Investigation

- Arm circumference/triceps skinfold thickness
- Serum albumin
- Full blood count
- Transferritin
- Retinol binding protein

Malnourished patients requiring elective surgery should be considered for pre and peri-operative feeding. This may include enteral supplements, nasogastric/nasoduodenal fine bore tube feeding, feeding gastrostomy/jejunostomy, or parenteral nutrition (peripheral or central).

Obesity

Obese patients are at increased risk of surgical complications for many reasons:

- Poor quality abdominal musculature predisposes to wound infection and dehiscence.
- Increased adipose tissue predisposes to haematoma formation and subsequent wound infection
- Obese patients are more prone to hyperglycaemia
- Surgery takes longer and is more difficult due to problems of access and obscuring of vital structures by intra-abdominal fat deposits
- Technical problems arise with intravenous cannulation and subsequent phlebitis
- Decreased chest wall compliance, inefficient respiratory muscles and shallow breathing cause an increased risk of pulmonary infections

For elective surgery in obese patients pre-operative assessment should include:

- Measurement of the patient's body mass index (BMI) (i.e. weight (kg)/height^2 (metres))
- Referral to a dietitian
- Blood glucose estimation and restoration of glycaemic control
- The measurement of blood gases – hypoxia and hypercarbia reflect respiratory impairment; and respiratory function tests – forced expiratory volume in one second (FEV$_1$)/forced vital capacity (FVC) of less than 75% in patients with obstructive pulmonary disease.

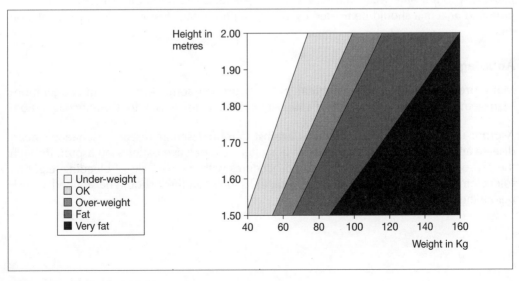

Body mass index for adults

2.7 Anaemia and anticoagulants

Anaemia

A pre-operative finding of anaemia (Hb <12g/dl in male, Hb <11g/dl in female) requires investigation. In emergency cases where there is no time for further pre-operative investigation, correction of anaemia (by transfusion) may be required to be part of resuscitation whilst surgical intervention is ongoing. (See blood transfusion in Peri-operative Management 2, section 3.4)

In elective cases a cause for anaemia should be sought.

History

- Acute or chronic blood loss e.g. menorrhagia
- Dietary
- Malignancy
- Chronic disorders

Examination

Investigations

- Differential blood count (macrocytic anaemia e.g. alcohol), folate deficiency (e.g. dietary), microcytic anaemia (e.g. chronic bleeding, iron deficiency)
- Investigation of GI tract (OGD, colonoscopy)
- Investigation of renal tract (IVU, cystoscopy)

Reversible causes of anaemia should be corrected before elective surgery. Mildly anaemic patients who are otherwise well may tolerate general anaesthesia and surgery well. More profound anaemia should be treated by consideration of transfusion, iron supplementation etc.

Anticoagulants

Many pre-operative elective surgical patients are on some form of anticoagulation. Management depends on the type of anticoagulation and the reason for the anticoagulation.

Aspirin: usually given as prophylaxis against cerebrovascular disease, ischaemic heart disease and peripheral vascular disease. It is often safe to leave patients on aspirin through the peri-operative period, but in certain procedures with special risks of bleeding, e.g. thyroidectomy, TURP it should be stopped. Due to its long half-life it should be stopped a week before the proposed date of surgery.

Heparin: low molecular weight heparin is usually given subcutaneously throughout the peri-operative period for DVT prophylaxis (see DVT prophylaxis, section 1.3). It may be stopped 24 hours before the proposed date of surgery in procedures with special risks of bleeding, or where the use of epidural anaesthesia is anticipated.

Intravenous heparin has a more profound anticoagulant effect, but a shorter half-life, and only needs to be discontinued 6 hours before a procedure.

Warfarin: has a more prolonged anticoagulation effect. It is usually given to patients with special risk of thrombosis e.g. artificial heart valves, thrombophilia, previous deep venous thrombosis or pulmonary embolism.

Warfarin effect is monitored by INR measurement

- INR = 0.8 – 1.2   Normal coagulation
- 1.2 – 2.0   Mild anticoagulation – moderate risk of surgical bleeding
- 2.0 – 3.5   Normal therapeutic range – severe risk of surgical bleeding
- >3.5   Severe anticoagulation – surgery should not be contemplated until INR reduced.

Elective surgery

Warfarin should be stopped 2–3 days prior to surgery, and the INR checked on the day of surgery. Patients with catastrophic consequences of thrombosis, e.g. artificial heart valve should be started on intravenous or subcutaneous heparin to maintain anticoagulation until the time of surgery.

Emergency surgery

Anticoagulation effects should be rapidly reversed, for example using fresh frozen plasma or vitamin K, prior to surgery.

2.8 Steroids and immunosuppression

Steroid therapy

Indications for peri-operative corticosteroid cover

- Pituitary-adrenal insufficiency on steroids
- Undergoing pituitary or adrenal surgery
- Patients on systemic steroid therapy of >7.5 mg for >1 week before surgery
- Patients who have had a course of steroids for >1 month in the last year

Complications of steroid therapy in the peri-operative period

- Poor wound healing
- Increased risk of infection
- Addisonian crisis with vomiting and cardiovascular collapse
- Side-effects of steroid therapy (e.g. impaired glucose tolerance, osteoporosis, muscle wasting, fragile skin and veins, peptic ulceration)
- Mineralocorticoid effect, i.e. sodium and water retention, potassium loss and metabolic alkalosis
- Masking of sepsis/peritonism

Management
This depends on the nature of the surgery to be performed:

- Minor: 50 mg hydrocortisone IM/IV pre-operatively
- Intermediate: 50 mg hydrocortisone IM/IV with pre-med and 50 mg hydrocortisone every 6 hours for 24 hours
- Major: 100 mg hydrocortisone IM/IV with pre-med and 100 mg hydrocortisone every 6 hours for at least 72 hours after surgery.

Equivalent doses of steroid therapy: hydrocortisone 100 mg; prednisolone 25 mg; dexamethasone 4 mg.

3. THE OPERATING THEATRE ENVIRONMENT

3.1 Theatre design

Position – theatres ideally should be close to the surgical wards, ITU, sterile supplies unit, A&E and radiology/CT.

Layout – clean areas/corridors should be separate from dirty areas/sluices etc. Anaesthetic rooms should be adjacent to theatre. Adequate space is required for storage, staff recreation etc.

Environment – Ideal temperature of 20–22°C to maintain patient and staff comfort.

- Humidity control
- Clean filtered air – enters via ceiling, leaves via door flaps. Higher pressure in ultra clean/clean areas, lower in dirty areas.
- Power, piped gas, anaesthetic gas scavaging system, suction
- Adequate lighting

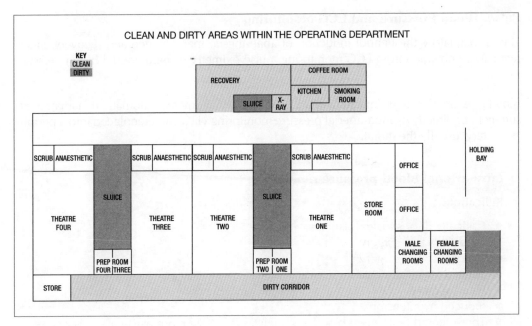

Theatre design

3.2 Care and monitoring of the patient in theatre

This starts on entering the theatre complex.

Pre-induction – correct identification of patient, operation, site, side, starved (if for GA), allergies, blood available (if required).

Recommendations for standards of monitoring of the Association of Anaesthetists of Great Britain and Ireland.

- Continuous presence of an adequately trained anaesthetist and clinical observation
- Regular arterial pressure and heart rate measurements (recorded)
- Continuous display ECG throughout anaesthesia
- Continuous analysis of gas mixture oxygen content (with audible alarm)
- Oxygen supply failure alarm
- Tidal/minute volume measurement
- Ventilator disconnection alarm
- Pulse oximeter
- Capnography with moving trace
- Temperature measurement available

Pulse, Blood Pressure and ECG Monitoring

This is mandatory throughout induction of anaesthesia, maintenance and recovery. Heart rate can be obtained from ECG monitoring, pulse oximetry or intra-arterial blood pressure monitoring.

Blood pressure can be estimated by manual sphygmomanometry, automatic dynamap measurement or directly by intra-arterial pressure monitoring via a catheter placed into a peripheral artery, usually the radial.

Intra-arterial blood pressure monitoring

Indications

- Critically ill or shocked patients
- Cardiothoracic surgery
- Major vascular surgery
- Surgery for phaeochromocytomas
- Neurosurgery
- Induced hypotension
- Those requiring frequent blood gas analysis (i.e. severe pre-existing lung disease undergoing any major operation)

Complications

- Embolization
- Haemorrhage
- Arterial damage and thrombosis
- Sepsis
- Tissue necrosis
- Radial nerve damage

Pulse oximetry

Pulse oximeters measure the arterial oxygen saturation (SaO_2), not the partial pressure of oxygen (PaO_2). Probes are attached to either fingers or ear lobes and contain two light emitting diodes (one red, one infra-red) and one detector.

The instrument pulses infra-red light of wavelengths 660 nm to 940 nm through the tissues. A constant 'background' amount is absorbed by skin, venous blood and fat, but a changing amount is absorbed by the pulsatile arterial blood. The constant amount is subtracted from the total absorbed to give the amount absorbed by arterial blood. Because oxygenated and deoxygenated Hb absorb differing amounts at the two wavelengths, the instrument is able to calculate a percentage of saturated Hb from the ratio of the two. Skin pigmentation does not affect the readings.

However, observation of the haemoglobin dissociation curve may show that a significant fall in the PaO_2 occurs before the SaO_2 decreases (15–20 sec delay).

Problems with pulse oximetry

- Delay: calculations are made from a number of pulses hence there is a delay of about 20 seconds between the actual and displayed values
- Abnormal pulses: atrial fibrillation; hypotension/vasoconstriction; tricuspid incompetence (pulsatile venous component)
- Abnormal Hb or pigments: CO poisoning (e.g smokers); methaemoglobinaemia; bilirubin
- Interference: movement/shivering; electrical equipment (e.g. diathermy); bright ambient light (e.g. in theatre)
- Poor tissue perfusion; nail varnish (coloured or not)

NB. Pulse oximetry only measures oxygenation, not ventilation. CO_2 content of blood is a reflection of ventilation (measured using a capnograph or ABGs).

Urine output

Renal perfusion is closely linked to cerebral perfusion. Urine output is a good indicator of renal perfusion and thus of overall fluid balance and adequate resuscitation in a sick patient.

Catheterization and hourly urine measurement is mandatory in

- Massive fluid or blood loss
- Shocked patients, whatever the cause
- Major cardiac/vascular/general surgery
- Surgery in jaundiced patients (hepatorenal syndrome)
- Pathology associated with major fluid sequestration 'third space loss' (e.g. bowel obstruction, pancreatitis)

Central Venous Pressure lines

CVP lines are useful for measuring the central venous pressure and for administering total parenteral nutrition (TPN) or toxic drugs (e.g. vancomycin). They should be placed with the tip in the superior vena cava if they are to provide a guide to circulating volume status.

They are indicated in critically ill patients and in major surgery if there is likely to be a complicated post-operative course, or in patients with a poor cardiac reserve where fluid balance may prove difficult to assess correctly.

The most common approaches are via the internal jugular or subclavian vein, the latter being more hazardous in a patient with chronic lung pathology where there is an increased risk of pneumothorax. An aseptic Seldinger technique is employed using a metal guide wire.

Complications of central venous lines

- **Common**
  Sepsis
  Pneumothorax
  Incorrect placement (position should be confirmed with a chest X-ray)

- **Less common**
  Brachial plexus injury
  Phrenic nerve injury
  Carotid or subclavian artery puncture
  Thoracic duct injury

- **Uncommon but potentially fatal**
  Tension pneumothorax
  Air embolism (head down position in ventilated patient) employed during
    insertion, aspirate blood prior to flushing lines)
  Haemothorax
  Lost guide wire

Pulmonary artery pressure catheters (Swan–Ganz catheters)

These may be required when the central venous pressure (CVP) does not correlate with pressure in the left atrium as in the following conditions:

- Left ventricular failure
- Interstitial pulmonary oedema
- Valvular heart disease
- Chronic severe lung disease

They are also of value for the calculation of cardiac output and systemic vascular resistance (e.g. use of inotropes following cardiac surgery).

Most catheters have at least four lumens:

- Distal lumen (at the tip) which should lie in a peripheral pulmonary artery
- Proximal lumen ~25 cm from the tip, which should lie in the right atrium
- Balloon lumen
- Thermistor lumen used to measure temperatures

The catheter is inserted into a central vein, connected to an oscilloscope and advanced into the right atrium (shown by the venous waveform). The balloon is then inflated with air and floated into the right ventricle and then into the pulmonary artery. Further advancement will occlude a branch of the pulmonary artery and show a typical 'wedging' waveform. When occluded there is a column of fluid from the end of the catheter to the left atrium and left arterial pressure can be measured. The balloon is then deflated to prevent pulmonary infarction.

Cardiac output can be measured indirectly by infusing a small amount of cold glucose solution through the proximal lumen and measuring the temperature with the thermistor. If the volume and temperature are known the degree of dilution can be determined and thus the cardiac output can be calculated.

3.3 Injury to the anaesthetized patient

This can be caused by general hazards e.g. transferring anaesthetised patients on and off the operating table, or by specific hazardous events e.g. use of diathermy/laser/tourniquet.

Pressure areas injury

- Risk factors: elderly, immobile, steroids, peripheral vascular disease
- Risk areas: sacrum, heels, back of head
- Prevention: padding, heel protectors

Joint injury

- Risk factors: lithotomy position, "breaking" the table
- Risk areas: prosthetic hip joints, cervical spine, limbs
- Prevention: co-ordinated lifting, head support, care with transfers

Eye injury

- Eyes should be closed and taped

Nerve injury

- Risk factors   : excessive arm abduction
- Risk areas   : brachial plexus
- Prevention   : abd <80° pronate hand and turn head

- Risk areas   : ulnar nerve causing claw hand
- Prevention   : excessive flexion, avoid full flexion trauma with poles from stretchers

- Risk areas   : lat. popliteal causing foot drop
- Prevention   : padding nerve of fibula in lithotomy position

- Risk areas   : femoral nerve causing loss of knee extension
- Prevention   : avoid extension of hip

Skin injury

- Burns – may be due to diathermy earth, by patient touching metal on operating table or by use of flammable skin preparation, which may be ignited by diathermy.

- Allergies – to dressings or skin preparations
- Explosions – may be caused by flammable skin preparations, or ignition of anaesthetic or colonic gases

Muscle injury

- Compartment syndromes may occur after prolonged surgery e.g. in lithotomy position

3.4 Diathermy

Principles

- Passage of high-frequency alternating current through body tissue
- No stimulation of neuromuscular tissue at frequencies above 50 kHz
- Safe passage of currents up to 500 mA at frequencies of 400 kHz to 10 MHz
- Locally concentrated currents (high density) generate local temperatures of up to 1000°C

Settings

Cutting

- Continuous output
- High local temperature causes tissue disruption, some vessel coagulation and vaporization of water

Coagulation

- Pulsed output of high-frequency current at short intervals
- Tissue water vaporization and vessel coagulation

Blend

- Continuous sine wave current with superimposed bursts of higher intensity

Monopolar

- High power unit (400 W) generates high-frequency current
- Current passes from active electrode (HIGH current density), (held by surgeon) through body, returning via patient plate electrode (LOW current density) to generator
- Forceps point, spatula or diathermy scissors commonly used
- Alternate return pathway if patient touching earthed metal objects (may cause burns in older machines). Most modern diathermy machines do not have earth-referenced generators.

Patient plate electrode

- Good contact on dry, shaved skin; kinking must be avoided
- Contact surface area at least 70 cm^2 – minimal heating

- Away from bony prominences and scar tissue (poor blood supply means poor heat distribution)
- Normally on patient's thigh or back

NB. Incorrect placement is the most common cause of accidental diathermy burns. Most systems have an alarm system if there is a fault.

Bipolar

- Lower power unit (50 W)
- Current passes between two limbs of diathermy forceps only
- No need for patient plate electrode
- Inherently safer BUT no use for cutting or touching other instruments to transfer current (buzzing)
- Useful for surgery to extremities: scrotum, penis or on digits

Use with pacemakers

Diathermy may

- Affect pacemaker function or cause myocardial burn
- Bipolar wherever possible, with careful ECG monitoring

If using monopolar:

- Away from heart – short bursts (<2 secs) at long intervals

Diathermy safety

- Ensure patient not touching earthed metal (older machines)
- Pooling of inflammable agents (alcohol, inflammable gases)
- Pedal
- Lowest practicable power setting
- Active electrode in contact with target tissue and in view
- Do not use too close to important structures (skin, blood vessels, nerves)
- No monopolar on narrow pedicles (penis, digits, dissected tissue block, spermatic cord)
- Place plate away from metallic implants (e.g. prosthetic hips)

Causes of diathermy burns

- Incorrect plate electrode placement
- Careless technique e.g. using spirit based skin preparation fluid, not replacing electrode in a quiver after use
- Use of diathermy on appendages (e.g. penis) where a high current can persist beyond the operative site
- Use of diathermy on large bowel should be avoided as explosions have been reported

3.5 Tourniquets

Used to prevent bleeding in limb surgery or isolate limb for perfusion (e.g. Bier's block). Should not be used as a first aid measure to arrest bleeding.

Application

Simple tourniquets e.g. elastic tourniquet for phlebotomy, rubber tourniquet for digital surgery e.g. ingrowing toenail.

Limb tourniquets: check monitor or cuff before application. Ensure application to correct limb and adequate breadth tourniquet (too thin may cause pressure necrosis). Apply tourniquet before skin preparation, avoiding vital structures e.g. testicles. Place plenty of padding beneath tourniquet.

Inflate appropriately to 50 mm/Hg over systolic pressure in upper limb, 100 mmHg over systolic pressure in lower limb for adults. Note the time of applications.

The cuff should be deflated to allow reperfusion every 90 mins (upper limbs) or 120 mins (lower limb).

Complications of tourniquets

- Damage to skin, soft tissues or joints during application
- Chemical burns due to skin preparation getting under tourniquet
- Pressure necrosis from overtight tourniquet, insufficient padding on prolonged application
- Distal ischaemia, venous or arterial thrombosis
- Haemorrhage following release

3.6 Lasers

LASER – **L**ight **A**mplification by the **S**timulated **E**mission of **R**adiation

Lasers produce light by high voltage stimulation of a medium, causing it to emit photons which are then reflected around the medium exciting other particles, which release further photons in phase with the initial photons. This process is repeated until a very high density of inphase photons is achieved (coherent light), some of which is allowed to escape through a partially reflected mirror (the beam).

Action of the beam at cellular level

- Vaporize tissue by evaporating water: for cutting or ablation
- Coagulating proteins: for haemostasis

Advantages of lasers

- Access: can reach difficult areas as the beam can be projected through narrow spaces, or down endoscopes
- Selective effects: e.g. argon lasers selective absorption of red pigments e.g. blood vessels
- Precision: very fine beams can be used for cutting and/or coagulation
- Minimal damage to surrounding tissues

Dangers of lasers

- Retinal or corneal damage
- Fire risk
- Damage to structures beyond the target if burns through target
- Burns (patient or operator)
- The beam may be invisible

Examples of uses:

- Argon-beam laser – eye surgery, endoscopic ablations
- CO_2 (Carbon Dioxide) laser – ENT ablation surgery, cervical ablation surgery
- Nd YAG laser – Endoscopic debulking surgery or GI bleeder coagulation, laparoscopic surgery

3.7 Precautions in Hepatitis and HIV Patients

Protection of the patient from sources of infection in the operating theatre is covered in Section 6.

Surgeons, anaesthetists, theatre nurses, operating department assistants and other theatre personnel also need protection from potentially infectious agents.

Sources of infection

- Contact - blood, saliva, urine, tears, CSF, stool
- Airborne – following use of power tools
- Inoculation – via needle stick injuries, scalpel injuries

Universal precautions

Refers to the precautions taken to protect theatre staff from infection with all cases. e.g. surgical gloves, gowns, masks, no touch surgical technique.

Special precautions

These are used for high risk surgical patients e.g. Hepatitis and HIV patients. In an ideal world all procedures would be performed using special precautions, but in practice the level of precaution is limited by expense, time etc.

- Disposable drapes and gowns
- Double-gloving and use of 'indicator' glove systems
- Face visors
- Use blunt suture needles
- Pass instruments in a kidney dish
- 'No-touch' technique
- Minimize theatre staff
- Only vital equipment in theatre
- Some of the special precautions should be undertaken with all patients (e.g. high-risk patients or areas)

Special precautions are also used for infective cases to prevent spread of infection to other patients e.g. MRSA.

4. ANAESTHESIA

4.1 Principles of anaesthesia

Definition: *The rendering of part (local anaesthesia [LA]) or all (general anaesthesia [GA]) of the body insensitive to pain or noxious stimuli.*

GA induces

- Narcosis (unconsciousness)
- Analgesia
- Muscle relaxation

in a controlled and reversible manner, so the patient suffers no pain and has no recollection of the experience, and the surgeon has ideal operating conditions.

Includes

- Pre-operative assessment and preparation
- Induction
- Maintenance and monitoring
- Recovery
- Post-operative monitoring and transfer

ASA Classification

ASA Grading (American Society of Anesthesiologists) classification of physical status

- **Class 1**
  Normal healthy individual

- **Class 2**
  Patient with mild systemic disease

- **Class 3**
  Patient with severe systemic disease that limits activity, but is not incapacitating

- **Class 4**
  Patient with incapacitating disease that is a constant threat to life

- **Class 5**
  Moribund patient not expected to survive with or without an operation

4.2 Local and regional anaesthesia

Characteristics of local anaesthetics

- Work by altering membrane permeability to prevent passage of nerve impulses
- Stored as acidic salt solutions. Following infiltration the base is released by the relative alkalinity of the tissue (hence LA ineffective in acidic conditions e.g. infected wounds)
- Dosage 1% = 10 mg/ml therefore 2% is 20 mg/ml etc.
- Often used in combination with GA, to reduce opiate analgesic and GA requirements
- Ideal LA has low toxicity, high potency, rapid onset, long duration

Complications of LA

Toxicity

- May occur from overdosage, inadvertent intravenous administration, or cuff failure in Bier's block
- Causes perioral tingling and paraesthesia, anxiety, tinnitus, drowsiness, unconsciousness, seizures, coma, apnoea, paralysis and cardiovascular collapse
- Management of toxicity: stop administration of LA, then ABC resuscitation – protect airway, intubate and ventilate if necessary. IV fluids, consider inotropic support.

LOCAL ANAESTHESIC AGENTS

	Max. dose	+Adrenaline	Use
Lignocaine (Lidocaine)	3 mg/kg	5 mg/kg infiltration	Infiltration Nerve blocks Epidurals
Bupivacaine (Marcain)	2 mg/kg	3 mg/kg nerve blocks	Infiltration Epidurals Spinals – high cardiotoxic
Prilocaine	6 mg/kg	6 mg/kg	Regional nerve blocks, Bier's block, high cardiotoxic
Cocaine			ENT
Ropivacaine			Like Bupivacaine but less cardiotoxic

Local anaesthetics should be used at their lowest concentration and warmed to body temperature to decrease pain on injection. Adrenaline may be used with local anaesthetics to slow systemic absorption and prolong duration of action. NB. Never use near end-arteries (e.g. digits, penis) as may result in ischaemic necrosis.

Routes of administration

Topical (e.g. EMLA cream before cannulation in children, Lignocaine gel before urethral catheterization, Xylocaine spray before gastroscopy).

Direct infiltration (e.g. removal of skin lesions).

Field block (e.g. inguinal hernia repair).

Ring block (for digits or penis).

Individual nerve block (e.g. femoral nerve block for fractured shaft femur, sciatic block, ankle block. May be given using nerve stimulator to identity nerve).

Plexus block (e.g. brachial plexus block).

Intravenous regional anaesthesia (e.g. Bier's block for Colles' fracture of wrist).

Epidural (extradural): injection into the extradural space with a large bore needle – includes caudal block – injected into epidural space via sacral canal.

Spinal (subarachnoid block): injection into the subarachnoid space with a fine bore needle.

Bier's block

- Intravenous regional anaesthesia
- Usually upper limb

Technique: Intravenous access – both arms!
                Exsanguinate limb (e.g. Eschmark bandage)
                Apply double cuff tourniquet (with padding)
                Inflate upper cuff to approximately 300 mmHg
                Inject approximately 40 ml 0.5% prilocaine IV into isolated arm
                Inflate lower cuff (over anaesthetized segment)
                Release upper cuff (reduces cuff pain and acts as safeguard)

Spinal anaesthesia

- Introduced via fine bore needle into spinal (subarachnoid space)
- Low dose, low volume, rapid (<5mins) onset.
- Duration 3–4 hours
- Mainly used for peri-operative pain relief

Complications

- Toxicity
- Hypotension (avoid in severe cardiac disease)
- Headache, meningism, neurological disturbance
- Urinary retention

Epidural anaesthesia

- Introduced via large bore needle or catheter into extradural space
- High dose, high volume, delayed (>5 mins) onset
- Duration: continuous infusion – up to a few days
- Can be used for peri and post-operative pain relief

Complications

- Dural tap
- Backache
- Infection
- Haematoma
- Urinary retention

4.3 Premedication and sedation

Premedication: objectives

- Anxiolytic
- Sedation and enhancement of hypnotic effect of general anaesthetic
- Amnesia
- Drying of secretions
- Antiemetic
- Increase vagal tone

Sedation – administration of drug(s) to alleviate discomfort and distress during diagnostic and therapeutic interventions, but with maintenance of patient responsiveness and protective reflexes.

Benzodiazepines – sedative, anxiolytic and amnesic.

e.g. **Midazolam** can be used for:

- Induction of anaesthesia
- Sedation during endoscopy and procedures performed under LA
- As a hypnotic
- For premed
- In the treatment of chronic pain
- Water soluble, short duration, rapid clear-headed recovery
- Dose 0.05–0.1mg/kg by slow IV injection
- May cause oversedation or respiratory depression
- Can be reversed with Flumazenil (which may itself cause seizures)
- All patients having Midazolam sedation should have IV access, pulse oximetry, ECG monitoring, resuscitation facilities available and should not drive or operate machinery for 24 hours afterwards.

Temazepam: 10–20 mg oral (1 hour) pre surgery.

Diazepam: oral or IV. Longer duration and more difficult to reverse.

Droperidol: a Butyrophenone. Antiemetic, neuroleptic, alpha-blocker. Prolonged duration action and 'locked in' syndrome may cause problems. Rarely used.

Opioids: analgesic and sedative.

e.g. Papaveretum (Omnopon®) 20 mg IM, Morphine 10 mg IM. Can be reversed with Naloxone (Narcan).

Anticholinergics: competitive acetylcholine antagonists at muscarinic receptors.

Dry secretions, prevent reflex bradycardia.
e.g.   Atropine, 300–600 microgram IV pre induction.

Glycopyrronium: less chronotropic effect. Doesn't cross blood brain barrier, 200–400 micrograms IV/IM pre induction.

Hyoscine (Scopolamine®): as Atropine, but more sedative and antiemetic. May cause bradycardia, confusion, ataxia in elderly, 200–600 micrograms SC/IM 60 min pre induction.

Antacids: used to prevent aspiration of gastric contents (Mendelson's syndrome) in patients at risk e.g. pregnancy, trauma patients (not starved), obese, hiatus hernia.

e.g. Cimetidine 400 mg oral   1–2 hours pre surgery
      Ranitidine 50 mg IV or 150 mg oral   1–2 hours pre surgery
      Omeprazole 20 mg oral   12 hours pre surgery

4.4 Induction agents

Induction – administration of drug(s) to render patient unconscious prior to commencement of surgery. May be intravenous or inhalational (see section 4.6). Intravenous route is quicker, but requires IV access, so inhalation induction may be method of choice in children.

Intravenous induction agents are liquid soluble, and thus hydrophobic. Intravenous induction agents are also used for maintenance of anaesthesia, by slow IV infusion.

Thiopentone sodium is a commonly used induction agent. It is a barbiturate which appears as a pale yellow powder with a bitter taste and a faint smell of garlic. It is given in an alkaline solution (pH 10.8) and thus is irritant if injection occurs outside the vein. It causes a smooth and rapid induction but has a narrow therapeutic window and overdose may cause cardiorespiratory depression. It is a negative inotrope and can result in a drop in blood pressure. There is often associated respiratory depression. It sensitizes the pharynx and cannot be used with laryngeal airways.

Propofol is more expensive than thiopentone but has the advantage of a slight antiemetic effect. It is a phenol derivative which appears as a white aqueous emulsion, and may cause pain on injection. It gives a rapid recovery without a 'hangover' and has a lower incidence of laryngospasm which makes it the agent of choice if using a laryngeal mask. It causes vasodilatation and is a negative inotrope resulting in a drop in blood pressure therefore not recommended for hypovolaemic patients.

Etomidate: Less myocardial depression, so better used in cardiovascularly unstable patients.

Complications of induction agents

- Hypotension
- Respiratory depression
- Laryngeal spasm
- Allergic reactions
- Tissue necrosis from perivenous injection

Effects especially pronounced in hypovolaemic patients.

Contraindications: previous allergy/porphyria.

4.5 Muscle relaxants

Depolarizing muscle relaxants – work by maintaining muscle in depolarized (or relaxed) state. Main example Suxamethonium.

Suxamethonium has a structure similar to two acetylcholine molecules and acts in the same way at the neuromuscular junction. The rate of hydrolysis, by plasma cholinesterase, is however much slower, thus depolarization is prolonged resulting in blockade. Its action therefore cannot be reversed. Because it acts on the acetylcholine receptor there is an initial period of muscle fasciculation which may be painful and distressing to the patient.

It is the most rapid-acting of all the muscle relaxants and is therefore useful when rapid tracheal intubation is required (crash induction). It has a duration of 2–6 minutes in normal individuals, but some people have a deficiency of plasma cholinesterase and thus have prolonged response (scoline apnoea).

Depolarizing muscle relaxants

Complications and contraindications of depolarising muscle relaxants

- **Complications**
  Muscle pain
  Hyperkalaemia
  Myoglobinaemia
  Bradycardia
  Hyper- or hypotension
  Malignant hyperpyrexia

- **Contraindications**
  Patients prone to hyperkalaemia, especially burns victims
  History or family history of malignant hyperpyrexia
  History or family history of bronchospasm

Non depolarizing muscle relaxants

All have slower onset than Suxamethonium, but longer duration.

Atracurium or benzylisoquinolinium – intermediate duration.

Atracurium undergoes non-enzymatic metabolism independent of hepatic or renal function and thus has a safety net advantage for critically ill patients. It does, however, cause significant histamine release in some people, which can cause cardiovascular problems or redness at the site of injection.

Other benzylisoquinolinium   Cisatracurium
    Gallamine

Vecuronium   An aminosteroid. Intermediate duration.
Other aminosteroids   Pancuronium

Reversal agents: Neostigmine is used to reverse nondepolarising neuromuscular blockade, but the resulting muscarinic action may induce a profound bradycardia and is therefore given with atropine or glycopyrronium.

Factors causing prolonged neuromuscular blockade

- Hypothermia
- Acidosis
- Hyperkalaemia
- Increasing age
- Concurrent use of suxamethonium
- Inhalational anaesthetics

Myasthenia gravis patients have a lower number of post-synaptic receptors due to auto-antibodies against them, which therefore makes the patient more sensitive to nondepolarizing muscle relaxants but resistant to suxamethonium.

4.6 Inhalational anaesthetics

Usually used for maintenance of anaesthesia, after IV induction, but can be used for induction e.g. in children.

Halothane is a volatile liquid anaesthetic of the halogenated hydrocarbon class. Inhalation is well tolerated and non-irritant, which means that it rarely causes the patient to cough or hold their breath. It is a very potent anaesthetic. Halothane causes respiratory depression resulting in the retention of carbon dioxide. In addition, it is a negative inotrope, resulting in a decrease in heart rate and blood pressure. It is also a mild general muscle relaxant.

The major disadvantage of halothane is its association with severe hepatotoxicity (1 in 30,000) with a 50% mortality. The risk is increased with repeated exposures over a short period of time and is known to occur in theatre personnel where there have been inadequate or faulty gas exhaust systems.

Like all inhalational anaesthetics, apart from nitrous oxide, it is also associated with malignant hyperthermia.

Contraindications:

- Pyrexia following administration of halothane or a history of jaundice is an absolute contraindication to its use.

Enflurane is a halogenated ether volatile liquid anaesthetic. It causes respiratory and myocardial depression resulting in a decrease in cardiac output and a rise in $PaCO_2$. It is best avoided in epilepsy as it has been shown to cause EEG changes. It may cause hepatotoxicity and hyperthermia but less commonly than halothane. Free fluoride ions are a product of metabolism and may result in the very rare complication of fluoride-induced nephrotoxicity.

Isoflurane is the inhaled anaesthetic of choice for most surgical procedures and is also a halogenated ether. It is an isomer of enflurane but only an insignificant amount is metabolized by the patient. Hepatotoxicity is rare and malignant hyperthermia is as common as with other agents. Respiration is depressed and respiratory tract irritation may occur. There is a decrease in systemic vascular resistance due to vasodilatation and blood pressure falls. This may result in an increase in heart rate and rarely in 'coronary steal' syndrome.

Sevoflurane is a recently introduced volatile liquid anaesthetic. It produces a rapid induction and recovery which means that post-operative pain relief must be planned well.

Nitrous oxide is a potent analgesic but only a weak anaesthetic. This would therefore require greater than atmospheric pressure to produce effective anaesthesia. It does, however, potentiate the effect of other inhalational anaesthetic agents allowing a reduction in the dose required. A mixture of 50% nitrous oxide and oxygen (entonox) is used for analgesia, especially in obstetrics and emergency departments. Nitrous oxide will diffuse into any air-containing space. It diffuses more rapidly than nitrogen, and can lead to distension of the bowel. It must not be used in those who have recently been diving, exposed to high atmospheric pressures or who are suspected of having a gas-filled space (e.g. pneumothorax or pneumocephalus).

Exposure to nitrous oxide for prolonged periods of time causes suppression of methionine synthetase which leads to myelosuppression and a megaloblastic anaemia. Prolonged exposure should therefore be avoided.

4.7 Complications of anaesthesia

Malignant hyperpyrexia

This condition may be triggered by all inhalational anaesthetics, except nitrous oxide, and also by suxamethonium. It is a rare life-threatening condition (1 in 150,000) which requires recognition and treatment.

It is a familial disorder thought to be of autosomal dominant inheritance in which there appears to be a rapid influx of Ca^{2+} into muscle cells resulting in actin/myosin activation and muscle rigidity.

Signs include hyperthermia, muscle rigidity, tachycardia, tachypnoea and DIC. There is an increase in oxygen demand and carbon dioxide production leading to a metabolic acidosis, as well as hyperkalaemia.

Treatment
Dantrolene sodium 1 mg/kg by rapid IV injection, repeated to a maximum dose of 10 mg/kg. Surface cooling and cool IV fluids may be administered. Hyperventilation will help reduce $PaCO_2$. The patient will need to be nursed on ITU and carefully monitored for signs of renal failure. The patient and family must be counselled as to further risks and the possibility of genetic inheritance.

5. PRINCIPLES OF SURGERY

5.1 Techniques of biopsy

Definition – Retrieval of part or all of tissue or organ for histological evaluation to ascertain future management. Specifically to:

- Determine tissue diagnosis where clinical diagnosis in doubt e.g. Tru-cut® liver biopsy for cirrhosis of unknown aetiology
- Ascertain whether benign or malignant e.g. gastric ulcer biopsy
- Ascertain extent of spread of disease e.g. sentinel node biopsy in melanoma
- Determine different therapeutic pathways e.g. lymph node biopsy in lymphoma
- Excise whole skin lesion for histological analysis and local treatment e.g. excision biopsy for rodent ulcer

Biopsy is merely a form of special investigation and should be interpreted in the light of the clinical picture.

Fine needle aspiration biopsy for cytology (FNAC)

Is performed by inserting a fine bore needle into a lesion, aspirating cells and performing a smear on a slide to allow cytological examination.

It can be performed:

- Directly into a lump e.g. thyroid lump FNAC
- Under ultrasound control e.g. breast lump FNAC
- Under CT guidance e.g. liver lesion FNAC

Advantages

- Simple and minimally invasive
- Easily repeatable
- Cheap

Disadvantages

- Gives cytological, but not architectural histology
- Potential for spread of malignant cells
- Sample may be insufficient, or only blood may be aspirated
- May alter morphology of lesion for subsequent imaging
- Depends on expertise of cytologist – may be operator dependent

Brush cytology

Is performed by collecting exfoliated cells usually using a brush, from intraluminal lesions and performing a smear on a slide to allow cytological examination.

It can be performed

- Endoscopically for gastroduodenal lesions
- At ERCP for biliary or pancreatic lesions
- Bronchoscopically for pulmonary or bronchial lesions

Advantages/disadvantages as for FNAC, except in addition false negatives may occur as the tumour may not be reached, or may not shed sufficient cells.

Core biopsy

Uses a circular cutting device to retrieve a core of tissue, either manually or with a trigger device (Tru-cut®, Bioptigun®). As FNAC may be direct, ultrasound or CT controlled. Useful for breast, liver and lymph node biopsy.

Advantages

- Simple, easily repeatable
- Provides a core of tissue architectural and cytological evaluation

Disadvantages

- Insufficient sample
- May cause bleeding
- May be painful or distressing to patient
- Potential for spread of malignant cells
- May alter morphology of lesion for subsequent imaging

Endoscopic biopsy e.g. gastrointestinal tract, airways and sinuses, bladder, uterus.

Advantages

- Avoids open surgery

Disadvantages

- Operator dependent – lesions may not always be seen or reached
- Bleeding
- Perforation
- Small samples – malignant areas may be missed

Excisional biopsy

Is performed when the whole lesion is excised to give histological diagnoses. Usually applies to skin tumours e.g. basal cell carcinoma, melanoma.

Incisional biopsy

Is where part of a lesion is removed to allow histological diagnosis.

- May be performed laparoscopically or open
- May be useful when other biopsy techniques have failed
- Performed when the lesion is too big or too fixed to allow complete excision

Frozen section

Is where fresh tissue is sent for rapid histological assessment, during the course of an operative procedure, to allow therapeutic decisions to be made at the time of surgery. The tissue is frozen in liquid nitrogen then rapidly sectioned and examined, and the result phoned back to the theatre.

Uses

- Assess operability e.g. to examine lymph nodes in pancreatico-duodenectomy
- Localize tissues e.g. parathyroids
- Assess tumour margins
- Assess malignant status where pre-operative diagnosis is in doubt and more radical surgery may be required

Disadvantages

- Operator and histologist dependent
- Occasional false positive and false negatives
- May delay surgical procedure

5.2 Excision of cysts and benign tumours of skin and subcutaneous tissues

Many skin and subcutaneous lumps can be left alone. Reasons for consideration of excision:

- Diagnosis – when histology required e.g. risk of malignancy
- Pain
- Enlargement – small lesions are easier to excise than large
- Infection – e.g. ingrowing toenail
- Cosmesis

Techniques

Many skin and subcutaneous lumps can be removed using local anaesthesic. Skin lesions are best excised with elliptical incisions around the lesion. Subcutaneous lesions may be excised through linear incisions over the lesion. (NB. Epidermal cysts are skin lesions and are best excised with elliptical incisions including the punctum). Incisions should be along or parallel to Langer's lines, tension lines or skin creases.

Benign lesions can be excised with small margins, approximately 1 mm. Malignant lesions require bigger margins, 5–10 mm for basal cell carcinomata or squamous cell carcinomata depending on site. Margins for excision of malignant melanomata is a topic of some debate and depends on the thickness of the melanoma, which may not be known until after it has been excised. It is sometimes necessary to excise superficial melanoma with a 2–3 mm margin, and be prepared to return for wider excision depending on the histology and thickness of the lesion.

Closure can be with subcuticular, continuous or interrupted suture, or with glue (see section 5.6). Closure may be easier if the edges are undermined to relieve tension. Infected wounds may be left open, or closure delayed.

Complications

- Incomplete excision – may lead to recurrence
- Infection
- Dehiscence
- Scarring (including hypertrophic scars and keloid)
- Damage to surrounding structures – especially nerves

Special considerations

- Suspected malignant lesions are often best treated in specialist units where other modalities of treatment may be considered
  e.g. basal cells carcinomata can be considered for radiotherapy
  e.g. malignant lymph nodes require other investigations after excision

- Lesions in difficult anatomic positions may need specialist techniques
  e.g. lesion close to the eye by ophthalmic surgeons
  e.g. lesions on the face by plastic surgeons
- Children may require general anaesthesia

5.3 Drainage of abscesses

Definition: Abscess – a localized collection of pus – is a normal response of the body to infection. Left alone many abscesses will drain spontaneously.

Diagnosis
Abscess may be difficult to distinguish from cellulitis. The former requires surgical drainage, the latter may respond to antibiotics. Abscess may be inferred if the area is pointing or the centre is fluctuant. If in doubt needle aspiration or ultrasound may help.

Treatment
Superficial skin abscesses may be lanced. Deeper abscesses require general anaesthesia. A cruciate incision is made, pus is released, some is sent for microbiological analysis, the cavity may be irrigated or curetted and is then gently packed. Packs are changed frequently until the cavity closes. Antibiotics are not usually indicated.

Complications

- Inadequate drainage (especially loculated abscesses)
- Damage to adjacent structures
- Persistent cellulitis – may require antibiotics

Special cases

- Neck abscesses – may be due to simple abscess, furuncle, infected epidermal cysts or branchial cysts, abscess in lymph node, dental abscesses, actinomycosis or TB (cold abscess)
- Perianal abscesses – is usually infection in the anal glands. Other causes include fistulae, Crohn's, tumours and HIV.
- Breast or axillary abscesses are occasionally related to underlying malignancy
- Groin abscesses may be due to suppurating lymph nodes, TB, or psoas abscess (tracking down from the kidney or lumbar spine)

5.4 Basic principles of anastomosis

Gastrointestinal and genitourinary anastomosis require

- Good blood supply
- Good size approximation (avoid mismatch) and accurate apposition
- No tension
- No holes or leaks (good surgical technique)

Good surgical technique includes:

- Do not perform anastomoses in 'watershed' areas
- Adequate mobilization of the ends
- Inversion of the edges to discourage leakage
- Consideration of pre-operative bowel preparation to prevent mechanical damage to the anastomosis
- Consideration of the type of suture material (absorbable v non-absorbable, continuous v interrupted v stapled
- Prophylactic antibiotics – to cover bowel organisms including anaerobes
- Single layer v double layer – ischaemia of ends v leak rate

Factors leading to anastomotic dehiscence:

- Poor surgical technique
- Premorbid factors e.g. malignancy, malnutrition, old age, sepsis, immunosuppression, steroids, radiotherapy

In the presence of the above conditions, or if the bowel is of dubious viability or there is great size disparity it may be worth considering a defunctioning colostomy proximal to the anastomosis.

Vascular anastomoses

- May be between arteries, veins, prosthetic materials or combinations of these
- Everted edges to prevent intimal disruption
- Prophylactic antibiotics – especially antistaphylococcal cover
- Use smallest needles and suture strong enough to hold anastomosis
- Usually continuous non-absorbent suture, which pulls through easily e.g. Proline®

5.5 Minimal access surgery

Surgical procedures performed through incisions or via orifices, smaller than or remote from those required for conventional surgery.

Examples

- General surgery –
  laparoscopic procedures e.g. laparoscopic cholecystectomy
  laparoscopic appendicectomy
  laparoscopic assisted colectomy
- Urological procedures
  e.g. cystoscopy, transurethral resection of prostrate (TURP) or bladder tumour (TURBT), retroperitoneoscopic nephrolithotomy, ureteroscopic lithotripsy laparoscopy for undescended testicle
- Orthopaedic procedures
  e.g. arthroscopic meniscectomy
  arthroscopic cruciate ligament repair
- Thoracic procedures
  e.g. thoracoscopic sympathectomy
- Vascular procedures
  e.g. transluminal angioplasty
  retroperitoneoscopic sympathectomy

- Gynaeological procedures   e.g. hysteroscopic evacuation of the retained products of conception (ERPC)
  laparoscopic sterilization

Advantages

- Smaller wounds/less tissue trauma/fewer wound complications
- Short hospital stay
- Quicker return to normal activities/shorter rehabilitation
- Reduced analgesic requirement
- Reduced post operative adhesions
- Television screen pictures facilitates teaching

Disadvantages

- Requires sophisticated and expensive equipment
- Learning curve
- Complication rate – damage to other structures, e.g. small bowel in laparoscopic surgery, bladder perforation in TURBT
- Loss of tactile feedback
- May be difficult to control bleeding
- May take longer
- Laparoscopic surgery may be impractical due to previous adhesions

5.6 Suture and ligature materials

Features of ideal suture material:

- Monofilament
- Strong
- Easy handling
- Minimal tissue reaction
- Holds knots well
- Predictable absorption

Classification

- Absorbable   v   non-absorbable
- Monofilament   v   multifilament
- Synthetic   v   natural

Types of sutures

Absorbable
- Catgut   Biological origin from sheep or ox intestine; twisted, monofilament, undyed and uncoated
- Collagen   Biological origin from ox achilles tendon; rolled monofilament, undyed and uncoated

- Polyglycolic acid   Man-made homopolymer; braided multifilament, dyed or undyed, coated or uncoated; trade name *Dexon*
- Polygactin 910   Man-made copolymer; coating is calcium stearate, glycolide and lactide
- Polyglecaprone   Man-made copolymer, monofilament, dyed or undyed; trade name *PDS* (polydioxanone sulphate)
- Polyglyconate   Man-made copolymer; monofilament, dyed or undyed; trade name *Maxon*

Non-absorbable
- Silk   Biological origin from silk worm; braided multifilament, dyed or undyed, coated or uncoated; coating is wax
- Linen   Biological origin from flax plant; twisted multifilament, dyed or undyed, uncoated
- Cotton   Biological origin from cotton seed plant; twisted multifilament, dyed or undyed and uncoated
- Polyester   Man-made; multifilament; dyed or undyed, coated or uncoated; trade name *Ethibond* or *TiCron,* and *Mersilene* or *Dacron* (uncoated)
- Polyamide   Man-made, monofilament or multifilament, dyed or undyed, trade name *Ethilon* or *Dermalon* (monofilament) and *Nurolon* (braided) or *Surgilon* (braided nylon)
- Polypropylene   Man-made, monofilament, dyed or undyed; trade name *Prolene*
- PVDF   Man-made, monofilament, dyed or undyed, trade name *Novafil*
- Steel   Man-made, monofilament or multifilament

Selection of suture materials

- Absorbable sutures for tissues which heal quickly (e.g. bowel anastomosis)
- Non-absorbable sutures for tissues which heal more slowly (e.g. abdominal wall closure)
- Smooth (monofilament) sutures for running stitches (e.g. vascular surgery)
- Braided sutures for knotting properties (e.g. ligating pedicles)
- Smaller sutures for fine stitching (e.g. 6.0 or 7.0 proline for tibial arteries)
- Larger sutures for strong stitching (e.g. 1 nylon for abdominal wall closure)

6. SURGICAL INFECTION

6.1 Pathophysiology of the body's response to infection

Inflammation is the body's response to injury. Injury may be traumatic, infective, neoplastic, autoimmune etc. The purpose is to remove, destroy or isolate the cause of the injury, and repair the damage.

Acute inflammation

Rapid onset, limited duration response to injury.

Features

- Local vasodilatation
- Fluid and plasma protein exudation
- Leucocyte migration (mainly neutrophils) and activation
- Calor (heat), rubor (redness), tumor (swelling), dolor (pain) and loss of function

Chronic inflammation

Longer duration response to continued injury, with ongoing repair.

Features

- Blood vessel and connective tissue proliferation
- Lymphocyte and macrophage migration and activation
- Fibrosis, repair
- In some cases granulomata formation

Surgical infections may be due to

- Pathogenic organisms
- Infection with normal body commensals
- Infection with saprophytic organisms from soil, plants etc.

Pathogenicity of surgical infections depends on the

- Virulence of the pathogen
- Level of host defence
- Nature of the infection

Conventional infections – affect previously healthy individuals
Conditional infections – require predisposing factor
Opportunistic infections – immunosuppressed host

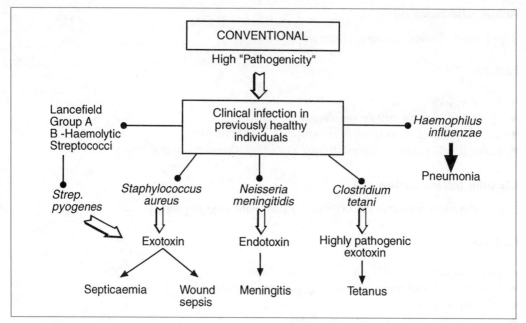

Conventional pathogens

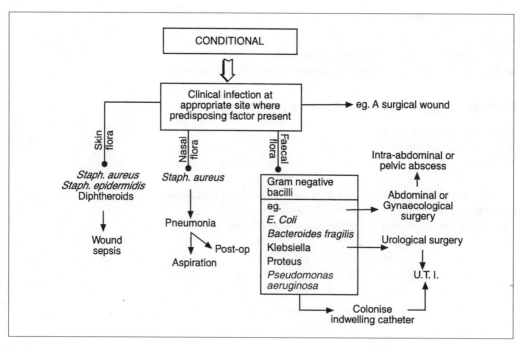

Conditional pathogens

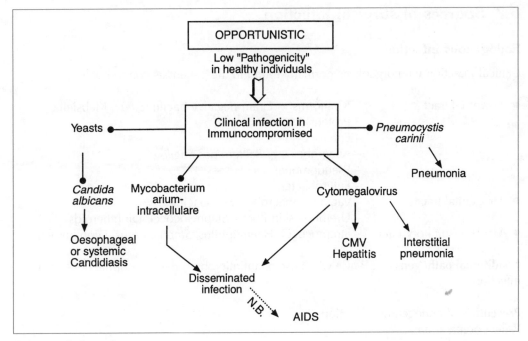

Opportunistic pathogens

Mechanisms of virulence

Exotoxins

- Usually Gram-positive bacteria e.g. Clostridia
- Highly toxic, highly antigenic polypeptides
- Specific target sites
- Excreted by living bacteria
- Neutralised by anti-toxins
- Include enterotoxins e.g. *S. aureus, E. coli*

Endotoxins

- Lipopolysaccharide molecules in outer layer of Gram-negative cell walls
- Stimulate non-specific release of mediators from inflammatory cells
- Severe endotoxaemia is life-threatening

Capsules

- Capsule enhances invasiveness
- Increased resistance to phagocytosis
- Reduced effectiveness of bacterial killing within macrophages and polymorphs

6.2 Sources of surgical infection

Endogenous infection

Clinical infection with organisms normally found in the patient as commensals.

- Lower GI tract
  - 'Coliforms' = Gram-negative bacilli (*E.coli*, Klebsiella, Proteus)
  - Enterococci
  - Anaerobes e.g. *Bacteroides fragilis*
  - Pseudomonas
  - Enterobacter
- Urogenital tract
  - Vagina – anaerobes, lactobacilli
  - Urethra – skin flora – Staphylococci, Diphtheroids
- Upper respiratory tract
  - Streptococci, Haemophilus, *Staph. aureus*, Diphtheroids

Conditional pathogens – colonise when use of antimicrobials destroy normal flora – 'super-infection'.

Prevention of endogenous infection
Patient preparation:

- Disinfect skin
- Bowel preparation
- Appropriate antibiotic prophylaxis

Avoid disrupting normal flora: antibiotics only for specific infection.

Treat sepsis with full course antibiotics not prophylaxis (inadequately treated infections encourage bacterial resistance).

Exogenous infection

Clinical infection acquired from an external source, incidence is low (2%):

- Hospital staff
- Hospital environment
- Other patients

Wound sepsis

- Asepsis = no organisms present during surgery; truly aseptic environment needed in immunocompromised patients
- Antisepsis = prevention of sepsis; total abolition of organisms not achieved

Clean wounds

- Incision through non-inflamed tissue
- No entry into genitourinary/GI/respiratory tracts

Contamination: <2% (exogenous sepsis)

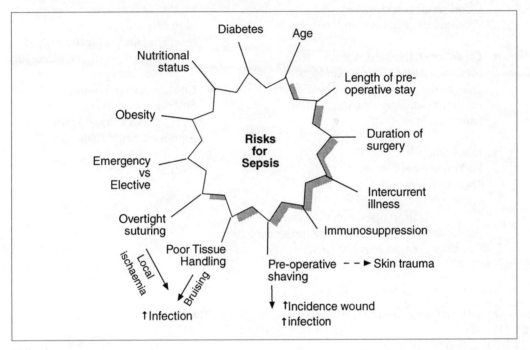

Risks for sepsis

Clean–contaminated wounds

- Entry into a hollow viscus other than the colon with minimal, controlled contamination
Contamination: 8–10%

Contaminated wounds

- Breaching of hollow viscus with more spillage: opening the colon, open fractures, penetrating animal or human bites.
Contamination: 12–20%

Dirty wounds

- Gross pus, perforated viscus (e.g. faecal peritonitis) or traumatic wounds >4 hours.
Contamination: >25%

Prevention of wound sepsis

- **Exogenous infection**
  Control of operative conditions
  Sterilization: air, instruments
  Aseptic technique
  Good surgical technique
  Preparation of patient and surgeon

- **Clean–contaminated wounds**
  Measures as for clean wounds, plus:
    single-shot antibiotic prophylaxis
  Minimize spillage – swabs, suction
  Saline lavage

- **Dirty wounds**
  Full course antibiotics
  Thorough removal of pus
  Thorough lavage
  Simplest shortest operation (life-saving)
  Avoid anastomosis (e.g. Hartmann's procedure)
  Consider delayed primary closure

- **Clean wounds**
  No touch technique
  Careful, gentle dissection
  Careful haemostasis
  Minimize duration
  Skin preparation
  Prophylactic antibiotics only if
    insertion of prosthetic material

- **Contaminated wounds**
  Full course antibiotics
  Debride devitalized tissues
  Remove foreign material
  Clean tissues
  Lavage

6.3 Surgically important micro-organisms

Classification of bacteria:

Gram-positive

Stain blue/purple/black

Gram-positive cocci

Aerobic
Staphylococci (clusters)

Presence of coagulase enzyme = virulence factor:

- Coagulase-positive *S. aureus*
- Coagulase-negative skin flora; *S. epidermidis*

Streptococci (chains/pairs)

Virulence: ability to lyse red blood cells:

- Alpha-haemolytic: partial lysis of RBCs; altered haemoglobin causes green colour around each colony on blood agar: *S. pneumoniae* = diplococcus; *S. viridans* group

- Beta-haemolytic: complete lysis of RBCs around each colony

Lancefield grouping

- Used mainly for beta-haemolytic streptococci
- Based on specific polysaccharide antigen extracted from streptococcal cell walls
- Lancefield group A *S. pyogenes*
- Lancefield group B *S. faecalis*
- Other groups C, G
- Gamma-haemolytic no lysis of RBCs: *S. faecalis* (most common); *S. bovis*

Anaerobic

Anaerobic streptococci:

- Gut flora
- Enterococcus faecalis

Gram-positive bacilli

Aerobic

Diphtheroides:

- *C. diphtheriae*
- *L. monocytogenes*
- Bacillus spp.

Anaerobic

Clostridial species – spore-forming:

- *C. botulinum* (botulism)
- *C. perfringens* (gas gangrene)
- *C. tetani* (tetanus)
- *C. difficile* (pseudomembranous colitis)

Actinomycetes – non spore-forming ('sulphur granules'):

- *A. israelii* (actinomycosis: cervicofacial, pulmonary, pelvic)

Gram-negative

Stain pink/red

Gram-negative cocci

Aerobic

Neisseria (pairs):

- *N. meningitidis* (meningococcus): meningitis and septicaemia
- *N. gonorrhoeae* (gonococcus): gonorrhoea

Moraxella:

- *M. catarrhalis* (atypical pneumonia)

Gram-negative bacilli

This is a large group.

Aerobic
Pseudomonas:

- *P. aeruginosa* (immunocompromised host, hospital acquired infection, associated with respirators, drainage tubes, catheters).

Vibrios:

- *V. cholerae*

Campylobacter:

- *C. jejuni* (human infection of small bowel)

Parvobacteria:

- *Haemophilus influenzae*
- *Yersinia enterocolitica* (gastroenteritis)
- *Yersinia pseudo-tuberculosis* (mesenteric adenitis)
- *Bordetella pertussis*
- Brucella spp.

Legionella:

- *L. pneumophilia*
- Enterobacteria ('coliforms') (gut flora)

Lactose fermenters 'facultative anaerobes' – can grow without oxygen:

- *Escherichia coli*
- Klebsiella spp.
- Enterobacter spp.
- Shigella spp. (late lactose fermenter)
- Citrobacter spp.

Non-lactose fermenters:

- Proteus spp.
- Salmonella spp.

Anaerobic
Bacteroides:

- *B. fragilis*

Methicillin-resistant *Staphylococcus aureus* (MRSA)

During the last 20 years the prevalence of MRSA in hospitals has fluctuated. It is now 5–10% in UK hospitals.

Beta-lactam antibiotics inhibit bacterial cell wall synthesis by inactivating penicillin-binding proteins (PBP). MRSA strains produce an alternative PBP (mecA gene) thus allowing continued cell wall synthesis.

Management

- Determine if all infective organisms are of same strain – may identify single source
- May need to screen all ward staff and patients: hand, brow, nasal, axilla, and perineum
- May require appropriate antibiotics if from sterile site (i.e. blood – vancomycin)

Colonization

- Preventative measures (handwashing etc.)
- Isolation of patients (barrier nursing)
- Removal of any colonized catheters
- Eradication of carriage – nasal: Mupirocin; chlorhexidine hair and body wash; hexachlorophene powder

Systemic infections

- Glycopeptide alone or in combination with gentamicin or rifampicin/fusidic acid (better diffusion into bones, joints, endocarditis, meningitis)
- Re-swab after 5–7 days' treatment
- Need three clear swabs

Helicobacter pylori

Gram-negative spiral, motile microaerophilic bacteria.

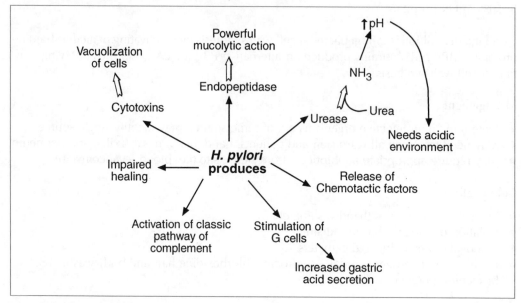

Pathogenesis of *H. pylori* infection

Epidemiology

- 70–90% prevalence in developing countries
- 25–50% prevalence in developed countries
- Acquired in childhood
- Male:female ratio is equal
- Lower socio-economic status

Transmission

- Faecal–oral
- Oral–oral
- Iatrogenic: endoscopes and endoscopists

How does it evade host immunity?

- Urease production against acid environment
- Disguises with host antigens
- Protected by mucous layer of stomach

Associations

- Type B antral gastritis: 100%
- Duodenal ulcer: 90–95%
- Gastric ulcer: 60–80%
- Also: B cell MALT lymphoma, gastric cancer, non-ulcer dyspepsia (unclear relationship)

Diagnostic tests for H. *pylori* infection

- Urea breath test: labelled CO_2 is rapidly expired if stomach is infected; limited availability
- Histopathological examination
- Serology: serum or saliva
- Mucosal biopsy (CLO test)
- Culture

Eradication therapy

- Dual therapy: two-week course, ranitidine plus clarithromycin – 88% eradication
- Triple therapy: one-week course, proton-pump inhibitor plus two of amoxicillin/clarithromycin/metronidazole – 85–90% eradication
- Quadruple therapy: one-week course, proton-pump inhibitor plus tetracycline plus metronidazole plus bismuth – 95% eradication

Very low recurrence of *H. pylori* after effective eradication. Fewer DU/GU recurrence after successful eradication.

DIAGNOSTIC TESTS FOR *H. PYLORI* INFECTION

Test	Sensitivity	Specificity	Relative cost	Comments
Non-invasive				
14C-urea breath test	90–100	95–100	++	Well tolerated Small radiation dose
13C-urea breath test			++	Well tolerated Non-radioactive
Serology	94–99	91–100	+	Cannot distinguish active and past infection Not for confirmation of eradication
Invasive				
Histology	85–100	85–100	+++	'Gold standard' two biopsies
Culture	50–95	100	+++	Technically demanding Reserve for suspected resistant organism
Rapid urease biopsy (CLO test)	75–95	75–100	+	Rapid results Endoscopic method of choice

Necrotizing fasciitis

- Infection that spreads along fascial planes
- Secondarily affecting muscle, subcutaneous tissue and skin

Aetiology

- Typically polymicrobial: streptococci; haemolytic staphylococci; *Bacteroides;* coliforms
- Post-op
- Trauma
- Ignored perineal wound
- Contaminated needle

Pathology

- Appears benign in initial stages
- Untreated: massive subcutaneous oedema dermal gangrene
- Fournier's gangrene: dermal gangrene of scrotum and penis

Management

- Rapid aggressive resuscitation
- Broad-spectrum antibiotics
- Skin incisions down to fascia
- Massive debridement of soft tissue with excision of necrotic tissue
- Colostomy if perineal area is involved
- Nutritional support
- Mortality: 30%

6.4 Sterilization and disinfection

Sterilization

Definition: *complete destruction of all viable micro-organisms, including spores and viruses. Inanimate objects only (e.g. not skin, damages tissue).*

Autoclave

- Saturated steam at high pressure
- Kills ALL organisms, including TB, viruses, heat-resistant spores
- Holding times depend on temperature and pressure (e.g. 134°C at 30 lb/in^2: 3 min holding time; 121°C at 15 lb/in^2: 15 min holding time)
- Wrapped instruments: porous load autoclave – steam penetration monitored with Bowie–Dick test
- Unwrapped instruments: Little Sister II – portable autoclave
- Fluids: bottle autoclaves

Dry heat

- Sterilization by hot-air ovens
- For moisture-sensitive instruments (no corrosion) – non-stainless metals – surgical instruments with fine cutting edges
- Able to process airtight containers and non-aqueous liquids
- Effective BUT inefficient 160°C for at least 2 hours kills ALL micro-organisms
- Monitoring: Brownes tubes III

Ethylene oxide

- Highly penetrative gas
- Kills vegetative bacteria, spores and viruses
- Effective at ambient temperatures and pressures
- Effective as a liquid or a gas
- Efficient for heat-sensitive equipment (e.g. rubber, plastics, electrical equipment, lenses), used for sutures and single-use items
- Flammable if vapour >3% in air
- Toxic, irritant, mutagenic, carcinogenic
- Limited availability and expensive – predominantly industrial process

Low-temperature steam and formaldehyde

- Physico-chemical method
- Kills vegetative bacteria, spores and viruses
- 73°C for heat-sensitive items
- NOT suitable for sealed, oily or greasy items

Irradiation

- Use of gamma rays limited to industry
- Large batches of single-use items: catheters, syringes

Disinfection: reduction in the number of viable organisms. Some viruses and bacterial spores may remain active.

Inanimate objects

- Low-temperature steam
- Boiling water
- Formaldehyde gas

Antiseptics = disinfectants used in living tissue.

Alcohols

- Broadest spectrum at 70% concentration
- Rapidly effective against Gram-positive and Gram-negative bacteria; some anti-viral activity
- No residual activity
- Relatively inactive against spores and fungi
- Denature proteins

Uses: skin preparation. (NB. ensure dryness before using diathermy – explosions and pooling may irritate sensitive areas, e.g. groin.)

Diguanides

Chlorhexidine

- Good activity against *S. aureus*
- Moderate activity against Gram-negative bacteria
- Some activity against *P. aeruginosa*, although may multiply in deteriorating solutions
- Non-toxic to skin and mucous membranes
- Poor activity against spores, fungi and viruses
- Inactivated by pus, soap and some plastics
- Causes bacterial cell wall disruption

Uses:

- In local antisepsis
- 4% chlorhexidine in detergent (Hibiscrub)
- Chlorhexidine-cetrimide mixture (Savlon) for some dirty wounds
- 0.5% chlorhexidine in 70% alcohol

Iodophors and iodine

- Broad spectrum of activity: bacteria, spores, fungi and viruses, including hepatitis B and HIV
- Easily inactivated by blood, faeces and pus
- Need optimum freshness, concentration and pH <4
- Stains skin and fabrics; irritant; may cause local hypersensitivity

Uses:

- Pre-operative skin disinfection
- Wound antisepsis

Hydrogen peroxide

- Only weak bactericidal activity

Aldehydes

Glutaraldehyde and formaldehyde

- Rapidly active against vegetative bacteria and viruses, including hepatitis B and HIV
- Slowly effective against spores
- Only fair activity against tubercle bacilli
- Exposure of at least 3 hours to kill ALL microbes; most bacteria killed in less than 10 minutes
- Toxic; sensitivity reactions in skin, eyes, lungs (glutaraldehyde safer)

Endoscopes:

- Heat-sensitive
- Disinfected by immersion in 2% glutaraldehyde

Cleaning: physically removes contamination does NOT necessarily destroy micro-organisms.

6.5 Prevention of surgical infection – asepsis and prophylaxis

Wound sepsis

- Asepsis = no organisms present during surgery; truly aseptic environment needed in immunocompromised patients
- Antisepsis = prevention of sepsis; total abolition of organisms not achieved

Clean wounds

- Incision through non-inflamed tissue
- No entry into genitourinary/GI/respiratory tracts

Contamination: <2% (exogenous sepsis)

Surgical infection can be prevented by

- Environmental factors – see operating theatre design section 3.1
- Patient factors
- Surgeon factors
- Prophylactic antibiotics – see antibiotics section 6.6

Preparation of the patient

Pre-op skin preparation

'High risk' areas:

- Perineum
- Groin
- Axilla

Alcoholic antiseptics are more effective than aqueous but pooled areas on the skin may ignite if using diathermy.

Plain soap washing and pre-op shaving:

- Causes skin abrasion
- Disrupts deeper flora layers; increased bacterial count on skin surface
- Increased tendency to post-op wound sepsis

Therefore shave immediately pre-op with surgical clippers or use depilatory cream before theatre.

Adhesive wound drapes:

- Do not prevent contamination
- Reported to reduce wound contamination by 50% BUT no decrease in wound infection
- Trapped bacteria may multiply

In theatre

Control of air quality
Aim: decrease number of airborne particles carrying bacteria from skin flora.
Positive pressure filtered ventilation (PPFV) prevents bacteria gaining entry to the air.
Laminar flow plus ultra-clean air systems: two-fold reduction in post-op wound infection.

Scrub-up
Aim: decrease bacterial skin count.
Chlorhexidine gluconate or povidone-iodine solutions: stiff brushes damage the epidermis; use on fingernails only. One nail scrub at beginning of operating list is sufficient.

Clothing
Cotton gowns reduce the bacterial count in the air by only 30%. Bacteria-impermeable fabrics may reduce bacterial air counts by 40–70%. No evidence of reduced wound infection.

Caps: useful as *S. aureus* can be carried on the scalp. Also prevents hair from falling in the wound.

Masks

- Deflect forceful expirations which carry bacteria; normal speech does not expel bacteria
- May rub off bacteria-carrying skin squames from the face
- No effect on infection rates
- Prudent use in implant surgery

Gloves

- Glove punctures or tears do not affect incidence of wound infection
- Effective hand disinfection

Plastic overshoes are not proven to reduce wound infection.

6.6 Antibiotics

Mode of action

Bactericidal
(e.g. beta-lactams, vancomycin, aminoglycosides, chloramphenicol)

Indications for bactericidal antibiotics:

- Life-threatening sepsis
- Infective endocarditis
- Opportunistic infections in immunocompromised patients

Bacteriostatic
(e.g. tetracycline, erythromycin, clindamycin, chloramphenicol). Bacteria can multiply again. Final elimination of pathogens depends upon host defence mechanisms with effective phagocytosis.

Mechanisms of action
Inhibition of cell wall synthesis. Leads to osmotic lysis of bacteria with defective peptidoglycan molecules in the cell wall.

Bactericidal action

- Beta-lactams (e.g. penicillin, ampicillin, cephalosporin)
- Mono-bactams
- Vancomycin

Inhibition of protein synthesis
At following sites:

- Transfer RNA: amino acid attachment (tetracyclines, bacteriostatic)
- Translocation (chloramphenicol, erythromycin (static at low concentrations), clindamycin, fusidic acid (cidal at high concentrations))
- mRNA attachment to ribosome (aminoglycosides, bactericidal)

Inhibition of nucleic acid synthesis

Bactericidal action

- Decreased RNA replication (sulphonamides, trimethoprim, quinolones (e.g. ciprofloxacin, nalidixic acid), metronidazole)
- Decreased mRNA (rifampicin)

ANTI-MICROBIALS: SPECTRUM OF ACTIVITY

Drug	Gram-negative cocci	Gram-negative bacilli	Gram-positive cocci	Gram-positive bacilli	Others
Beta-lactams: Benzylpenicillin Penicillin V First generation Cephalosporins	*N.meningitides* *N.gonorrhoeae*	Produces beta-lactamases	Streptococci: *Strep. pyogenes* *Strep. viridans* Anaerobic cocci	*C.perfringens* *S.pyogenes* *S. viridans* Anaerobic cocci	*T.pallidum*
Anti-staphylococcal penicillins: Methicillin Cloxacillin Flucloxacillin			*S. aureus* (produces beta-lactamase)		
Aminoglycosides: Gentamicin Tobramycin		*E. coli* Klebsiella Proteus 'Coliforms' *P. aeruginosa*	*S. aureus* (especially gentamicin)		
Macrolides: Erythromycin		Campylobacter spp.	Streptococci, including *S. pneumoniae* (may produce beta-lactamase) *S. aureus*	*C. diphtheriae*	*M. pneumoniae*
Vancomycin			*S. aureus*	*C. difficile*	
Metronidazole activze only against anaerobic protozoa and bacteria		Bacteroides spp.	Anaerobic cocci	Clostridium spp.	

BROAD-SPECTRUM ANTIBIOTICS

Drug	Gram-negative cocci	Gram-negative bacilli	Gram-positive cocci	Gram-positive bacilli	Others
Aminopenicillins: Amoxycillin Ampicillin Clavulanic acid	*N. meningitides* *N. gonorrhoeae*	*E. coli* and other coliforms (**not** Klebsiella) *H. influenzae*	Streptococci, including *S. pneumoniae* (beta-lactamase-producing)	Clostridium spp.	*T. pallidum*
Broad-spectrum penicillins: Piperacillin		*P. aeruginosa* Coliforms			
Cephalosporins: (second generation, beta-lactamase-stable) Cefuroxime Ceftazidime	*N. gonorrhoeae*	*E. coli* and other coliforms, including Klebsiella	Streptococci Staphylococci	Clostridium spp.	
Tetracyclines	*N. gonorrhoeae*	*H. influenzae*	Streptococci Staphylococci	Clostridium spp.	*M. pneumoniae* Chlamydia
Ciprofloxacin	*N. gonorrhoeae*	Haemophilus *P. aeruginosa* Coliforms	*S. aureus* and some streptococci		

Alteration of cell membrane function

Bactericidal action

- Polymyxin – against Gram-negative bacilli

Which antibiotic?

Narrow spectrum selected for specific infections. Narrow spectrum antibiotics cause less disturbance of normal flora:

- Reduced risk of superinfection
- Fewer resistant strains
- Use of broad-spectrum antibiotics associated with acquiring *Clostridium difficile* (pseudo-membranous colitis)

Hence:

- Penicillin V for simple streptococcal infections
- Flucloxacillin for *S. aureus* (non-beta-lactamase-producing)
- Erythromycin for beta-lactamase-producing Staphylococcus and Streptococcus (usually given to penicillin-allergic patients)

Broad spectrum for Gram-negative bacilli

- Aminopenicillins
- Cephalosporins

Synergistic combinations

- Penicillin plus gentamicin damages bacterial cell wall

Drug combinations

- Trimethoprim plus sulphonamides: co-trimoxazole (Septrin)
- Amoxicillin plus clavulanic acid: augmentin

Antibiotic prophylaxis

Issues

- Is it needed?
- What pathogen and where?
- Route of administration?
- Immunocompromised?

Aim

- Prevent bacteria from multiplying without altering normal flora

Indications

- Where procedure commonly leads to infection (e.g. colectomy)
- Proven value in reducing post-op infections from endogenous sources
- Where results of sepsis would be devastating, despite low risk of occurrence e.g. vascular or other prostheses
- No value in clean procedures (risk of sepsis from exogenous source <2%)

Administration

- Choice of antibiotic: bacteriostatic or bactericidal (immunocompromised)
- Short courses: <24 hours
- Single dose: (used if 3–6% post-op infection rate) versus
- Multiple dose: (used if 6% post-op infection rate)
- Timing: within one hour pre-op or at induction (15–20 minutes before skin incision or tourniquet inflation); second dose IF operation >4 hours to maintain adequate tissue levels

Beware

- Toxicity
- Side-effects
- Routes of excretion
- Allergies

7. SUGGESTED FURTHER READING

Clinical surgery in general, Kirk RM, Mansfield AO, Cochrane JPS, 1999, Churchill Livingstone.
Seeking patient's consent: The ethical considerations, 1997, General Medical Council booklet.
Suitability for consideration of day case surgery, Royal College of Surgeons of England booklet.

Chapter 2

Peri-operative Management 2

CONTENTS

Peri-operative Management 2

1. PATHOPHYSIOLOGY OF THE BODY'S RESPONSE TO TRAUMA

1.1 Acute inflammation

Inflammation is the essential response of living tissue to trauma. It destroys and limits the effect of the injurious agent and is intimately related to the process of repair. It is therefore an essential, integral component of the body's defence mechanisms, and without it there would be no defence against foreign organisms and no wound healing.

Acute inflammation is usually beneficial, although can occasionally be harmful (e.g. anaphylaxis, acute lung injury, systemic inflammatory response syndrome).

The characteristic features are:

- Heat (calor)
- Erythema (rubor)
- Oedema (tumor)
- Pain (dolor)
- Loss of function (functio laesa)

Two main pathways of acute inflammation

- Changes in microcirculation
- Activities of phagocytic cells

Changes in microcirculation

- Arteriolar smooth muscle relaxation and therefore increased local blood flow
- Increased vascular permeability and exudation of fluid and plasma proteins

Cellular events

Initially neutrophils, and later macrophages, rapidly migrate to the injured area. Their subsequent activities involve the following steps.

- **Margination**: as blood flow decreases, leucocytes move from the centre of the vessel to lie against the endothelium (pavementing).
- **Leucocyte adhesion**: adhesion molecules on leucocytes bind to corresponding molecules on the endothelium. Expression of these adhesion molecules is enhanced by specific inflammatory mediators (C5a, IL-1, TNF).
- **Emigration**: adherent leucocytes pass through interendothelial junctions into the extravascular space. Neutrophils are the predominant cell type in the first 24 hours, after which monocytes predominate.
- **Chemotaxis**: leucocytes move to the injury site along a chemical gradient assisted by chemotactic factors (bacterial components, complement factors, LT, B4).
- **Phagocytosis and intracellular degradation**: opsonized bacteria (opsonins – IgG and C3b) attach via Fc and C3b receptors to the surface of neutrophils and macrophages. The bacteria/foreign particle is then engulfed to create a phagosome. This then fuses with lysosomal granules to form a phagolysosome. The contents of the lysosome degrade the ingested particle.

1.2 Pharmacological mediators of inflammation

The inflammatory response to trauma is mediated by chemical factors present in the plasma and produced by the inflammatory cells.

Inflammatory mediators	
● **Plasma**	● **Cells**
Complement system	Vasoactive amines (e.g. histamine)
Kinin system	Lysosomal enzymes
Coagulation pathway	Prostaglandins
The fibrinolytic system	Cytokines (e.g. TNFα, interleukins)

The complement system

The complement system

- Consists of 20+ component proteins
- The classic pathway is initiated by antigen-antibody complexes
- The alternative pathway is activated by endotoxins, complex polysaccharides and aggregated immunoglobulins
- Both pathways convert C3 to C3a and C3b
- C3b initiates the lytic pathway which produces the membrane attack complex (MAC), which forms destructive pores in the membranes of target cells
- C3a and C5a increase vascular permeability by causing release of histamine from granulocytes, mast cells and platelets; C5a is also chemotactic.

The biological functions of complement are as follows:

- Yields particles which coat micro-organisms and function as adhesion molecules for neutrophils and macrophages (opsonins)

- Leads to lysis of bacterial cell membranes via the MAC
- Yields biologically active fragments which influence capillary permeability and chemotaxis

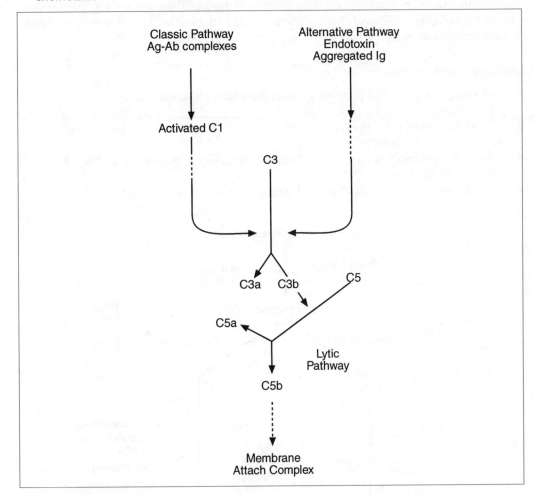

The Kinin system

Activation of coagulation factor XII produces factor XIIa. This converts prekallikrein into the active enzyme, kallikrein, which produces bradykinin from high-molecular-weight kininogen.

Bradykinin is a potent vasodilator and increases vascular permeability.

Arachidonic acid metabolism

Arachidonic acid is a 20–carbon polyunsaturated fatty acid present in cell membranes. Following activation, arachidonic acid is released from the membrane by phospholipases. It is then metabolized via two main pathways: the cyclo-oxygenase pathway and the lipoxygenase pathway. Prostaglandins (PGE2 and PGI2) are generated which cause vasodilatation and increased vascular permeability. E series prostaglandins are hyperalgesic, see diagram below.

Aspirin and other non-steroidal anti-inflammatory drugs block the cyclo-oxygenase system thereby suppressing PGE2 and PGI2. They are therefore effective as antipyretic, analgesic and anti-inflammatory agents.

Histamine and serotonin

- Mast cells, basophils and platelets contain the amines histamine and 5–hydroxytryptamine (5–HT, serotonin)
- Release from mast cells granules is stimulated by C3a and C5a, IgE immunological reactions and interleukin-1
- Release from platelets is caused by contact with collagen, thrombin, ADP and by platelet activating factor
- Both amines cause vasodilatation and increased vascular permeability

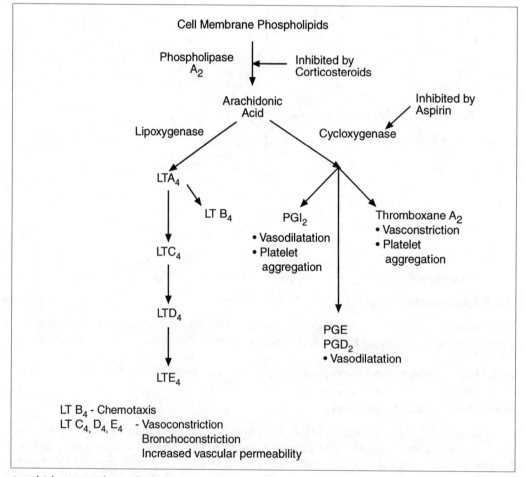

Arachidonic acid metabolism

Interleukins, cytokines and monokines

- **Polypeptides**: produced by activated monocytes (monokines), lymphocytes (lymphokines) and other inflammatory cells.
- **Interferons**: viral infection induces the synthesis and secretion of interferons. They confer an anti-viral state on uninfected cells.
- **Interleukins**: **IL-8** is a chemokine produced by monocytes, T-lymphocytes, endothelial cells and platelets, which mediates the rapid accumulation of neutrophils in inflamed tissues. **IL-1** is secreted by numerous cell types (monocytes, macrophages, neutrophils, endothelial cells). It promotes T- and B-cell proliferation, tissue catabolism and the acute phase response, and also acts as a pyrogen. (See Section 1.4, *Immunology*)
- **Tumour necrosis factor α (TNFα)**: produced by monocytes and macrophages, particularly if stimulated by bacterial endotoxin. Plays an important part in host defence against Gram-negative sepsis. When endotoxin present at a low dose, TNFα enhances macrophage killing, activation of B lymphocytes and cytokine production. When endotoxin is present at a high dose TNFα is an extremely potent mediator in the pathogenesis of endotoxin-related shock.

Platelet activating factor (PAF)

- A wide variety of cells produce PAF, including mast cells, neutrophils, platelets and macrophages
- It increases vascular permeability, leucocyte aggregation and exudation

Leucocyte constituents (released from lysosomes)

- **Cationic proteins**: increase vascular permeability and act as chemotactants
- **Acid proteases**: most active at a pH~3
- **Neutral proteases**: degrade extracellular matrix

1.3 Outcome of acute inflammation

- Resolution with restoration of normal cellular and tissue function
- Scar formation (repair versus regeneration)
- Chronic inflammation

Chronic inflammation results from:

- Persistence of the acute inflammatory stimulus (e.g. cholangitis leading to chronic liver abscess)
- Deranged inflammatory response (e.g. autoimmune conditions such as rheumatoid arthritis or systemic lupus erythematosus)
- Recurrent episodes of acute inflammation (e.g. recurrent cholecystitis or pyelonephritis)

Features of chronic inflammation

- Prolonged presence of macrophages, lymphocytes and plasma cells
- Angiogenesis

- Fibrosis
- Tissue damage

Non-specific chronic inflammation

Acute inflammation fails to end in resolution or repair, as a result of:

- Persistence of injurious agent (e.g. chronic osteomyelitis, peptic ulcer due to *Helicobacter pylori*)
- Failure of removal of pus and foreign material (e.g. undrained abscess)
- Inadequate blood supply or drainage (e.g. ischaemic or venous ulceration)
- Inadequate drainage of a exocrine gland (e.g. chronic sialoadenitis)

Granulomatous inflammation

Characterised by small collections (granulomas) of modified macrophages called 'epithelioid cells'. It is usually a low-grade smouldering response occurring in the following settings:

- Persistent infection by intracellular organisms (e.g. *Mycobacterium tuberculosis*)
- Prolonged exposure to non-degradable substances (e.g. pulmonary asbestosis)
- Immune reactions, particularly autoimmune disorders (e.g. rheumatoid arthritis)

1.4 Immunology

Exposure to certain infectious disease leads to a reduction in subsequent susceptibility to that disease in the future. This acquisition of increased resistance to a specific infectious agent is known as acquired specific immunity, and forms the basis to many immunisation programmes.

The primary function of the immune system is to eliminate infectious agents and to minimise the damage they cause.

Immune system

- **Non-specific defences**
  Skin and mucus membranes
  Lymphocytes
  Commensal organisms
  Bactericidal body fluids (gastric acid)
  Complement system
  Neutrophils
  Natural killer cells

- **Specific immunity**
  Lymphocytes
  Features:
    specificity
    adaptation
    memory

Non-specific defences

Complement system and neutrophils
Pharmacological mediators of inflammation (see Section 1.3).
Concerned with the initial elimination of foreign micro-organisms.

Natural killer cells

- A class of cytotoxic lymphocytes which carry the marker CD16
- Lyse virus-infected cells and tumour-derived cells
- No immunological memory
- Actions enhanced by interferons and interleukin-2

Specific immunity

Acquired specific immunity provides the ability to:

- Recognise the difference between self and non-self
- Mount a response that is specific to foreign material
- Remember previous responses so that a subsequent response to previously encountered foreign material will be faster and larger

Antigen presentation

An antigen is a substance capable of inducing a specific immune response. When a host encounters an antigen two things may occur:

- Antibody formation by plasma cells
- Proliferation of T-lymphocytes

Dendritic cells and macrophages process antigens and present peptide fragments in association with class II MHC molecules. These are usually recognised by CD4+ helper T-cells.

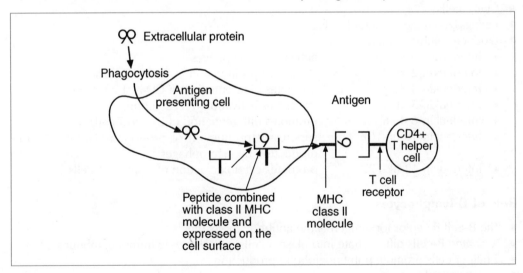

Activation of CD4+ T-lymphocytes

All nucleated cells express MHC class I molecules. Peptides derived from viruses or intracellular bacteria may be expressed in association with class I MHC molecules. These complexes are recognised by CD8+ cytotoxic T-cells.

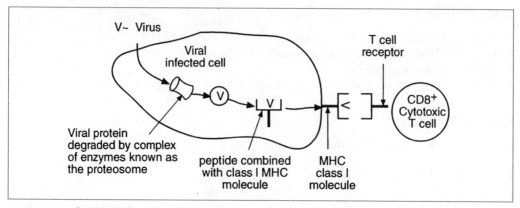

Activation of CD8+ T-lymphocytes

Role of T-lymphocytes

Cytotoxic T-lymphocytes

- CD8+ cells
- Recognize antigen + class I MHC
- Kill cells infected with viruses or intracellular bacteria
- Memory cytotoxic T-cells persist after recovery

Helper T-lymphocytes

- CD4+ cells
- Recognize antigen + class II MHC
- Produce soluble mediators:
    - Interferon-g (IFN-g)   activates macrophages
    - Interleukin-2 (IL-2)   stimulates proliferation of B- and T-cells
    - Interleukin-4 (IL-4)   promotes differentiation of CD4+ T-cells and B-cells
    - Interleukin-5 (IL-5)   stimulates activation of eosinophils
    - Interleukin-6 (IL-6)   promotes differentiation of B- and T-cells
    - Interleukin-10 (IL-10) suppresses production of pro-inflammatory cytokine production by macrophages
    - Interleukin-12 (IL-12) promotes cytotoxic action of T- and NK-cells

Role of B-lymphocytes

- The B-cell receptor for antigen is the antibody molecule
- Activated B-cells differentiate into plasma cells which secrete immunoglobulins
- T-helper cells promote immunoglobulin production
- All have similar monomeric structure except IgM – pentameric structure

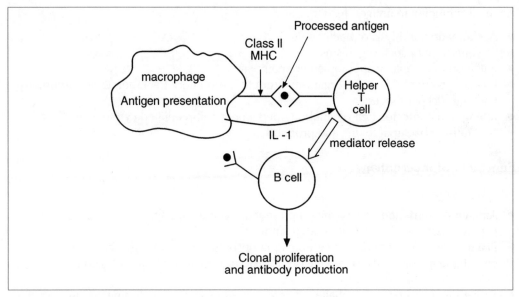

T- and B-cell interaction

Immunoglobulin

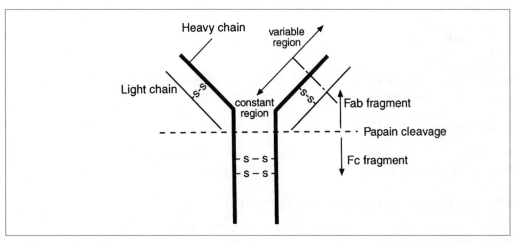

Antibody structure

- An immunoglobulin molecule is a 4 polypeptide chain structure with two heavy and two light chains linked covalently by disulphide bonds
- Digestion with papain produces antigen binding fragments (Fab) and one Fc fragment, which is involved with complement and macrophage binding
- Light chains are either kappa or lambda
- There are five main classes of immunoglobulin, based on the Fc fragment of the heavy chain IgG – Gamma, IgM – Mu, IgA – Alpha, IgD – Delta, IgE – Epsilon

Antibodies binding to antigen lead to:

- Agglutination and lysis of bacteria (IgM)
- Opsonisation of such organisms
- Initiation of the classical complement pathway
- Blocking entry of the micro-organisms from the respiratory tract, gut, eyes and urinary tract into deeper tissues
- Killing of the infected cell by antibody-dependent cell-mediated cytotoxicity
- Neutralising bacterial toxins and products

Functions of macrophages

Present in most tissues:

- **Antigen presentation**: macrophages present antigen to T-lymphocytes as processed peptides associated with class II MHC molecules
- **Phagocytosis**: macrophages ingest bacteria opsonised by immunoglobulin and/or complement. This leads to the release of toxic molecules into the phagosome and death of the micro-organism.
- **Secretion**: activated macrophages secrete numerous factors, including neutral proteases, lysozyme, cytokines, chemotactic factors, arachidonic acid metabolites and complement components

Cell mediated immunity has the following roles:

In bacterial infection

- Specific recognition of antigen by T-cells
- Non-specific lymphokine production, which upregulates macrophages and activates cytotoxic T-cells and B-cells

In viral infections

- Upregulation of macrophages and killer cells for cell killing
- Producing interferons

The major histocompatibility complex (MHC)

- Important set of genes on the short arm of chromosome 6
- The genes code for the human leucocyte antigens which are present on cell membranes and are specific to each individual
- The human leucocyte antigen (HLA) system is the most polymorphic genetic system in humans
- The recognition by the recipient's immune system of human leucocyte antigens on the surface of donor cells forms the basis of rejection following organ transplant
- Based on their structure, distribution and function, the MHC gene products are classified into three groups

MHC gene products

- **Class I antigens**
  Found on all nucleated cells and platelets
  Coded by three loci designated HLA-A, HLA-B and HLA-C
- **Class II antigens**
  Found on dendritic cells, macrophages, B-lymphocytes and activated T-cells
  Coded for in a region known as HLA-D
  Antigens are HLA-DR, -DQ and -DP
- **Class III proteins**
  Components of the complement system coded for within the MHC

All Class I antigens and most of the Class II antigens evoke the formation of the antibodies in genetically non-identical individuals.

Management of splenectomy patients

Such patients are particularly susceptible to encapsulated bacteria (pneumococcus, Haemophilus influenzae, and meningococcus), and these infections may be life-threatening.

- Pneumococcal vaccine must be given at least 2 weeks before splenectomy, or immediately after surgery if carried out as an emergency
- The patient must be reimmunised in 5–10 years
- The patient must be on prophylactic antibiotics (penicillin-V or erythromycin) for at least 2 years

1.5 Immune system disorders

- **Hypersensitivity**: tissue damage results from an inappropriate immune response to an exogenous antigen
- **Autoimmunity**: immune response against the host's own antigens
- **Immune deficiency**: inadequate immune response, may be due to a congenital or acquired defect
- **Neoplastic proliferations** of various elements of the immune system

Hypersensitivity

Gell and Coombs' classification

Type I hypersensitivity (anaphylactic or immediate)

Exposure to allergen leads to formation of IgE. IgE binds to mast cells and basophils, and then re-exposure to allergen leads to release of mediators from mast cells and basophils.

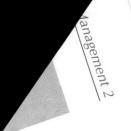

ial constriction, increased vascular permeability and
cretion)
d E4 are 1000× more potent than histamine)
phil chemotactic factors
ses
t activating factor

Examples: hayfever, asthma and food allergies, anaphylactic shock

Sodium cromoglycate and steroids are thought to inhibit mediator release by stabilising lysosomal membranes.

Type II hypersensitivity (cytotoxic)
Mediated by antibodies against intrinsic or extrinsic antigens absorbed on the cell surface or on other components. Tissue damage results from:

- Complement-dependent reactions. Antibody complexes with antigen present on the cell surface activate the complement system. The cell then becomes susceptible to phagocytosis by the antibody or C3b present on the cell surface. In addition, cellular damage may be secondary to the formation of the membrane attack complex.

Examples: transfusion reaction, autoimmune thrombocytopenia and drug reactions.

- Antibody-dependent cell-mediated cytotoxicity. Cells complexed with antibody are lysed by non-sensitized cells (natural killer cells, neutrophils and monocytes).

Examples: parasitic infections and graft rejection.

Type III hypersensitivity (immune complex-mediated)
Mediated by immune complexes (antigen-antibody) formed either in the circulation or at extravascular sites.

- Immune complex leads to complement activation and thence to neutrophil activation with release of lysosomal enzymes, resulting in tissue damage

Examples: SLE and acute glomerulonephritis.

Type IV hypersensitivity (cell-mediated/delayed)
Mediated by sensitized T-lymphocytes.

- Sensitised T-cells lead to cytotoxic T-cell activation plus release of lymphokines from T-helper cells, and thence to recruitment and activation of macrophages and monocytes, resulting in cell damage

Examples: TB and transplant rejection.

Type V hypersensitivity (stimulatory)

- Antireceptor antibodies lead to stimulation of cell function

Examples: Graves' disease and myasthenia gravis.

Autoimmunity

Autoimmune disorders result from a defect in self-tolerance. This may result from:

- Defects in suppressor cell number or function
- Micro-organisms eliciting antibodies that cross-react with self-antigens
- Alteration of self-antigens by drugs or micro-organisms, exposing new antigenic sites
- T-cell-independent emergence of B-cells that are capable of mounting an autoimmune response
- Autoimmunity may be tissue-specific or systemic

Major autoimmune diseases

Disease	Autoantibodies present against
Organ-specific	
Hashimoto's thyroiditis	Thyroglobulin, thyroid microsomes
Graves' disease	TSH receptor (thyroid stimulating Igs)
Atrophic gastritis	Parietal cells
Pernicious anaemia	Intrinsic factor
Goodpasture's syndrome	Basement membrane (lungs and kidneys)
Myasthenia gravis	Acetylcholine receptor
Non-organ-specific	
SLE	Nuclear antigens, DNA, smooth muscle
Rheumatoid arthritis	IgM
Scleroderma	Centromere

Immune deficiency

Can involve specific pathways of the immune system, and non-specific effector mechanisms (e.g. complement system and bacterial phagocytosis).

Primary immunodeficiency

Hereditary disorders which typically manifest between six months and two years of age as maternal antibody protection is lost.

Secondary immunodeficiency

Altered immune response secondary to malnutrition, ageing, infection, irradiation, splenectomy, chemotherapy or immunosuppression. Recurrent, persistent or atypical infections suggest an immune deficiency disorder.

X-linked agammaglobulinaemia of Bruton

- X-linked primary immunodeficiency disorder
- Lack of mature B-cells and nearly no Ig
- T-cell function and numbers are normal
- Recurrent bacterial infections
- Most viral and fungal infections are handled appropriately

IgA deficiency

- Common disorder – one in 600 people affected
- Congenital or acquired following viral infection
- Usually asymptomatic
- Recurrent pulmonary and GI infections
- 40% have antibodies to IgA

Common variable immune deficiency

- Congenital or acquired
- Hypogammaglobulinaemia, especially IgG
- ? disorder of T-cell regulation of B-cell function
- Typically presents after the first decade of life with recurrent pyogenic infections
- Prone to autoimmune diseases and lymphoid malignancies

di George syndrome

- Congenital disorder due to fetal damage to the third and fourth pharyngeal pouches
- Syndrome – thymic hypoplasia/aplasia, parathyroid hypoplasia, congenital heart disease and dysmorphic facies
- T-cell deficiency – prone to viral and parasitic infections
- B-cells and Ig levels normal

Severe combined immunodeficiency disease (SCID)

- Group of autosomal or X-linked recessive disorders
- Characterised by lymphopenia and defects in T- and B-cell function
- Death usually occurs within one year from opportunistic infection

Complement factor deficiencies

- C3 deficiency predisposes to bacterial infections
- C2 deficiency increases risk of autoimmune connective tissue disorders
- C5–8 defects lead to recurrent Neisserial infections

Acquired immunodeficiency syndrome (AIDS)

- Caused by the human immunodeficiency virus (HIV), a retrovirus
- The HIV membrane contains the glycoprotein gp120, which has a high affinity for the CD4 antigen on T-helper cells, monocytes and macrophages

- HIV complexes with T-helper cell, the virus invades cell, its single-stranded RNA genome is copied as double-stranded DNA by the viral reverse transcriptase system, and viral DNA integrates into the host genome
- Viral propagation occurs (via the viral protease system) with subsequent T-cell activation
- Most anti-HIV drugs inhibit either reverse transcriptase or protease synthesis
- CD4+ T-cell depletion increases susceptibility to opportunistic infections and malignancies
- Mean time from infection with HIV to diagnosis of a major opportunistic infection or tumour is 11.2 years; mean time to death is approximately 18–24 months after this; however, the course of infection depends on viral and host factors
- The routine HIV test is an enzyme-linked immunosorbent assay (ELISA) that detects antibody directed towards HIV
- HIV is classified on the basis of clinical conditions and CD4 count:

Class A: acute seroconversion illness, asymptomatic disease, persistent generalised lymphadenopathy
Class B: asymptomatic disease
Class C: AIDS; the class is further characterised by a CD4 count-related suffix: 1 = >500, 2 = 200–499, 3 = <200

- Natural history of infection

Seroconversion: Class A
Initial infection is usually asymptomatic. Following an incubation period of 2–6 weeks, there is a phase of viraemia. At this stage HIV antibody tests are often negative.

Asymptomatic disease: Class B
CD4 count 350–800 $\times$ 10^6/l: most patients are asymptomatic at this stage. Mild generalised lymphadenopathy is common.

Symptomatic disease – AIDS: Class C
CD4 count 200–350 $\times$ 10^6/l: infections with common organisms begin to occur. Particularly *S. pneumoniae, H. influenzae, M. tuberculosis* and Candida. Patients may present with weight loss, diarrhoea, fever, fatigue and myalgia.

CD4 count <200 $\times$ 10^6/l: increased risk of opportunist infections and tumours. Common conditions – *P. carinii* pneumonia (incidence decreasing with use of prophylaxis), cerebral toxoplasmosis, Kaposi's sarcoma and candidosis.

CD4 count <50 $\times$ 10^6/l: multiple, concurrent infections with organisms of low virulence are common. Common conditions – atypical mycobacterial infections, systematic fungal infections, CMV infection, AIDS dementia complex and lymphoma.

2. SKIN AND WOUNDS

2.1 Skin anatomy and physiology

A core knowledge of skin anatomy and physiology is essential to understand fully the processes involved in wound healing. The skin is an enormously complex organ acting both as a highly efficient mechanical barrier and also as a complex immunological membrane. It is constantly regenerating with a generous nervous, vascular and lymphatic supply, and has specialist structural and functional properties in different parts of the body.

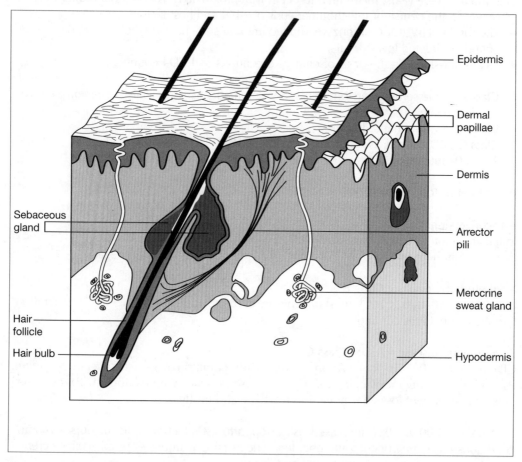

Skin anatomy

All skin has the same basic structure, although varies in thickness, colour and the presence of hairs and glands in different regions of the body. The external surface of the skin consists of a keratinised squamous epithelium called the epidermis. The epidermis is supported and nourished by a thick underlying layer of dense, fibro-elastic connective tissue called the dermis which is highly vascular and contains many sensory receptors. The dermis is attached to underlying tissues by a layer of loose connective tissue called the hypodermis or subcutaneous layer which contains adipose tissue. Hair follicles, sweat glands, sebaceous glands and nails are epithelial structures called epidermal appendages which extend down into the dermis and hypodermis.

The four main functions of the skin are:

Protection   against ultraviolet light, and mechanical, chemical and thermal insults. It also prevents excessive dehydration and acts as a physical barrier to micro-organisms.

Sensation   various receptors for touch, pressure, pain and temperature

Thermoregulation   insulation, sweating and varying blood flow in dermis

Metabolic functions the subcutaneous fat is a major store of energy, mainly triglycerides. Vitamin D synthesis in dpidermis

Skin has natural tension lines, and incisions placed along these lines tend to heal with a narrower and stronger scar, leading to a more favourable cosmetic result. These natural tension lines lie at right angles to the direction of contraction of underlying muscle fibres, and parallel to the dermal collagen bundles. On the head and neck they are readily identifiable as the 'wrinkle' lines, and can easily be exaggerated by smiling, frowning and the display of other emotions. On the limbs and trunk they tend to run circumferentially, and can easily be found by manipulating the skin to find the natural skin creases.

2.2 Pathophysiology of wound healing

All surgeons deal with wounds and it is essential to understand fully the exact pathophysiological mechanisms involved in wound healing, how this may be optimised and how it may be compromised, leading to wound dehiscence, delayed healing and incisional hernia formation.

The aims of wound healing are a rapid restoration of tissue continuity and a rapid return to normal function. Wound healing consists of three phases:

- Acute inflammatory response
- Cell proliferation and deposition of extracellular matrix (proliferative phase)
- Remodelling of the extracellular matrix (maturation phase)

Acute inflammatory response

- Injured blood vessels lead to platelet activation and initiation of the coagulation and complement cascades, leading to clot formation
- Vasodilatation and increased vascular permeability
- Influx of inflammatory cells and fibroblasts
- Neutrophils are the predominant cell type in the first 24 hours; they initiate phagocytosis
- Macrophages become the predominant cell type after 48 hours; they continue the process of phagocytosis and secrete growth factors (cytokines) which are instrumental in extracellular matrix production.

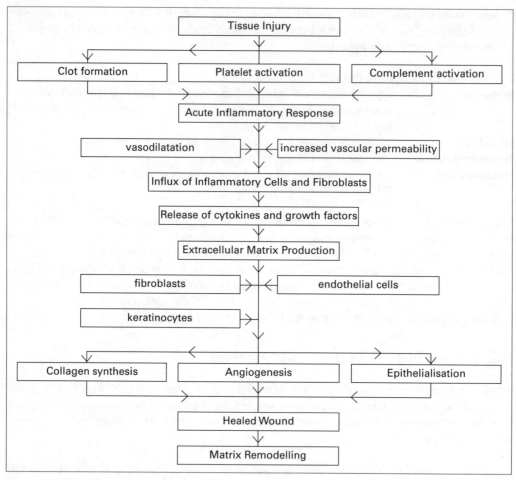

Wound healing

Extracellular matrix production

- Within hours of injury epithelial cells at the margins of the wound begin to migrate across the defect; epithelial closure is usually complete by 48 hours
- Fibroblasts migrate into the wound, proliferate and synthesise extracellular matrix components; after 4–5 days collagen fibrils begin to appear
- Angiogenesis occurs simultaneously with fibroplasia. Endothelial cell proliferation and migration, essential for this, depend upon the presence of matrix metalloproteinases, for which zinc is an essential cofactor.
- Granulation tissue is a temporary structure which consists of a rich network of capillary vessels and a heterogeneous population of cells (fibroblasts, macrophages and endothelial cells) within the stroma of the extracellular matrix. It has a characteristic pinkish, granular appearance.
- The wound contracts secondary to the action of myofibroblasts

Matrix remodelling

- This stage lasts for many months after the wound is clinically healed
- The scar becomes less vascular – hence the change in colour
- Scar tensile strength increases as the orientation and cross-linkage of collagen fibrils is modified; the maximum tensile strength regained is 80% of normal tissue.

Cell types involved in wound healing and timing of appearance in wound

- Platelets   Immediate
- Neutrophils   0–1 day
- Macrophages   1–2 days
- Fibroblasts   2–4 days
- Myofibroblasts   2–4 days
- Endothelial cells   3–5 days

Important cytokines

- Transforming growth factor (TGFβ) – collagen deposition, chemotaxis
- Basic fibroblast growth factor(bFGF) – angiogenesis, chemotaxis
- Platelet factor 4 (PF4) – chemotaxis
- β-Thromboglobulin (βTG) – chemotaxis
- Vascular endothelial growth factor (VEGF) – angiogenesis, chemotaxis
- Platelet-derived growth factor (PDGF) – chemotaxis, cytokine synthesis
- Monocyte chemotactic protein 1 (MCP-1) – chemotaxis
- Keratinocyte growth factor (KGF) – chemotaxis, mitogenic
- Epidermal growth factor (EGF)
- Fibroblast growth factor (FGF)

Different tissues heal in a remarkably similar way, albeit at different rates – the scalp and face heal very quickly, at least in part because of increased vascularity. Healing rates are quickest early in life, and decline with advancing years. Some tissues, such as liver and bone, possess the ability to regenerate their specialised cells following injury, with the result that significant tissue loss can be replaced by regenerated specialised cells, with no, or minimal, loss of function. Conversely, some tissues have no regenerative ability (for example cardiac and nervous tissue) and wounds heal by simple scar formation – significant tissue loss will result in significant loss of function.

2.3 Classification of wound healing

First/primary intention

Usually in uncontaminated wounds with minimal tissue loss and when the wound edges can easily be approximated with sutures, staples or adhesive strips, without excessive tension. The wound usually heals by rapid epithelialisation and formation of minimal granulation tissue and subsequent scar tissue.

Second/secondary intention

Usually in wounds with substantial tissue loss, when the edges cannot be apposed without excessive tension. The wound is left open and allowed to heal from the deep aspects of the wound by a combination of granulation, epithelialisation and contraction. This inevitably takes longer, and is accompanied by a much more intense inflammatory response. Scar quality and cosmetic result are poor.

Wounds which may be left to heal by secondary intention:

- Extensive loss of epithelium
- Extensive contamination
- Extensive tissue damage
- Extensive oedema leading to inability to close
- Wound reopened e.g. infection, failure of knot

Third/tertiary intention

The wound is closed several days after its formation. This may well follow a period of healing by secondary intention, for example when infection is under control or tissue oedema is reduced.

Surgical procedures may be classified according to the risk of **wound contamination:**

- Clean   hernia repair
- Clean contaminated   cholecystectomy
- Contaminated wound   colonic resection
- Dirty wound   laparotomy for peritonitis

Ideal conditions for wound healing

- No foreign material
- No infection
- Accurate apposition
- No excess tension
- Good blood supply
- Good haemostasis, preventing haematoma

2.4 Classification of wounds

Superficial wounds

Involve only the epidermis and dermis and heal without formation of granulation tissue and true scar formation. Epithelial cells (including those from any residual skin appendages such as sweat or sebaceous glands and hair follicles) proliferate and migrate across the remaining dermal collagen.

Examples: Superficial burn
                      Graze
                      Split skin graft donor site.

Deep wounds

Involve layers deep to the dermis and heal with the migration of fibroblasts from perivascular tissue and formation of granulation tissue and subsequent true scar formation. If a deep wound is not closed with good tissue approximation, it heals by a combination of contraction and epithelialisation, which may lead to problematic contractures, especially if over a joint.

Examples:
- **Incised wounds** – surgical or traumatic (knife, glass)
- **Laceration** – an epithelial defect due to blunt trauma or tearing, and results from skin being stretched leading to failure of the dermis and avulsion of the deeper tissues. It is usually associated with adjacent soft tissue damage, and vascularity of the wound may be compromised (for example pretibial laceration in elderly women).
- **Degloving injury** – a form of laceration when shearing forces parallel tissue planes to move against each other leading to disruption and separation. Although the skin may be intact, it is often at risk due to disruption of its underlying blood supply.
- **Burns**

2.5 Surgical access, incisions and wound closure

The figure overleaf shows all commonly used incisions, and the table overleaf shows different routes of access to different organs.

The commonest reason for a difficult operation is inadequate access. This may be because the organ is difficult to access (oesophagogastric junction, gastrosplenic ligament, lower rectum), the body shape is unfavourable or the wrong incision has been used. The surgeon can affect only the last of these, and it is extremely important therefore to plan the incision before the operation, having considered the likely course of the operation.

If it is considered that different incisions may give identical access, then that incision which leads to better healing and cosmesis should be used. As a general rule, transverse incisions heal better than vertical ones.

Abdominal incisions can be closed either in layers or by a mass closure technique. The mass closure includes all layers of the abdominal wall except subcutaneous fat and skin, and has been shown to be as strong as a layered closure with no greater incidence of later wound complications such as dehiscence or incisional hernia formation. This is now the preferred closure method of most surgeons. The 1 cm rule should be obeyed – each bite of the abdominal wall should be a minimum of 1 cm, and adjacent bites must be a maximum of 1 cm apart. Skin can be closed using staples, subcuticular or 'over and over' suturing. There is no evidence that any different form of skin closure leads to a better cosmetic result in the long-term, and the choice is usually down to cost and surgeon's preference. Cross hatching of scars is not a problem as long as the sutures or staples are not left in too long.

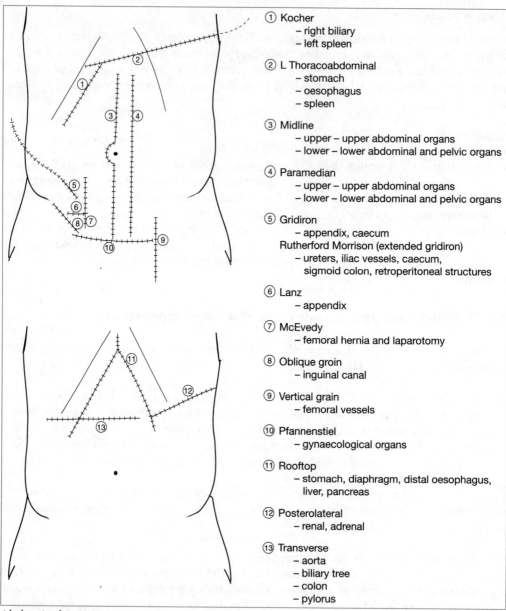

① Kocher
   – right biliary
   – left spleen

② L Thoracoabdominal
   – stomach
   – oesophagus
   – spleen

③ Midline
   – upper – upper abdominal organs
   – lower – lower abdominal and pelvic organs

④ Paramedian
   – upper – upper abdominal organs
   – lower – lower abdominal and pelvic organs

⑤ Gridiron
   – appendix, caecum
   Rutherford Morrison (extended gridiron)
   – ureters, iliac vessels, caecum,
        sigmoid colon, retroperitoneal structures

⑥ Lanz
   – appendix

⑦ McEvedy
   – femoral hernia and laparotomy

⑧ Oblique groin
   – inguinal canal

⑨ Vertical grain
   – femoral vessels

⑩ Pfannenstiel
   – gynaecological organs

⑪ Rooftop
   – stomach, diaphragm, distal oesophagus,
        liver, pancreas

⑫ Posterolateral
   – renal, adrenal

⑬ Transverse
   – aorta
   – biliary tree
   – colon
   – pylorus

Abdominal incisions

Organ		Approach
Oesophagus	Cervical	Cervical
	Upper thoracic	Right 4/5 posterolateral thoracotomy
	Mid thoracic	Right 5/6/7 posterolateral thoracotomy
	Lower thoracic	Right 5/6/7 posterolateral thoracotomy
		Left 6/7 posterolateral thoracotomy
		Left thoracoabdominal
	Abdominal	Left thoracoabdominal
		Rooftop
		Upper Midline
Stomach		Left thoracoabdominal
		Rooftop
		Upper Midline
Liver		Right thoracoabdominal
Biliary tree		Rooftop
		Upper Midline
		Right paramedian
		Kocher
		Transverse
Pancreas		Rooftop
Duodenum		Upper Midline
		Right paramedian
		Kocher
		Transverse
Small intestine		Midline
		Paramedian
		Transverse
Colon	Right	Midline
		Right paramedian
		Right transverse
		Rutherford Morrison
		Gridiron
	Appendix	Gridiron
		Lanz
	Left	Midline
		Left paramedian
		Left transverse
	Rectum	Midline
		Left paramedian
		Left transverse
		Perineal
Uterus, ovaries		Midline
		Pfannenstiel
Aorta		Midline
		Transverse
Iliac Vessels		Midline
		Transverse
		Rutherford Morrison
Bladder		Lower midline
		Pfannenstiel
Kidney		Midline
Adrenal glands		Kocher
		12th rib incision

Good surgical technique will optimise wound healing and cosmesis.

- Eliminate all dead tissue and infection
- Avoid haematoma
- Incise along natural tension lines
- Good apposition of tissues
- Avoid excess wound tension
- Ensure good blood supply
- Handle tissues gently
- Use appropriate suture material
- Choose appropriate closure technique

2.6 Delayed wound healing, wound dehiscence and incisional herniae

Predisposing factors

- **Local risk factors**
  Wound infection
  Haematoma
  Excessive mobility
  Foreign body
  Dead tissue
  Dirty wound
  Surgical technique
  Ischaemia a) acute damage to blood supply
             sutures too tight
          b) chronic previous irradiation
             diabetes
             atherosclerosis
             venous disease

- **General risk factors**
  Elderly
  Cardiac disease
  Respiratory disease
  Anaemia
  Obesity
  Renal or hepatic failure
  Diabetes mellitus
  Malnutrition – see below
  Malignancy
  Steroid or cytotoxic drugs
  Other immunosuppressive disease or drugs

Nutritional factors

- Proteins: essential for extracellular matrix formation and effective immune response
- Vitamin A: required for epithelial cell proliferation and differentiation

- Vitamin B6: required for collagen cross-linking
- Vitamin C: necessary for hydroxylation of proline and lysine residues; without hydroxyproline, newly synthesised collagen is not transported out of fibroblasts; in the absence of hydroxylysine, collagen fibrils are not cross-linked
- Zinc: essential trace element required for RNA and DNA synthesis and for the function of some 200 metalloenzymes
- Copper: plays a role in the cross-linking of collagen and elastin

On occasions the patient may be in such a poor condition (e.g. elderly, septic shock, on steroids) and the circumstances of the operation so hostile (emergency, faecal contamination, malignancy) that the chance of good wound healing would be very low. Under these circumstances, the surgeon would not carry out a primary bowel anastomosis, but would bring out a stoma, and maybe leave the skin and subcutaneous fat open, for delayed primary closure.

Wound dehiscence is the partial or total disruption of any or all layers of the operative wound.

Evisceration is rupture of all layers of the abdominal wall and extrusion of the abdominal viscera (usually preceded by the appearance of blood-stained fluid 'pink fluid sign').

Wound dehiscence without evisceration should be repaired by immediate elective reclosure. Dehiscence of a laparotomy wound with evisceration is a surgical emergency with a 25%+ mortality rate. Management involves resuscitation, protection of the organs with moist sterile towels and immediate closure, usually with deep tension sutures.

Incisional herniae are still common despite modern suture materials. Treatment depends on symptoms and size of defect.

2.7 Contractures and scars

As a scar forms, the strength increases rapidly within a period of 7–10 days, and it is at this stage that sutures are normally removed. It is usually many months, however, before the scar regains full strength. As fibrous tissue is laid down, this tissue is continually digested to modify the shape of the scar, and these two competing influences are usually in balance. If too little fibrous tissue is laid down, or excessive breakdown takes place, the wound will fail to heal adequately leading to wound dehiscence (early) or hernia formation (late). Conversely, if excessive scar tissue is laid down, the scar may be hypertrophic or keloid. Furthermore the scars may shorten, leading to contractures. Wounds made along natural tension lines (Langer's lines) or skin creases are much less likely to cause such problems.

Contractures

- These occur as the scar shortens. They may lead to distortion of adjacent structures (e.g. near the eye) or limit flexibility in joints. Contractures can be both prevented and treated by using a Z-plasty to break up the scar. Physiotherapy, massage and even splintage can be used to prevent contractures when scars cross joint surfaces.

97

Hypertrophic scars

- Most wounds become red and hard for a while but after several months spontaneous maturation leads to a pale soft scar. Occasionally this excessive scar tissue remains, but is *limited* to the site of the original wound
- Due to fibroblast overactivity in the proliferative phase; eventually this is corrected (usually by one year) and a more normal scar results

Keloid scars

- Excessive scar tissue which *extends* beyond the original wound
- Intense fibroblast activity continues into the maturation phase
- Complications – cosmetic, contractures and loss of function
- Prevention – use Langer's lines, meticulous wound closure without undue tension, avoidance of infection, and the use of pressure garments

Risk factors for hypertrophic and keloid scars

- Young age
- Male sex
- Dark pigmented skin
- Genetic predisposition
- Site – sternum, shoulders, head and neck
- Tension on wound
- Delayed healing

Treatment of hypertrophic and keloid scars

- Excision – will usually lead to recurrence
- Excision and radiotherapy – not always successful, and cannot be repeated
- Intralesional steroid injection – variable response rates
- Pressure garments
- Silastic gel treatment
- Carbon dioxide laser – variable response rates

Malignant change in scar

Rarely squamous cell cancers can form in scars (so-called Marjolin ulcer). Any unusual ulceration or appearance in a scar should be biopsied.

2.8 Dressings

Dressings can make a huge contribution to the healing of a wound. The optimum healing environment for a wound is:

- Moist
- Free of infection, with minimal slough
- Free of chemicals and foreign bodies (e.g. fibres from dressing)

- At the optimum temperature
- Minimal number of dressing changes
- The correct pH

Different dressings are appropriate for different stages of the wound healing, and therefore good wound management necessitates a flexible approach to the selection and use of dressings.

Requirements from a dressing

- Protection from infection and trauma
- Debrides, both mechanically and chemically
- Absorbent and removes excess exudates, whilst keeping wound moist
- Maintains temperature and gaseous exchange
- Comfortable and cosmetically acceptable
- Stimulate healing
- Inexpensive and easy to change

Commonly used dressings

Traditional dressings such as gauze and 'Gamgee' have few indications for the modern treatment of wounds. Modern dressings can be classified thus:

Hydrocolloids

- Available in pastes, granules and wafers
- Consist of mixture of carboxymethylcellulose, pectins, gelatins and elastomers
- Forms a gel on contact with wound secretions, which absorbs secretions
- e.g. Granuflex

Hydrofibre

- Consists of carboxymethylcellulose spun into a fibre
- Forms a gel on contact with wound secretions, which absorbs secretions
- Good for heavily exudating wounds
- e.g. Aquacel

Hydrogels

- Consist of insoluble polymers, water and propylene glycol
- Absorb large volumes of exudates and effective at desloughing/debriding
- Available in sheets or gels

Semipermeable film dressings

- Clear polyurethane film coated with an adhesive
- Not suitable if excessive exudate

Alginates

- Extracted from seaweed

- Absorb secretions to form gel to optimise moist wound healing
- Available in sheet form or ribbon for packing
- e.g. Kaltostat, Sorbsan

Foam dressings

- Consist of polyurethane or silicone foam
- Very absorbent
- For flat and cavity wounds – the latter in two forms: liquid foam polymer and hydrocellular cavity dressing

Antimicrobial dressings

- Usage has declined in recent years
- Little evidence of benefit
- e.g. Inadine, bactigras

Artificial and living skin equivalents

- Increasing interest in recent years
- These can facilitate cell proliferation, production of extracellular matrix components and increase concentrations of growth factors in the wound
- Epidermal components e.g. Vivoderm
- Dermal components e.g. Dermagraft
- Composite grafts (epidermal and dermal components) e.g. Apligraf

2.9 Drains

Drains are used for a variety of purposes, and overall the use of drains is reducing.

Indications

- To minimise dead space in a wound and prevent fluid collecting (e.g. following axillary nodal clearance, mastectomy, thyroidectomy)
- When risk of leakage (e.g. pancreatic surgery, bowel anastomosis)
- To drain actual fluid collections (e.g. radiologically placed drain for subphrenic abscess)
- To divert fluid away from blockage or potential blockage (e.g. biliary T-tube, suprapubic urinary catheter, ventricular CSF drain)
- To decompress and allow air to escape (chest drain)

Types

- Drains can be open (into dressings) or closed (into container) systems, and suction or non-suction (passive gravity drainage)
- Suction drains provide better drainage, but may damage adjacent structures, e.g. bowel, precipitating a leak
- Closed systems reduce the risk of introducing infection

Examples

- Suction drains (closed) – Redivac drain, suction chest drain
- Non-suction drains (open) – Penrose drain, corrugated drain
- Non-suction drains (closed) – Robinson drain, T-tube, urinary catheter, chest drain

Complications

- Infection via drain track
- Lets in air (e.g. chest drain)
- Injury to adjacent structures by drain or during placement e.g. bowel
- Anastomotic leakage – see below
- Retraction of the drain into the wound
- Bleeding by erosion into blood vessel
- Pain, e.g. chest drain irritating diaphragm
- Herniation at the drain site

Routine drainage of a bowel anastomosis is not recommended. They may cause more problems than they solve. They can directly damage the anastomosis, and can prevent formations of adhesions to adjacent vascular structures through which the anastomosis would expect to gain an extra blood supply. If the anastomosis is not watertight (e.g. biliary or urological) a drain is usually used to prevent build-up of a collection which may hinder healing.

3. SURGICAL HAEMATOLOGY

3.1 Haemostasis

Haemostasis is the physiological cessation of bleeding. It involves a series of complex interrelated events.

Key events

- Vascular injury with exposure of subendothelial tissue factor and collagen
- Vasoconstriction
- Platelet adherence and aggregation at the injury site (platelet plug)
- Platelet degranulation
- Activation of the coagulation cascade
- Platelet plug stabilised with cross-linked fibrin
- Fibrinolysis and vasodilatation
- Regulatory feedback mechanisms achieve a balance between haemostasis and fibrinolysis

Endothelial cell role in haemostasis

Endothelial cells form a barrier between their enveloping connective tissues and the blood. They also produce thrombotic and antithrombotic factors.

Role of endothelial cells in haemostasis

● Factor	● Action
Antithrombotic	
Prostacyclin (PGI2)	Inhibitor of platelet aggregation and vasodilator
Thrombomodulin	A glycoprotein bound to the endothelial cell membrane; on complexing with thrombin it activates protein C, (cofactor protein S), which degrades factors Va and VIIIa; it thus reduces fibrin formation
Nitric oxide	Vasodilator and inhibitor of platelet aggregation and adhesion
Tissue plasminogen activator (tPA)	Regulates fibrinolysis
Thrombotic	
von Willebrand's factor (vWF)	Cofactor for platelet adhesion and factor VIII
Platelet activating factor	Platelet aggregation and activation
Plasminogen activator inhibitor	tPA inhibitor

Role of platelets

Platelets play a crucial role in haemostasis:

- At sites of vascular injury they bind, via vWF, to subendothelial collagen
- On activation they secrete the contents of their alpha and dense granules: fibrinogen and ADP induce aggregation and thromboxane A2 causes vasoconstriction
- Platelet aggregation forms a platelet plug
- Their cell membrane becomes procoagulant by providing binding sites for coagulation factors and fibrin
- The platelet plug becomes stabilised with cross-linked fibrin

Coagulation system

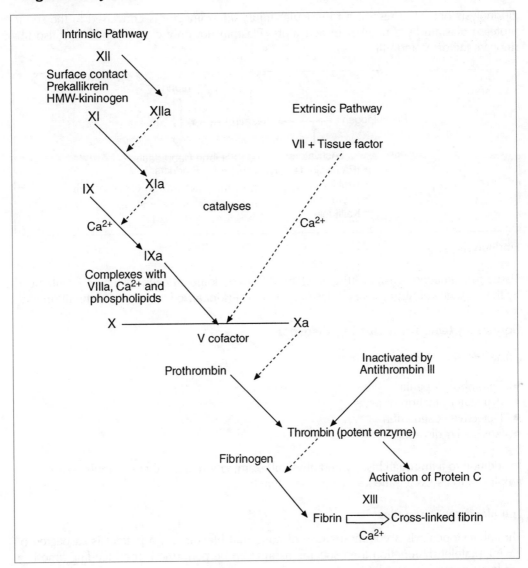

Coagulation system

Antithrombin III inactivates thrombin in the presence of heparin. It also inactivates factors VIIa, IXa, Xa, XIa, kallikrein and plasmin.

Fibrinolysis

Fibrinolysis occurs in response to vascular injury. Plasminogen is converted to the serine protease plasmin by a number of activators. Plasmin not only cleaves fibrin but also fibrinogen, factors V and VIII.

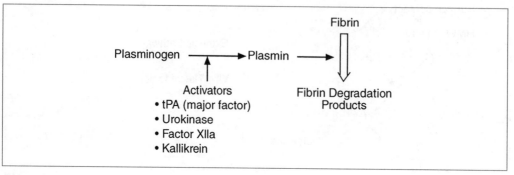

Fibrinolysis

Tissue plasminogen activator (tPA) is released from endothelial cells. Its action is enhanced by the presence of fibrin, hence, plasmin formation is localised to the site of the fibrin clot.

Screening tests for a clotting disorder

Defective haemostasis may result from:

- Thrombocytopenia
- A platelet function disorder
- Defective coagulation
- A vascular disorder

In addition to a thorough history and physical examination, a number of simple tests can be employed to assess a patient's haemostatic function.

Full blood count and film

Thrombocytopenia is a common cause of abnormal bleeding. If a patient is suspected of having platelet dysfunction then specific assays can be performed. The bleeding time is a crude assessment of platelet function.

Activated partial thromboplastin time (APTT)
Measures the intrinsic as well as the common pathway factors (X to fibrin). Normal time is about 30–40 seconds.

Prothrombin time (PT)
Assesses the extrinsic system factor (VII) as well as the common pathway factors. It is often expressed as the international normalised ratio (INR).

Thrombin time (TT)
This detects deficiencies of fibrinogen or inhibition of thrombin. Normal clotting time is 14–16 seconds.

Specific coagulation factor tests
For example, in haemophilia (Factor VIII), Christmas disease (Factor IX).

Fibrinogen and FDP levels
Useful for detection of on-going intravascular coagulation (e.g. disseminated intravascular coagulation (DIC)).

Results of common bleeding disorders

	PT	APTT	TT	Platelet count
Liver disease	Inc	Inc	Usually N	Dec
Warfarin	Inc	Usually N	N	N
Heparin	Usually N	Inc	Inc	N
Factor VII deficiency	Inc	N	N	N
Factor VIII deficiency	N	Inc	N	N
Factor IX deficiency	N	Inc	N	N
Disseminated intravascular coagulation (DIC)	Inc	Inc	Inc	Dec

Inc = increased, Dec = decreased, N = normal.

3.2 Bleeding disorders

Congenital bleeding disorders

Haemophilia A
Haemophilia A is an X-linked recessive disorder that results from a deficiency or an abnormality of the coagulation factor VIII. It affects 1 in 10,000 males (females can also rarely be affected) and up to 30% of cases are due to spontaneous mutations. It is characterised by bleeding into soft tissues, muscles and weight-bearing joints, the onset of which may be delayed by several hours after the injury. The functional level of factor VIII determines the severity of the disorder:

- **Severe disease**: <1% factor VIII
  Frequent bleeding after minor trauma
- **Moderate disease**: 1–5% factor VIII
  Less frequent bleeding
- **Mild disease**: 5–25% factor VIII
  Persistent bleeding usually secondary to trauma

105

The majority of affected individuals have factor VIII levels below 5%. Approximately 10–20% of patients develop antibodies to factor VIII. Treatment depends on the severity of the disorder and the proposed surgery. Factor VIII concentrate may have to be given repeatedly or continuously to maintain factor VIII levels. Desmopressin can be used transiently to raise the factor VIII level in patients with mild haemophilia.

Haemophilia B
Haemophilia B, also known as Christmas disease, is an X-linked disorder, which is clinically indistinguishable from haemophilia A. It occurs in 1 in 100,000 male births and is due to a defect or deficiency in factor IX. Treatment involves either prothrombin complex concentrate, which contains all of the vitamin K-dependent clotting factors, or factor IX concentrate.

von Willebrand's disease
von Willebrand's disease is the *most common* of the congenital bleeding disorders, occurring in as many as 1 in 800–1000 individuals. von Willebrand factor (vWF) is a plasma glycoprotein, which has two main functions. It aids platelet adhesion to the subendothelium at sites of vascular injury and serves as the plasma carrier protein for factor VIII. Three main disease subtypes have been described:

- Type I: (most common) autosomal dominant (quantitative reduction of vWF)
- Type II: variably inherited (qualitative defects in vWF)
- Type III: (very rare) autosomal recessive (almost no vWF)

Patients with the disease develop mucosal bleeding, petechiae, epistaxis and menorrhagia similar to patients with platelet disorders. Treatment depends on the symptoms and the underlying type of disease. Cryoprecipitate, factor VIII concentrate or desmopressin can be used.

Acquired bleeding disorders

Thrombocytopenia

- Normal platelet count 150–400 $\times$ 10^9/l
- Spontaneous bleeding uncommon 40–100 $\times$ 10^9/l
- Spontaneous bleeding often severe <10 $\times$ 10^9/l

Causes of thrombocytopenia

- Decreased production (marrow aplasia, marrow infiltration, uraemia and alcoholism)
- Decreased survival (drugs, ITP)
- Increased consumption (DIC, infection, heparin therapy)

Vitamin K deficiency
Vitamin K is a fat-soluble vitamin that is absorbed in the small intestine and stored in the liver. Serves as a cofactor gamma-carboxylase in the production of the coagulation factors II, VII, IX and protein C and protein S. The normal liver contains a 30–day store of the vitamin, but the acutely ill patient can become deficient in 7–10 days.

Causes of vitamin K deficiency

- Inadequate dietary intake
- Malabsorption
- Lack of bile salts
- Hepatocellular disease
- Cephalosporin antibiotics

Parenteral vitamin K produces a correction in clotting times within 8–10 hours. Fresh frozen plasma (FFP) should be administered to patients with ongoing bleeding.

Hepatic failure

Hepatocellular disease is often accompanied by impaired haemostasis.

Causes:

- Decreased synthesis of coagulation factors (except factor VIII)
- Decreased synthesis of coagulation inhibitors: protein C, protein S and antithrombin III
- Reduced clearance of activated coagulation factors, which may cause either DIC or systematic fibrinolysis
- Impaired absorption and metabolism of vitamin K
- Splenomegaly and secondary thrombocytopenia

Renal failure

Causes a decrease in platelet aggregation and adhesion.

Acquired vascular defects

A heterogeneous group of conditions characterised by bruising after minor trauma and spontaneous bleeding from small blood vessels.

- Senile purpura: due to atrophy of perivascular supporting tissues
- Scurvy: defective collagen due to vitamin C deficiency
- Steroid purpura
- Henoch–Schönlein syndrome
- Ehlers–Danlos syndrome: hereditary collagen abnormality

Congenital prothrombotic disorders

Antithrombin III deficiency

- Rare autosomal dominant disorder
- Antithrombin III inactivates thrombin, factors VIIa, IXa, Xa, XIa, kallikrein and plasmin
- Antithrombin III level measured by immunological assay
- Less than 70% of normal value increases risk of venous thrombosis
- Deficiency also associated with liver disease, DIC, nephrotic syndrome and heparin therapy
- Prophylaxis and treatment involves antithrombin III concentrate and anticoagulation

Protein C and protein S deficiencies

- Autosomal dominant disorders with variable penetrance
- Protein C is activated by thrombin binding to thrombomodulin, a glycoprotein bound to the endothelial cell membrane; this causes a reduction in fibrin formation by the degradation of factors Va and VIIIa; protein S acts as a cofactor
- Protein C and S levels can be assessed by immunoassay techniques
- Treatment involves replacement protein C or S and anticoagulation

Acquired prothrombotic disorders

Disseminated intravascular coagulation (DIC)

DIC is a systemic thrombohaemorrhagic disorder. It is the pathological response to many underlying disorders.

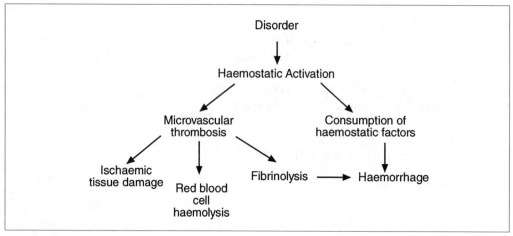

Disseminated intravascular coagulation

Conditions associated with DIC

- Malignancy
- Massive tissue injury and trauma
- Obstetric complications (e.g. placental abruption, septic abortion, intrauterine fetal death and amniotic fluid embolism)
- Infections (especially Gram-negative bacteria)
- Miscellaneous (e.g. acute pancreatitis, drug reactions, transplant rejection and ARDS)

The clinical presentation is extremely variable. Most patients present with easy bruising and haemorrhage from venepuncture and intramuscular injection sites. This may progress to profuse haemorrhage from mucous membranes and shock. Although haemorrhage is the most common presentation, about 10% present with widespread thrombosis and resultant multiorgan failure.

Laboratory features

- Thrombocytopenia
- Prolonged PT, APTT and TT
- Increased fibrin degradation products (also increased after surgery)
- Reduced fibrinogen level
- Fragmented red blood cells

Management

- Diagnosis and treatment of the underlying disorder
- Shock exacerbates DIC therefore adequate fluid resuscitation is essential
- Use FFP, cryoprecipitate and platelet concentrates as required; be guided by regular laboratory screening
- The use of heparin is controversial; it has been given in an attempt to reduce thrombin formation via antithrombin III activation, but trials have shown little benefit; however, if thrombosis is the predominant feature, heparin should be used at a relatively early stage.

3.3 Anticoagulant drugs

- **Warfarin**   Blocks the synthesis of vitamin K dependent factors
  It prolongs the PT and may slightly elevate the APTT
  It is highly plasma protein bound, therefore caution must be exercised when giving other drugs, as these may potentiate its effects
  Treatment of major bleeding consists of the administration of vitamin K and FFP
  The dose is adjusted to maintain the International normalised ratio (INR – ratio of patient's PT to that of control plasma) at level between 1 and 4 according to the degree of anticoagulation required.
- **Heparin**   A potent anticoagulant that binds to and activates antithrombin III, thus reducing fibrin formation. Heparin is neutralised with intravenous protamine (1 mg protamine for every 100 units of heparin)
  Can only be given parenterally. The dose is monitored by measurement of the ratio of the patient's APTT to that of control plasma
- **NSAIDs**   Low-dose aspirin irreversibly acetylates the enzyme cyclo-oxygenase
  Affected platelets are therefore unable to synthesise thromboxane A2 and become inactivated throughout their seven-day life span
  Other NSAIDs cause a reversible effect that lasts 3–4 days

For elective surgical patients on oral anticoagulation, the challenge is to balance the risk of haemorrhage if the INR is not reduced, against the risk of thrombosis if the INR is reduced for too long or by too great an amount. For some patients it is reasonable to stop the warfarin a few days before the surgery, and then restart afterwards at the maintenance dose, since the risk of thrombosis is relatively low (e.g. atrial fibrillation). In others (e.g. prosthetic heart valves) this approach would be prohibitively risky, and it is necessary to admit the patient several days before surgery, stop the warfarin and fully heparinise the patient. The heparin is then stopped six hours before surgery, and restarted immediately after surgery has finished. This minimises the length of time of increased thrombotic risk.

3.4 Blood transfusion

The supply of blood and plasma is based entirely on the goodwill of voluntary, healthy blood donors.

Blood grouping and compatibility testing

Red cells carry antigens, which are typically glycoproteins or glycolipids, attached to the red cell membrane. Antibodies to the ABO antigens are naturally occurring, whereas antibodies to other red cell antigens appear only after sensitisation by transfusion or pregnancy. Compatibility testing entails suspension of group-compatible red cells from a donor pack with recipient serum, incubation to allow reactions to occur, and examination for agglutination to ensure that no reaction has occurred.

Over 90% of donated blood is separated into its various constituents to allow prescription of individual components and preparation of pooled plasma from which specific blood products are manufactured – see below.

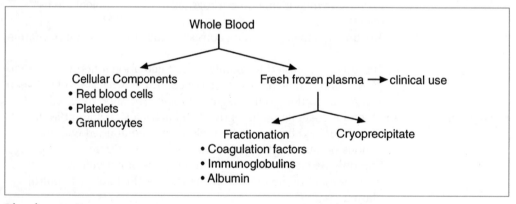

Blood components

Red blood cell concentrates

- In whole blood granulocytes and platelets lose function, many coagulation factors lose activity, and aggregates of dead cells, platelets, and other debris are formed unless it is used within a few days
- Red blood cell concentrates or packed cells consist of whole blood from which the plasma has been removed

- Red blood cells (RBCs) suspended in a solution (SAG-M) containing sodium chloride, adenine, glucose and mannitol
- Volume of one unit – 350 ml
- Shelf life of 35 days at 4°C
- Storage changes include increase in potassium and phosphate concentration, decrease in pH, haemolysis, microaggregation of dead cells, and loss of clotting factor VIII and V activity
- Washed RBCs are used in patients who cannot tolerate granulocyte and platelet debris normally present in RBC concentrates
- Units of rare blood types may be stored for up to 3 years at –65°C in glycerol containing media

Indications for transfusion

- Hb less than 7g/dl
- Red blood cell concentrates should simply be used to increase the oxygen-carrying capacity of the blood
- Whole blood should be used for transfusion when there is significant bleeding leading to hypovolaemia

Platelet concentrates

- Platelets suspended in plasma
- Shelf life of 5 days at room temperature

Indications for transfusion

- Thrombocytopenia prior to an invasive procedure
- Significant haemorrhage in the presence of thrombocytopenia
- Consumptive coagulopathy (e.g. DIC, significant haemorrhage)
- Prophylactic transfusion in patients with thrombocytopenia due to bone marrow failure, chemotherapy or radiotherapy
- Prophylactic or therapeutic transfusion in patients with primary platelet function disorders

Platelet concentrates should be ABO group compatible. Anti-D immunoglobulin should be given to premenopausal RhD-negative women to prevent sensitisation.

Granulocytes

- Very short shelf life of 24 hours at room temperature
- Prepared from a single donor or a pooled collection

Fresh Frozen Plasma (FFP)

- Prepared by centrifugation of donor whole blood within 6 hours of collection and frozen at –30°C
- Contains all coagulation factors

- Shelf life of 12 months at −30°C
- Unit volume approximately 250 ml
- Should be used within 1 hour of thawing
- Cryoprecipitate is produced by the slow thawing of FFP; this is rich in factors VIII and XIII, fibrinogen and vWF
- Individual clotting factors, immunoglobulins and plasma proteins may be isolated from plasma

Indications for FFP transfusion

- Prophylaxis or treatment of haemorrhage in patients with specific coagulation factor deficiencies for which the specific factor is unavailable
- DIC, in conjunction with cryoprecipitate and platelets
- Haemorrhage secondary to over-anticoagulation with warfarin (treatment with vitamin K or prothrombin complex and factor VII may be more effective)
- Following replacement of large volumes of blood (e.g. >4 units) where coagulation abnormalities often occur (guided by APTT)
- Thrombotic thrombocytopenic purpura

Not indicated in hypovolaemia, plasma exchange, nutritional support and immunodeficiency states.

Group compatible FFP should be used. To prevent Rh immunisation, RhD compatible FFP should be used in premenopausal women.

Albumin solutions
(See Section 8.5)

- Albumin should not be used as a general purpose plasma volume expander; it has no proven benefit over other colloid solutions
- In addition it should not be used as parenteral nutrition, or in impaired protein production or chronic protein loss disorders
- The only proven indication for the administration of 20% albumin is diuretic-resistant oedema in hypoproteinaemic patients

Coagulation factors

Cryoprecipitate
Used in haemorrhagic disorders with a fibrinogen deficiency (e.g. DIC).

Factor VIII concentrate
Treatment of haemophilia A and von Willebrand's disease.

Factor IX concentrate

Contains factors IX, X, and XI; it is used in the treatment of haemophilia B and congenital deficiencies of factors X and XI. When combined with factor VII concentrate it is more effective than FFP in the treatment of severe haemorrhage due to excessive warfarinisation and liver disease.

Other specific coagulation factors, including anticoagulant factors, protein C and antithrombin III, are available.

Autotransfusion

Due to concerns over the potential complications associated with blood transfusions, autotransfusion has become more popular. There are three methods of administering an autologous transfusion:

- **Pre-deposit**: blood is taken from the patient in the weeks prior to admission for elective surgery
- **Haemodilution**: blood is taken immediately prior to surgery and then reintroduced post-operatively
- **Intraoperative**: blood lost during the operation is processed and reinfused immediately. Contraindications are exposure of the blood to a site of infection, or the possibility of contamination with malignant cells.

Autologous transfusion (first two methods) is contraindicated in patients with active infection, unstable angina, aortic stenosis and severe hypertension. Due to patient restriction and high costs, autotransfusion has at present a limited role.

3.5 Complications of transfusion

- Immunological complications
- Infectious complications
- Miscellaneous

Immunological complications

Incompatible red cells

The mortality associated with the transfusion of blood products is approximately 1 per 100,000 units transfused. ABO incompatibility is the most common cause of death and is predominately due to clerical error.

Immunological complications

- **Immediate haemolytic transfusion reactions**
  Most severe haemolytic transfusion reactions are due to ABO incompatibility
  5–10 ml of blood is sufficient to cause reaction
  Symptoms: rigors, substernal pain and restlessness
  Signs: fever, hypotension, bleeding, haemoglobinuria, oliguria and jaundice
  Rhesus incompatibility does not cause complement activation and is
  usually milder

- **Delayed haemolytic transfusion reactions**
  Typically occurs 5–10 days after transfusion
  Occurs in approximately 1 in 500 transfusions
  Due to a secondary response; occurs in patients who have been immunised to a
  foreign antigen by a previous transfusion or pregnancy but in whom tests prior to
  the transfusion do not detect the low antibody concentration
  Signs: fever, progressive anaemia, jaundice and haemoglobinuria

Incompatible white cells

- Febrile reactions
- Relatively common in patients who have had previous transfusions or have been pregnant
- Symptoms: facial flushing and fever shortly after commencing the transfusion
- Due to the recipient's leucocyte antibodies complexing with donor leucocytes and causing the release of pyrogens from monocytes and granulocytes
- Most reactions respond to slowing the transfusion and giving aspirin or paracetamol

Transfusion-related acute lung injury (TRALI)

- Symptoms: fever, dyspnoea and cough; infiltrates on chest radiograph
- Result of incompatibility between donor antibodies and recipient granulocytes

Incompatible platelets

- Post-transfusion purpura may occur in patients who have been previously sensitised to a foreign platelet antigen; on subsequent exposure they mount a secondary response which causes destruction of the patient's own platelets.

Adverse reactions to plasma

- Urticaria results from a patient's IgE antibody complexing with a protein present in the donor's plasma; usually responds to slowing the transfusion rate and administering an antihistamine.
- Anaphylactic reactions rarely occur; they are usually due to anti-IgA antibodies in the patient's plasma binding to normal IgA in the donor's plasma; the incidence of anti-IgA individuals is approximately 1 in 1000.

Infectious complications

Blood donations in the UK are presently screened for hepatitis B surface antigen, antibodies to HIV, hepatitis C virus and to *Treponema pallidum* (syphilis). 'High risk' patients are excluded from donation.

Infections

- HIV: risk of transmission is less than 1 in 2 million units; previously (before screening) many haemophiliacs developed this disease
- Hepatitis: incidence of hepatitis B transmission is approximately 1 in 200,000 units transfused; the risk of hepatitis C transmission is between 1 in 150,000–200,000
- HTLV
- CMV
- Parvovirus: can cause aplastic crisis in a patient with sickle cell anaemia
- Bacteria: very uncommon; incidence less than 1 in 1 million units; *Y. enterocolitica* and *Pseudomonas spp.* are the most common; usually caused by delayed administration of donated blood (when stood at room temperature, blood is an excellent culture medium)
- Parasites: recent travel to regions where malaria is endemic is a contraindication to blood donation; because *P. malariae* has a long incubation period a few cases of transfusion-related malaria still occur.

Miscellaneous complications

- Fluid overload
- Air embolus
- Iron overload
- Immunosuppression. There is some evidence that blood transfusion results in a poorer prognosis in patients with colorectal cancer.
- Graft versus host disease (GVHD) – immunodeficient patients at risk

Massive transfusion

Defined as transfusion of the total blood volume in less than 24 hours.

Complications

- Cardiac abnormalities (ventricular arrhythmias) due to low temperature, high potassium concentration and excess citrate with low calcium concentration
- Hypothermia – use blood warmer
- Hyperkalaemia
- Hypocalcaemia
- Metabolic acidosis because of acid load in stored blood
- Coagulopathy due to lack of platelets and clotting factors in stored blood. FFP should be given prophylactically, and platelets if level less than $50 \times 10^9/l$
- Adult Respiratory Distress Syndrome/acute lung injury
- Disseminated Intravascular Coagulation

4. PAIN CONTROL

Pain is an unpleasant sensory and emotional experience associated with actual or potential tissue damage. It is a protective mechanism.

4.1 Harmful effects of under-treated acute pain

Harmful effects of under-treated acute pain

- **Cardiovascular**
  Tachycardia
  Hypertension
  Increased myocardial oxygen consumption
- **Respiratory**
  Splinting of the chest wall and therefore decreased lung volumes
  Atelectasis
  Inability to cough adequately, therefore sputum retention
  Infection
- **Gastrointestinal**
  Reduced gastric emptying and bowel movement
- **Genitourinary**
  Urinary retention
- **Musculoskeletal**
  Muscle spasm
  Immobility (therefore increased risk of DVT)
- **Psychological**
  Anxiety
  Fear
  Sleeplessness
- **Neuroendocrine**
  Secretion of catecholamines and catabolic hormones, leading to increased metabolism and oxygen consumption, and promotes sodium and water retention

4.2 Nociception

Four physiological processes are involved in the experiencing of pain, collectively called **nociception**:

- Transduction
- Transmission
- Modulation
- Perception

Transduction

The translation of a noxious stimulus into electrical activity at the sensory endings of nerves. A noxious stimulus can be mechanical, chemical or thermal. The pain receptors in the skin and other tissues are all free nerve endings. The noxious stimulus results in tissue damage and inflammation.

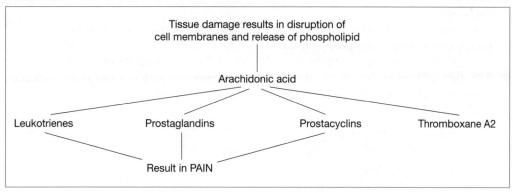

Events in tissue damage

Nociceptive neurones can change in their responsiveness to stimuli, especially in the presence of inflammation.

- In an area of damaged tissue the nociceptive threshold is decreased, i.e. normally noxious stimuli result in an exaggerated response (**primary hyperalgesia**); for example, the extreme sensitivity of sunburned skin
- In damaged tissue there can be a lower pain threshold in areas beyond the site of injury (**secondary hyperalgesia**)
- In damaged tissue normally innocuous stimuli, for example light touch, can cause pain (**allodynia**); for example, in peritonitis a light touch can cause severe pain
- In damaged tissue, pain is prolonged beyond the application of the stimuli (**hyperpathia**)

Transmission

Impulses travel in A (fast) and C (slow) fibres. A fibres transmit acute sharp pain, C fibres transmit slow chronic pain.
Due to this 'dual system' of pain transmission, a painful stimulus results in a 'double' pain sensation, a fast sharp pain followed by slow burning pain. 'Fast' pain involves a localised reflex flexion response, removing that part of the body from the injurious stimulus, therefore limiting tissue damage. Although C fibre pain is not well localised, it results in immobility which enforces rest and therefore promotes healing of the injured part.

- A fibres terminate at two places in the dorsal horn; laminae 1 and 5
- C fibres terminate in laminae 2 and 3 of the dorsal horn (this area is called the **substantia gelatinosa**)

- These primary afferent fibres synapse onto second-order neurones in the dorsal horn (the neurotransmitter here is **substance P**)
- The majority of these second-order neurones cross over in the **anterior white commissure** about one segment rostrally and ascend as the **lateral spinothalamic tract**; in the brainstem this is called the **spinal lemniscus**
- The second-order neurones eventually synapse in the thalamus (**ventral posterolateral nucleus**)
- From here the third-order neurone passes through the **internal capsule** to the **somaesthetic area** in the **postcentral gyrus** of the cerebral cortex, for conscious perception and localisation of the pain. This projection is **somatotopic**.
- Although A fibres project to the cortex, the C fibres nearly all terminate in the reticular formation, which is responsible for the general arousal of the CNS.

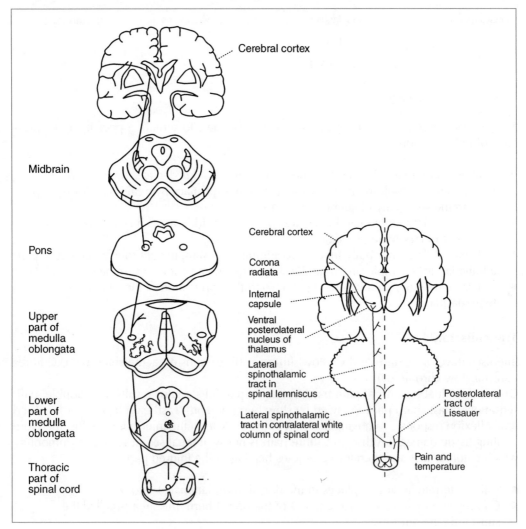

Pain and temperature pathways

Modulation

Central mechanisms

(Sometimes called the descending antinociceptive tract.)

- This originates in the periaqueductal grey and periventricular area of the midbrain, and descends to the dorsal horn of the spinal cord; here enkephalins are released which cause presynaptic inhibition of incoming pain fibres.
- Throughout the descending antinociceptive tract there are receptors which respond to morphine; the brain has its own natural opiates known as endorphins and enkephalins which act along this pathway; opiate analgesics act via these opioid receptors.

Spinal mechanisms

- Opioids act directly at the spinal laminae inhibiting the release of substance P, (the neurotransmitter involved between the primary and secondary afferent fibres) e.g. epidural injection.

Mechanical inhibition of pain

Stimulation of mechanoreceptors in the area of the body where the pain originates can inhibit pain by stimulation of large A fibres. (This is why rubbing the affected part or tran-scutaneous electrical nerve stimulation (TENS) induces analgesia.) TENS involves applying a small electrical current over the nerve distribution of pain. This activates the large sensory fibres and inhibits pain transmission through the dorsal horn. This is known as 'pain gating'.

Perception

This occurs in the thalamus and sensory cortex.

4.3 Referred pain

This pain is perceived as occurring in a part of the body topographically distinct from the source.

Branches of visceral pain fibres synapse in the spinal cord with some of the same second-order neurones which receive pain fibres from the skin. Therefore when the visceral pain fibres are stimulated, pain signals from the viscera can be conducted through second-order neurones which normally conduct pain signals from the skin. The person then perceives the pain as originating in the skin itself.

4.4 Visceral pain

- Viscera have sensory receptors for no other modality of sensation except pain. Localised damage to viscera rarely causes severe pain. Stimuli that cause diffuse stimulation of nerve endings in a viscus can cause pain which is very severe (e.g. ischaemia, smooth muscle spasm, distension of a hollow viscus, chemical damage to visceral surfaces).

- Visceral pain from the thoracic and abdominal cavities is transmitted through sensory nerve fibres which run in the sympathetic nerves. These fibres are C fibres (i.e. they transmit burning/aching type pain).
- Some visceral pain fibres enter the spinal cord through the sacral parasympathetic nerves, including those from distal colon, rectum and bladder.
- Note that visceral pain fibres may enter the cord via the cranial nerves (e.g. glossopharyngeal and vagus nerves) which transmit pain from the pharynx, trachea and upper oesophagus.

If a disease affecting a viscus spreads to the parietal wall surrounding the viscera, the pain perceived will be sharp and intense. The parietal wall is innervated from spinal nerves, including the fast A fibres.

Localisation of pain

Visceral pain is referred to various dermatomes on the body surface. The position on the surface of the body to which pain is referred depends on the segment of the body from which the organ developed embryologically. For example, the heart originated in the neck and upper thorax, therefore the visceral pain fibres from the surface of the heart enter the cord from C3 to T5. These are the dermatome segments in which cardiac pain may be perceived. Pain from organs derived from the foregut is felt in the upper abdomen, pain from organs derived from the midgut is felt in the mid-abdomen, and pain from organs derived from the hindgut is felt in the lower abdomen.

Parietal pain (e.g. from parietal peritoneum) is transmitted via spinal nerves which supply the external body surface.

Example: acute appendicitis

- A colicky umbilical pain appears to 'move' to the right iliac fossa and becomes constant
- Visceral pain is transmitted via the sympathetic chain at the level of T10; this pain is referred to the dermatome corresponding to this area, i.e. around the umbilicus; this is colicky pain associated with obstruction of a hollow viscus (the appendix)
- Where the inflamed appendix touches the parietal peritoneum, these impulses pass via spinal nerves to level L1–L2. This constant pain will be localised in the right iliac fossa (at McBurney's point, a third of the distance from anterior superior iliac spine to umbilicus).

4.5 Methods of assessing acute pain

Subjective measures

Verbal scale

- None
- Mild
- Moderate
- Severe

Visual analogue score

- Ranging from worst pain ever (10) to no pain at all (0)
- Smiley/sad faces

Objective measures

Most are indirect, e.g. blood pressure variations, vital capacity.

4.6 Management of post-operative pain

The realistic aim of pain relief is not to abolish pain completely, but to ensure the patients are comfortable and have return of function with a more rapid recovery and rehabilitation. Two fundamental concepts prevail:

- Preventing development of pain is more effective than treatment of established pain – pre-emptive analgesia, given prior to surgical trauma, using parenteral opioids, regional blocks or NSAIDS
- It is difficult to produce safe, effective analgesia for major surgery with a single group of drugs (monomodal therapy). Better analgesia will be achieved with combinations of drugs affecting different parts of the pain pathway (multimodal therapy) – usually a combination of local anaesthetics, opioids and non-steroidal anti-inflammatory drugs (NSAIDS).

NB. If possible choose the least painful incisions e.g. lower abdominal or transverse incisions.

Methods available to treat post-operative pain

Opioid analgesics

For example: morphine, diamorphine, fentanyl

- These cause analgesia, euphoria and anxiolysis
- Act centrally and peripherally at opiate receptors
- Three main types of receptor: mu/kappa/delta

Side-effects

Central

- Respiratory depression (act on respiratory centre)
- Nausea and vomiting (act on chemoreceptor trigger zone)
- Hypotension, especially if hypovolaemic or if taking vasodilating drugs (common cause of post-operative hypotension)
- Meiosis
- Tolerance and addiction

Peripheral

- Constipation
- Delayed gastric emptying
- Urinary retention

Routes of administration of opioid analgesics

Oral opioids

- Codeine phosphate, dihydrocodeine, codydramol, coproxamol
- Not useful immediately after major surgery, because of nausea and vomiting and delayed gastric emptying
- Very useful after day case surgery and 3–4 days after major surgery

Intramuscular opioids

- Commonest form of post-operative analgesia, despite the fact that it is ineffective in providing effective analgesia in up to 40% of patients
- There is a five-fold difference in peak plasma concentrations among different patients following administration of a standard dose of morphine, with the time taken to reach these levels varying by as much as seven-fold
- The minimum effective analgesic concentration (MEAC) may vary by up to four-fold between patients
- The 'standard' dose is likely to be optimal for a minority of patients

Intravenous opioids

- Continuous infusion leads to effective analgesia, but with significant risk of respiratory depression
- Patient-controlled analgesia – safest
- Epidural opioid analgesia – see below

Patient Controlled Analgesia (PCA)

- Now widely used for post-operative analgesia
- Administered via a special microprocessor-controlled pump which is connected to the patient via an intravenous line, and which is triggered by pressing a button in patient's hand
- A pre-set bolus of drug is then delivered, and a timer prevents the administration of another bolus for a specified period (lock-out interval)
- A loading dose of opioid must be given at the start to achieve adequate analgesia
- Patient titrates the level of analgesia
- e.g   Morphine 50 mg in 50 ml saline (1 mg morphine per ml)
  Bolus = 1 ml (1 mg morphine)
  Lock-out time = 5 mins
  4 hour limit = 30 mg morphine

Advantages

- Dose matches patient requirements
- Decreased nurse workload
- Painless (no IM injections)
- Placebo effect from patient autonomy

Disadvantages

- Technical error can be fatal
- Expense of equipment

Cautions

- A dedicated i.v. cannula should be used to ensure the drug from the PCA does not accumulate retrogradely
- Monitoring of respiratory rate and level of sedation
- Patient must be orientated and fully understand how to use the system for it to be effective; use may be difficult in some patients (e.g. those with rheumatoid arthritis)

Local anaesthetics

For example: bupivacaine (longest acting), lignocaine.

Side-effects
- Central nervous system   restlessness, convulsions
- Cardiovascular   hypotension, arrhythmias, cardiac arrest

Maximum safe dosage   bupivacaine 2 mg/kg
     lignocaine 3 mg/kg

Routes of administration

- Epidural block
- Local infiltration in wound:
  - Injection before incision (pre-emptive)
  - Injection at end of operation
  - Via catheter placed deep to skin incision for constant infusion

- Nerve/regional blocks:
  - Ilioinguinal nerve block for hernia repair
  - Penile block for circumcision
  - Ring block for Zadek's operation
  - Performed once anaesthetized before operation starts

Epidural anaesthesia

This is an extremely effective way of producing profound analgesia, by blocking afferent pathways.

Plain local anaesthetic solutions (usually bupivacaine 0.25%) can be administered into the epidural space intermittently via a catheter, or more usually continuously via an infusion pump. This is particularly good for major abdominal and thoracic operations.

Many hospitals now combine low-dose local anaesthetic (bupivacaine 0.1%) and opioid (e.g. fentanyl 0.0002%). Such low dose combinations are synergistic.

Side-effects

- Hypotension due to sympathetic blockade and peripheral vasodilatation. The treatment for this is fluid resuscitation, **not** reducing the epidural flow rate.
- Leg weakness and numbness
- Urinary retention
- Respiratory depression (particularly if opioid being used)
- Nausea and vomiting (opioid related)

Patients need to be closely monitored, ideally on a High Dependency Unit.

Paracetamol

- Mild analgesic and antipyretic
- No significant anti-inflammatory activity

Adverse effects: overdosage can cause liver damage.

Non-steroidal anti-inflammatory drugs (NSAIDs)

For example: diclofenac, ibuprofen.

- These have anti-inflammatory, analgesic and antipyretic action
- Mainly act peripherally but have some central action
- Mechanism of action is by inhibition of the enzyme cyclo-oxygenase; it therefore inhibits synthesis of prostaglandins; prostaglandins normally sensitise pain receptors to noxious stimuli.

Adverse effects:

- Prostaglandins are important in gastric mucous and bicarbonate production, therefore gastric irritation and peptic ulceration may result if their production is inhibited (especially in elderly patients)
- Nephrotoxic – chronic use can cause interstitial nephritis, papillary necrosis and urothelial tumours
- Increased bleeding because of decreased platelet adhesiveness due to inhibition of thromboxane production

- Bronchospasm in asthmatics (should be avoided)
- May cause gout (esp. indomethacin)
- May displace warfarin or other drugs from plasma proteins
- Aspirin overdosage causes metabolic acidosis and respiratory alkalosis

4.7 Strategies for effective post-operative analgesia

'Balanced analgesia' is the best method. This involves combining several therapeutic modalities to optimise pain relief and minimize unwanted adverse effects.

Keywords: **Pre-emptive analgesia**
 Multimodal therapy

- Initially use regular non-opioid analgesic (e.g. paracetamol or NSAID, if not contraindicated) for minor surgery
- Use regional or local analgesia techniques (e.g. epidural or peripheral nerve blocks); these techniques are especially effective in the immediate post-anaesthetic period
- In major surgery, opioids will be needed as an addition to the above to enhance analgesia; they are especially useful in the immediate post-operative period and are still the mainstay for routine post-operative pain relief. IV opioids preferred as dose-delivery of IM injections is erratic and has greater complications.
- Intravenous opioids are best administered in the form of Patient Controlled Analgesia

Acute Pain Service (APS)

Each hospital should have an acute pain service team who should be responsible for the day-to-day management of patients with post-operative pain. This is a multidisciplinary team using medical, nursing and pharmaceutical expertise. Anaesthetists have a major role to play, since they not only initiate post-operative analgesic regimes such as PCA and epidural infusions, but also are very familiar with the drugs and equipment. Protocols for the strict management of PCA and epidural regimes are essential.

5. VENOUS ACCESS

5.1 Peripheral venous access

In most patients requiring venous access for IV medication or fluids, a peripheral vein is the appropriate route. Peripheral venous cannulation may be a life saving procedure in hypovolaemic shock.

Cannula size ranges from 12G (largest, for rapid infusion in hypovolaemia) down to 24G (smallest, for children).

NB. Flow is proportional to radius^4

Indications

- Fluid/blood infusion
- Blood sampling
- Drug administration
- Central venous line via peripheral route
- Peripheral venous feeding

Contraindications

- Local sepsis
- Puncture of potential A-V fistula sites in haemodialysis patients

Complications

- Infection
- Thrombophlebitis – usually chemical e.g. erythromycin, cytotoxic agents
- Accidental arterial cannulation
- Subcutaneous haematoma
- Extravasation – may just cause oedema, but cytotoxic agents can cause considerable tissue damage

---

Common sites used for peripheral venous access

- Dorsum of hand
- Long saphenous vein at the ankle
  (avoid in patients with coronary artery disease)
- External jugular vein
- Femoral vein
- Median basilic, median cephalic, basilic veins at antecubital fossa (avoid in haemodialysis patients)
- Dorsum of foot
- Scalp veins in infants or neonates

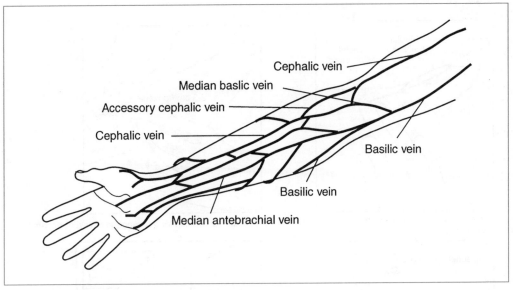

Cephalic vein

Median baslic vein

Accessory cephalic vein

Cephalic vein

Basilic vein

Basilic vein

Median antebrachial vein

Peripheral venous access – veins of the forearm

Patients in hypovolaemic shock often have collapsed peripheral veins resulting in difficult cannulation. In such circumstances rapid access can be gained by open cut down onto a vein and cannulation. The most common veins used for this are the antecubital veins or the long saphenous vein. Of the antecubital veins, the median basilic vein is most commonly used. It is found 2 cm medial to the brachial artery.

Technique of venous cutdown onto the long saphenous vein

- Prepare the ankle on the medial side with antiseptic and drapes
- Infiltrate local anaesthetic into the skin over the long saphenous vein (unless immediate access is required)
- Make a transverse incision 1–2 cm anterior to the medial malleolus
- Using blunt dissection isolate the vein and free it from surrounding tissue
- Ligate the distal end of the mobilised vein
- Pass a tie around the proximal aspect of the vein
- Make a small transverse venotomy
- Dilate this with closed haemostatic forceps
- Insert a large cannula and secure it with the proximal tie
- Close the wound with interrupted sutures and apply a sterile dressing

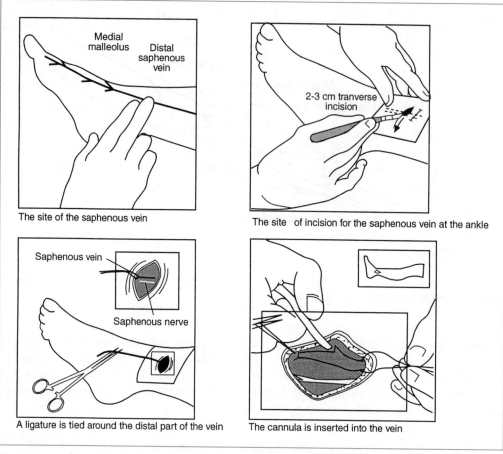

Venous cut-down into long saphenous vein

5.2 Central venous access

Indications

- Fluid infusion
- Drug infusion   – cytotoxic drugs which would damage peripheral veins
                             – inotropic drugs
- Total parenteral nutrition   – hypertonic solution would damage peripheral veins
- Pacemaker electrode insertion
- Monitoring of central pressures (e.g. CVP/pulmonary artery pressures)

Contraindications

- Local sepsis
- Severe coagulation disorders

Central venous cannulation is a potentially dangerous procedure, particularly in a hypo-volaemic patient, and should only be performed by or supervised by an experienced practitioner.

Central venous catheters may reach the superior vena cava (SVC) or right atrium via the basilic, cephalic, subclavian, external and internal jugular veins. The commonest sites are the subclavian and internal jugular veins. Insertion of catheters into the inferior vena cava via the long saphenous or femoral veins is associated with a high incidence of deep venous thrombosis and pulmonary embolism and should only be considered as a last resort.

Catheters are usually introduced with the 'through cannula' technique, whereby a short plastic cannula is first introduced into the vein:

- Needle introduced into the vein
- Cannula advanced over needle and needle withdrawn
- Catheter inserted through cannula and cannula withdrawn

The Seldinger technique uses a flexible metal guidewire as an intermediate step to prevent the catheter coiling up on itself inside the vein:

- Needle introduced into vein
- Guidewire advanced through needle and needle withdrawn
- Catheter advanced over guidewire and guidewire withdrawn

Catheters may be Teflon or silastic – the latter are more expensive, but induce less reaction, are more flexible, and are most suitable for long-term central venous access. Widebore silastic catheters (single, double or triple) (e.g. Hickman) suitable for long-term parenteral nutrition or chemotherapy are introduced percutaneously or surgically and skin tunnelled (to reduce catheter related sepsis) to an exit site on the chest wall.

Methods of central venous cannulation

Catheters are usually inserted percutaneously, but may be placed under direct vision after surgical exposure of the vein.

The axillary vein continues as the subclavian vein as it crosses the outer border of the first rib behind the clavicle, and it ends behind the sternoclavicular joint where it joins the internal jugular vein (IJV) to form the brachiocephalic vein. It is closely related to the subclavian artery above and behind it and to the dome of the pleura below and behind it. The thoracic duct enters the brachiocephalic vein at its origin on the left and cannulation of the right side is therefore probably safer.

The infraclavicular approach is the safest, as there is less chance of injuring the pleura (see figure on page 130).

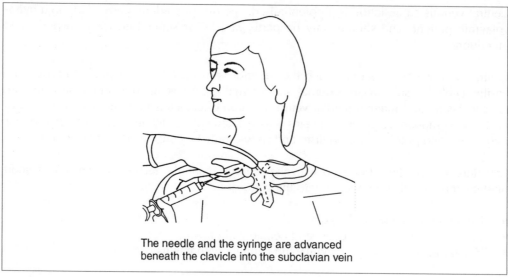

The needle and the syringe are advanced
beneath the clavicle into the subclavian vein

Subclavian vein

- The patient should be supine, with arms by the side, head turned to the opposite side, with the body head down, and the shoulders fallen back
- After infiltration of local anaesthesia, introduce the needle through the skin immediately below the junction of the lateral 1/3 and medial 2/3 of the clavicle and advance the tip towards the suprasternal notch, 'walking' the needle tip along the under surface of the clavicle
- Aspirate gently as the needle advances, until there is free aspiration of blood, indicating that the vein has been entered.

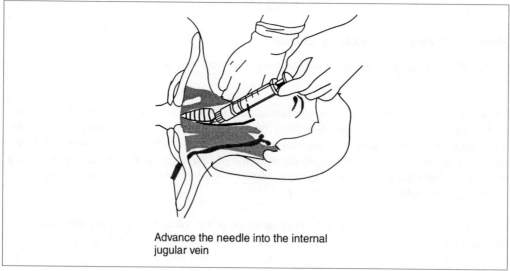

Advance the needle into the internal
jugular vein

Internal jugular vein

- Advance the guidewire through the needle, checking that it advances freely, with no obstruction, then remove the needle. Railroad the catheter over the guidewire, again checking that it advances freely with no obstruction, to its required length (usually about 20 cm).
- Remove guidewire, suture the catheter to the adjacent skin, and check that blood can be aspirated freely from all lumens
- Take a chest X-ray in expiration to exclude a pneumothorax and to check the catheter tip is in the optimal position – SVC or right atrium

As the IJV runs down in the neck, it comes to lie lateral to the internal and common carotid arteries deep to sternomastoid muscle and joins the subclavian vein to form the brachiocephalic vein behind the sternoclavicular joint. The vein may be punctured from three sites: posterior border of sternomastoid muscle, anterior border of sternomastoid muscle, and near its lower end between the two heads of sternomastoid muscle – the first route is most commonly used.

The right IJV is in line with the brachiocephalic vein and SVC and therefore cannulation of the right IJV is probably easier

- Position and prepare the patient as for subclavian vein cannulation
- Palpate the sternomastoid and introduce the needle through the skin at the midpoint of the posterior border of the muscle, whilst displacing the carotid artery medially with your finger
- With the needle at 30° to the skin surface, advance the tip towards the posterior aspect of the sternoclavicular joint, aspirating at regular intervals until the IJV is entered
- Complete as per subclavian line insertion

Complications of central venous catheterisation

- Catheter related sepsis
- Pneumothorax
- Haemothorax, due to laceration of intrathoracic vein wall
- Puncture of adjacent artery causing subcutaneous haematoma, A-V fistula or aneurysm
- Thoracic duct injury
- Brachial plexus damage
- Cardiac complications: arrhythmias, perforation of right atrium
- Malposition of the catheter e.g. into neck veins, axillary vein or contralateral veins
- Catheter occlusion
- Catheter embolisation, due to migration of detached catheter
- Central vein thrombosis

Subcutaneously implanted vascular access systems
Consist of a stainless steel (Port-a-Cath) or plastic (Infuse-a-Port) reservoir with a silicone septum buried in a subcutaneous pocket and connected to a silastic central venous catheter. Access to the reservoir is with a percutaneous needle which pierces the self-sealing septum without coring. Used for long-term antibiotics or chemotherapy.

5.3 Intraosseous puncture

This is an **emergency** technique.

Indication

Used in emergency situations in children aged 6 years or younger in whom venous access by other means has failed on two attempts.

Contraindications

- Local sepsis
- Ipsilateral fractured extremity

Complications

- Misplacement of the needle; this usually involves incomplete penetration of the anterior cortex or over penetration, with the needle passing through the posterior cortex
- Epiphyseal plate damage
- Local sepsis
- Osteomyelitis

Technique of intraosseous puncture

- Identify the puncture site – approximately 1.5 cm below the tibial tuberosity on the anteromedial surface of the tibia
- Clean and drape the area
- If patient is awake infiltrate the area with local anaesthetic
- Direct the intraosseous needle at 90° to the anteromedial surface of the tibia
- Aspirate bone marrow to confirm the position
- Inject with saline to expel any clot and again confirm the position; if the saline flushes easily with no swelling the needle is correctly placed
- Connect the needle to a giving set and apply a sterile dressing
- Discontinue as soon as reliable venous access has been established

---

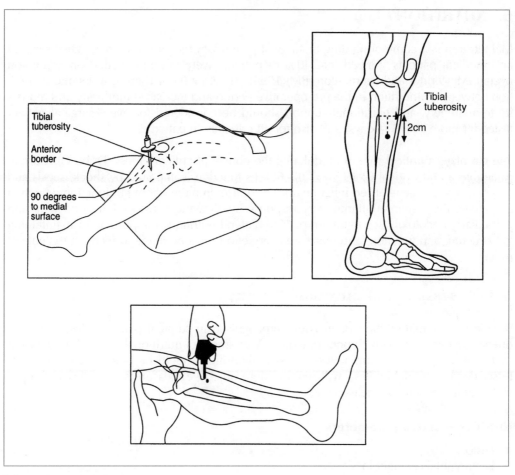

Intraosseous puncture

6. NUTRITION

Malnutrition is a common finding in surgical patients. A recent survey of elective surgical and medical patients showed that 40% of patients were undernourished on admission overall (McWhirter and Pennington; BMJ 1994; 308: 945–948). There is a definite correlation between malnutrition in the pre-operative period and increased morbidity and mortality from surgery, and nutritional support should be considered for every surgical patient fasted for more than 3–4 days, and also for all critically ill patients.

The gut plays a critical role in modulating the course of critical illness (Dobb GJ; Current Anaesthesia and Critical C; 1996: 7: 62–68). Its function is impaired by shock, sepsis and other causes of a generalised inflammatory response. Impairment of gut function may then perpetuate the systemic inflammatory response by allowing translocation of bacteria and particularly endotoxin (see figure on p. 135). Enteral nutrition is important for maintaining gut structure and function, and therefore every effort must be made to feed via the enteral route.

6.1 Assessment of nutritional status

Protein energy malnutrition often goes unrecognised in surgical patients, despite its frequency and association with poor outcome. Assessment of nutritional status should form a part of every physical examination. Gross malnutrition should be obvious clinically, but lesser degrees of malnutrition will require more objective measurements using anthropometric and biochemical measurements.

Nutritional status parameters

- History
  Dietary intake/weight loss
- Examination
  Muscle power, peripheral oedema, angular stomatitis, glossitis
- Anthropometric
  Triceps skin-fold thickness (index of fat store), mid-arm circumference (index of muscle mass)
- Body mass index: weight (kg)/height (m)^2

Normal 20–25	Mild malnutrition <20
Obese >25	Moderate malnutrition <18
Morbid obesity >30	Severe malnutrition <16

- Dynamometric
  Hand grip strength
  FEV^1/FVC ratio
- Biochemistry
  Serum albumin, but this is not a reliable indicator of nutritional state – (it often reflects underlying illness)
  Transferrin
  Retinol binding protein
  Thyroid binding pre-albumin

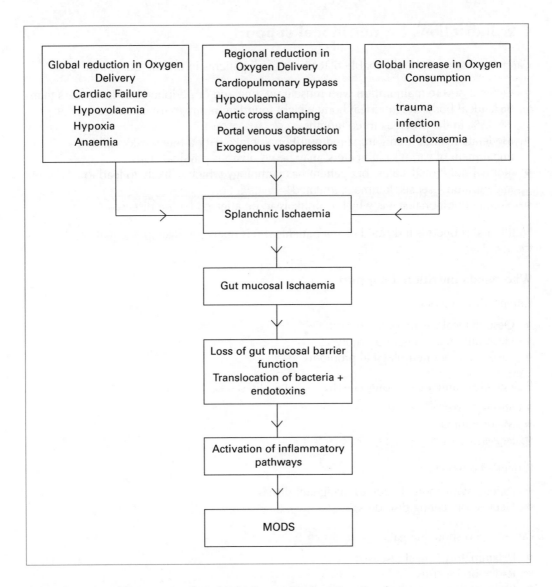

Role of Gut in Pathogenesis of Multiple Organ Dysfunction Syndrome

6.2 Indications for nutritional support

Careful assessment should enable placement of all patients in one of four groups:

- Obvious severe malnutrition with muscle wasting and/or peripheral oedema. Less than 85% ideal body weight (ideal body weight found on **nomogram**) or weight loss of 10–15% in the previous three months.
- Moderate malnutrition – impaired nutritional intake over a few weeks, mild impairment of various parameters, may be no obvious physical signs
- Normal nutritional status, but patient has pathology which is likely to lead to malnutrition – sepsis, trauma, ventilated
- Normal nutritional status which is unlikely to be affected by the disease

Nutritional support is indicated in any patient who is unable to take in adequate oral intake for 3–4 days.

Who needs nutritional support?

Patient who cannot eat:

- Oesophageal/gastric outlet obstruction
- Head and neck surgery or injury
- Stroke or other neurological problems

Patient who cannot eat enough i.e. hypermetabolic states:

- Severe burns
- Major trauma
- Sepsis

Patient who won't eat:

- Patients with anorexia due to malignant disease
- Depression, eating disorders

Patients who shouldn't eat:

- Inflammatory bowel disease
- Radiation enteritis
- Prolonged paralytic ileus
- Intestinal failure
- GI fistulae
- Severe pancreatitis (there is a growing body of opinion that these patients can receive enteral feeding)
- Bowel obstruction/leakage

Pre-operative nutritional support

There is no clear evidence of benefit from pre-operative nutritional support unless the pre-op weight loss >20%. Such feeding for less than 7 days is entirely ineffectual, and rarely should the surgery be delayed to allow for nutritional support.

6.3 Consequences of malnutrition in the surgical patient

- Poor wound healing
- Poor immune function
- Reduced muscle strength – respiratory muscles – atelectasis and pneumonia
  – poor mobilisation – increased DVT risk
- Psychological – apathy and depression
- Reduced gut barrier function – translocation of bacteria / endotoxin (see figure overleaf)

6.4 Nutritional requirements

Daily requirements

- Water   35 ml/kg/day
- Energy   30 kCal/kg/day
- Sodium   1–1.5 mmol/kg/day
- Potassium   1 mmol/kg/day
- Fat   3 g/kg/day
- Carbohydrate   2 g/kg/day
- Vitamins   Varied recommended daily allowance
- Minerals   Zn/Mg/phosphate/selenium
- Nitrogen   0.15–0.2 g/kg/day

In the critically ill, a postive nitrogen balance may be impossible to achieve until the primary pathology has been treated.

The proportion of energy provided from lipids is greater than that from carbohydrates. As there is an element of insulin resistance in trauma, carbohydrate is not used as well as lipid (50% of the energy requirement should be from lipid).

Sources of energy

- Fat   9.3 kCal/g
- Protein   5.3 kCal/g
- Carbohydrate   4.1 kCal/g

Zinc is important for wound healing and is thought to have an antibacterial action when secreted by the prostate. Selenium is involved in antioxidant defence.

If glucose is used as metabolic fuel, this produces more CO_2 than if fat is used. This would result in an increased respiratory workload for the critically ill patient.

Some glucose is required in all feeding regimes to prevent ketosis. Critically ill patients may require greater energy and nitrogen requirements.

6.5 Routes for nutritional support – enteral or parenteral

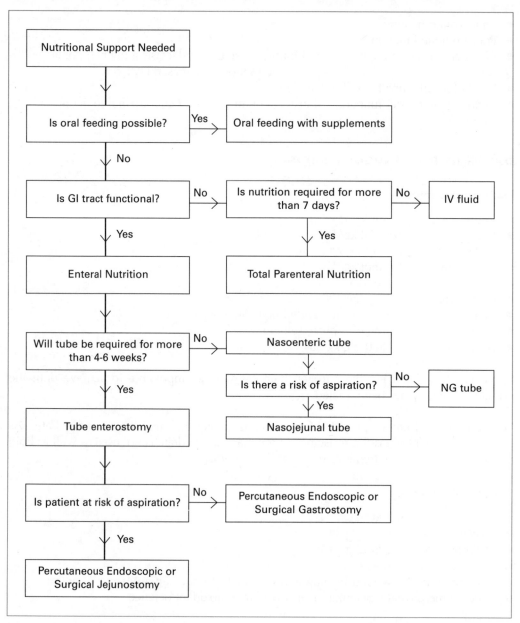

Nutritional support

If the gastrointestinal tract is functional and access can be obtained, then enteral nutrition should be used as it is cheaper, safer and has physiological advantages.

Luminal nutrition is the main stimulus for mucosal growth by a combination of mechanical desquamation, provision of specific nutrients (especially glutamine), stimulation of trophic hormones and increase in splanchnic blood flow. Consequently, starvation leads to mucosal atrophy, increased gut permeability, a decrease in gut-associated lymphoid tissue, changes in microflora and reduced gut barrier function. This may lead to translocation of bacteria and endotoxin into the portal and systemic circulation and consequent fuelling of the process leading to Multiple Organ Dysfunction Syndrome (MODS).

Enteral nutrition has been shown to maintain mucosal integrity, maintain the immune function of the gastrointestinal tract, reduce bacterial translocation and increase gut blood flow. Furthermore, it has been shown to improve survival in animal models of experimental haemorrhage and peritonitis.

Total parenteral nutrition has been shown to increase bacterial translocation, is immuno-suppressive and leads to a greater incidence of septic complications. In a meta-analysis of eight studies of abdominal trauma patients randomised to receive either enteral or par-enteral nutrition, there was a significantly lower incidence (18% v 35%) of septic complications in those receiving enteral nutrition compared to parenteral nutrition (Moore et al 1992; Annals of Surgery 216:172–183).

Gut function is conventionally assessed by the presence or absence of bowel sounds, the passage of flatus or stool and the amount of nasogastric drainage when a nasogastric tube is in place. These methods, however, predominantly assess stomach and colonic function and may tell us little about small bowel function. Small bowel peristalsis and absorptive function is maintained in the immediate post-operative period and in the critically ill surgical patient, and in the majority of patients the small bowel can be used safely for enteral nutrition.

Enteral nutrition

Contraindications
The only absolute contra-indication to enteral feeding is the absence of a gut!

- Intestinal failure
- Prolonged small bowel ileus
- Complete small bowel obstruction
- Small bowel fistula
- Intrinsic small bowel pathology e.g. Crohn's disease, radiation enteritis

It is now common practice to feed enterally patients with severe acute pancreatitis.

Routes

Oral
Patients who can eat normally may still benefit from oral supplementation.

Nasogastric
Best for short-term nutritional supplementation, via a fine bore NG tube.

Nasoenteric
If there is impaired gastric emptying (and consequent risk of aspiration), or jejunal feeding is required (e.g. pancreatitis). Can be placed at laparotomy, endoscopically or radiologically. There are an increasing number of well-designed nasojejunal tubes for endoscopic placement, both single lumen and double lumen for simultaneous gastric drainage and jejunal feeding.

Percutaneous endoscopic gastrostomy (PEG)
The best access for long-term feeding. It is a very safe technique carried out under sedation. Jejunal extension can be placed if post pyloric feeding is required.

Feeding jejunostomy
Placed at laparotomy directly into the jejunum, most commonly by the needle catheter technique (see below). Placement should always be considered at laparotomy when oral intake is not likely for seven or more days.

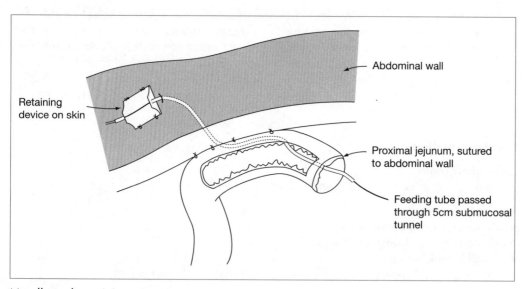

Needle catheter jejunostomy

Indications for feeding jejunostomy

- Major upper gastrointestinal resections
  - Oesophagectomy
  - Total gastrectomy
  - Pancreaticoduodenectomy
- Major abdominal trauma
- Abdominal surgery when malnourished
- When having post-operative chemotherapy or radiotherapy
- Emergency abdominal surgery when prolonged intensive care is anticipated

Technique of fashioning feeding jejunostomy

- 10–15 cm beyond ligament of Treitz
- Minimum 15 cm of feeding tube in bowel lumen
- Create tunnel (either intramural with needle catheter jejunostomy, or seromuscular 'Witzel' Tunnel
- Suture jejunum to parietal peritoneum
- Can start feeding immediately, once adequately resuscitated

Types of enteral diet

- **Polymeric**: used for the majority of patients with normal/near normal GI function.
- **Pre-digested/elemental**: used for severe exocrine pancreatic insufficiency in intestinal failure due to short bowel syndrome; intraluminal hydrolysis may be severely impaired therefore limiting diet assimilation.
- **Disease-specific diet:** used in, for example, patients with respiratory failure on ventilators. These patients need low carbohydrate diets to reduce CO_2 production, therefore the majority of energy requirement is from fat. Also for renal and liver failure.

Immuno-nutrition – may have some effect in enhancing immune function in critically ill:

- Glutamine
- Arginine
- Branched chain amino acids
- RNA Nucleotides
- Omega-3 fatty acids

Complications of enteral nutrition

Feeding tube related:

- Malposition (NG or nasoenteric tubes, e.g. into lungs)
- Blockage
- Aspiration
- Leak and peritonitis (feeding jejunostomies)
- Bowel obstruction (feeding jejunostomies)
- Tube displacement
- Fistula

Diet-related:

- Diarrhoea (10% of patients)
- Bloating
- Nausea/vomiting
- Cramps
- Pulmonary aspiration
- Vitamin, mineral, trace element deficiencies
- Drug interactions

Anti-emetics are used to treat nausea and vomiting. Bloating and cramps usually occur if feed is administered too rapidly.

Diarrhoea should be managed by excluding infection, adjusting volume load on the gut and using **loperamide** empirically.

6.6 Total parenteral nutrition (TPN)

Although enteral feeding is always the preferred route of feeding if possible, TPN plays an essential role in the management of some acutely ill patients, and in those without a normally functioning small bowel. It can be life saving.

Indications

- Intestinal failure
- Prolonged small bowel ileus
- Complete small bowel obstruction (not amenable to surgical treatment)
- Small bowel fistula
- Intrinsic small bowel pathology e.g. Crohn's disease, radiation enteritis
- Short bowel syndrome

There is good evidence that TPN is of no benefit (and may be deleterious) if given for less than 10 days. It should not be given, therefore, unless it is anticipated that it will be used for at least 10 days.

Contraindications

If the patient can receive nutritional support via the enteral route.

Route

Peripheral or central

TPN solutions have high osmolalities and can therefore result in thrombophlebitis if given into a peripheral vein. Central lines are usually tunnelled to exit the skin away from the point of vein penetration to decrease the risk of line sepsis (e.g. Hickman line).

There is little evidence demonstrating any benefit at all from peripheral parenteral nutrition (PPN). In order to reduce the osmolality of PPN (the cause of the thrombophlebitis) the lipid content is increased, and it is the lipid which is immunosuppressive. If parenteral nutrition is required, it should be given centrally, via a dedicated tunnelled line with full aseptic technique.

Complications of TPN

Line-related

- Complications of central line (see section 5.2)
- The most important is sepsis. (See also Chapter 4, *Intensive Care*)

Metabolic
- Hyperglycaemia
- Hypoglycaemia
- Fluid overload
- Excess Na/K/Ca
- Deficiency of Na/K/Ca
- Deficiency of folate, zinc, phosphate, magnesium, selenium, other trace elements, vitamins
- Deranged liver function and fatty liver, due to excess calorie administration
- Gall bladder stasis and biliary sludging

6.7 Monitoring during nutritional support

Checks during nutritional support

- **Daily**
  Full blood count
  Urea and electrolytes
  Random blood glucose
- **Weekly**
  Liver function tests including albumin
  Trace elements
- **Fortnightly**
  Vitamin B12/zinc/magnesium/selenium/copper/iron/transferrin/selenium

A multidisciplinary nutrition team ensures the optimum nutritional care of a patient. It should include line-insertion specialists, clinicians, dieticians, nurses, pharmacists and chemical pathologists.

In specialist centres it is now possible to maintain patients on long-term TPN as outpatients.

7. ACID-BASE BALANCE

Arterial blood-gas measurements are an important adjunct in the management of critically ill patients. They provide an assessment of oxygenation, carbon dioxide excretion, and of acid-base balance, and thus a measurement of respiratory, renal and cardiovascular function, including tissue perfusion.

Definitions:

- **Acid**: proton or hydrogen ion donor
- **Base**: proton or hydrogen ion acceptor
- **Acidaemia**: arterial blood pH <7.35
- **Alkalaemia**: arterial blood pH >7.45
- **Acidosis**: an abnormal condition which tends to decrease arterial pH
- **Alkalosis**: an abnormal condition which tends to increase arterial pH

Arterial blood gases: normal ranges

- pH   7.35–7.45
- H^+ 36–44 mmol/l
- pO_2 10–14 kPa (75–100 mmHg)
- pCO_2 4–6 kPa (35–42 mmHg)
- HCO_3^- 23–33 mmol/l

pH
The logarithm (to the base 10) of the reciprocal of the hydrogen ion concentration:

$$pH = \log_{10} 1/[H^+] = -\log_{10} [H^+]$$

pKa
The pH of a buffer at which half the acid modules are undissociated and half are associated.

Henderson–Hasselbach equation

$$pH = pKa + \log \frac{[base]}{[acid]}$$

i.e.

$$pH = pKa + \log \frac{[HCO_3^-]}{[H_2 CO_3]}$$

- This equation describes the relationship of arterial pH to Bicarbonate and $PaCO_2$
- It is derived from the reaction of carbon dioxide with water

$$CO_2 + H_2O \leftrightharpoons H_2CO_3 \leftrightharpoons H^+ + HCO_3^-$$

- The carbonic acid can be expressed as CO_2, i.e.

$$pH = pKa + \log \frac{[HCO_3^-]}{KpaCO_2}$$

pKa is a constant
K is a constant

This is a buffer system aiming to **minimise pH change**, i.e. if $PaCO_2$ goes up, HCO_3^- goes up; if $PaCO_2$ goes down, HCO_3^- goes down.

Acid base changes:

- Can be **alkalosis** or **acidosis**
- Can be **respiratory** or **metabolic**

The respiratory mechanism is a rapid response system that allows carbon dioxide to be transferred from pulmonary venous blood to alveolar gas and excreted in expired gas. Any dysfunction of the mechanics or control of ventilation will lead to retention of CO_2 and a rise in hydrogen ion (respiratory acidosis) or overexcretion of CO_2 and a fall in hydrogen ion (respiratory alkalosis).

The renal mechanism is a slower responding system that depends on the excretion of hydrogen ions in the urine by the distal nephron. Renal dysfunction (whether pre-renal, renal or post-renal) will prevent hydrogen ion excretion, resulting in a metabolic acidosis.

7.1 Respiratory acidosis

Respiratory acidosis results in a primary disturbance of increased pCO_2 leading to a decrease in pH and a compensatory increase in $[HCO_3^-]$.

Causes of respiratory acidosis

- **Depression of the respiratory centre**
  CVA
  Cerebral tumour
  Drugs (narcotics/sedatives)
  Encephalitis
- **Decreased chest wall movement**
  Neuromuscular disorder (e.g. myasthenia gravis)
  Trauma/surgery
  Ankylosing spondylitis
- **Pulmonary disease (known as type II respiratory failure)**
  COAD
  Pneumonia

7.2 Respiratory alkalosis

Respiratory alkalosis results from the primary disturbance of a decreased $PaCO_2$ leading to an increase in pH and a compensatory decrease in $[HCO_3^-]$.

Causes of respiratory alkalosis

- **Stimulation of the respiratory centre**
  CNS disease (e.g. CVA/encephalitis)
  Hypermetabolic state (e.g. fever/hyperthyroidism/sepsis)
  Exercise
  Hypoxia (e.g. pneumonia/pulmonary oedema/pulmonary collapse or fibrosis)
- **Excess mechanical ventilation (by patient or ventilator)**
  Anxiety
  Certain drugs (e.g. aspirin)

7.3 Metabolic acidosis

Metabolic acidosis results from the primary disturbance of a decreased $[HCO_3^-]$ or increased $[H^+]$ leading to a decrease in pH and a compensatory decrease in $PaCO_2$.

Causes of metabolic acidosis

- **Increased anion gap**
  Renal glomerular failure
  Overdose (e.g. salicylate – also causes respiratory alkalosis – see above)
  Lactic acidosis – inadequate tissue perfusion (hypovolaemia, ischaemic gut)
  Ketoacidosis – diabetic or alcoholic
  Renal tubular acidosis
  Acetazolamide therapy
  Ureterosigmoidostomy
- **Normal anion gap**
  Excess acid intake (e.g. parenteral nutrition)
  Bicarbonate loss (e.g. diarrhoea/fistulae/proximal renal tubular acidosis)

7.4 Metabolic alkalosis

Metabolic alkalosis results from the primary disturbance of an increase in $[HCO_3^-]$ or decrease in $[H^+]$ leading to an increase in pH and a compensatory increase in $PaCO_2$ (although clinically this effect is small).

> **Causes of metabolic alkalosis**
>
> - **Excess alkali intake**
>   Alkali abuse
>   Over treatment of acidosis
>
> - **Excess loss of acid**
>   Vomiting
>
> - **Increased urinary acidification**
>   Diuretics
>   Excess aldosterone
>   Hypokalaemia

Compensation

During a disturbance in the acid base status there is an attempt by the body to try to correct the disturbance.

There are two main mechanisms:

1. Manipulation of $PaCO_2$ by the respiratory system. This is rapid but not as effective as renal compensation.
2. Manipulation of $[HCO_3^-]$ by the kidneys. This is slow but more effective than respiratory compensation.

NB. Compensatory changes do not bring the pH to normal, they simply change the pH towards the normal range.

7.5 Interpretation of acid-base balance

From the Henderson–Hasselbach equation it can be seen that if a patient has a change in acid base status, three parameters also change:

- pH
- $[HCO_3^-]$
- $PaCO_2$

Blood gas machines measure pO_2, pH and pCO_2 directly. Bicarbonate is calculated from the Henderson–Hasselbach equation.

Other important variables given by the blood gas machine include:

- **Actual bicarbonate**: the concentration of bicarbonate measured in the blood sample at the $PaCO_2$ of the patient
- **Standard bicarbonate:** the concentration of bicarbonate in the blood sample when the $PaCO_2$ is normal (i.e. if there was no respiratory disturbance); therefore this gives information about metabolic changes.

Normal standard bicarbonate = 22–26 mmol. If greater than this = **metabolic alkalosis**; if less than this = **metabolic acidosis**.

- **Standard base excess**: the amount of acid/base needed to be added to the sample to return the pH to the normal range.

7.6 Anion gap

Normal = 10–16 mmol/l.

In the body, to maintain electrical chemical neutrality the number of cations equal the number of anions. The main cations in the body are sodium and potassium. The main anions in the body are chloride, bicarbonate, proteins, phosphates, sulphates and organic acids. Usually the ions which are measured are **sodium**, **potassium**, **bicarbonate** and **chloride**.

If the sodium and potassium ions (cations) are added and the chloride and bicarbonate ions (anions) are added, the values will not be the same.

The anion gap

Ion	Concentration (mmol/l)
Na^+	140
K^+	5
	The difference is 10 mmol/l
Cl^-	105
HCO_3^-	30

Therefore the anion gap is 10 mmol/l

This anion gap is made up of anions which are not usually measured.

Why is this important?

- An increased anion gap = **metabolic acidosis**
- The cause of this metabolic acidosis will be due to retention of acid other than HCl (e.g. lactic acid)

Buffers

These are substances which minimise the change in pH of a solution for a given addition of acid or alkali.

- 75% of buffer systems in the body are in cells (e.g. proteins/haemoglobin/bicarbonate buffer systems)
- 25% are in the extracellular fluid

8. FLUID BALANCE

8.1 Water distribution

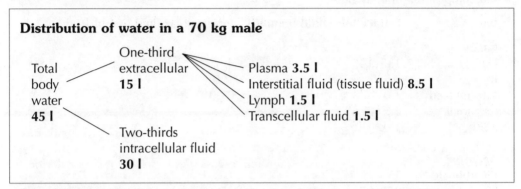

Distribution of water in a 70 kg male

Total body water 45 l
— One-third extracellular 15 l
  — Plasma **3.5 l**
  — Interstitial fluid (tissue fluid) **8.5 l**
  — Lymph **1.5 l**
  — Transcellular fluid **1.5 l**
— Two-thirds intracellular fluid 30 l

- **Total body water (TBW)** = 60% of total body weight (increased in children)
- **Intracellular fluid (ICF)** = fluid inside the cells = TBW – ECF
- **Extracellular fluid (ECF)** = fluid outside the cells
- **Plasma** = blood minus cells; it contains proteins
- **Transcellular fluid** = defined as being separated by a layer of epithelium; it includes CSF, intraocular, pleural, synovial, digestive secretions and gut luminal fluid; volume is relatively small.
- **Intravascular volume** = fluid within vascular compartment
- **Interstitial fluid** = fluid within tissues = ECF – intravascular volume

If the transcellular compartment is very large, it may be called the 'third space', because fluid in this compartment is not readily exchangeable with the rest of the extracellular fluid.

8.2 Ion composition of body fluids

Ion composition of body fluids		
Ion	**Extracellular fluid (mmol/l)**	**Intracellular fluid (mmol/l)**
Cations		
Na⁺	135–145	4–10
K⁺	3.5–5	150
Ca²⁺ ionized	1.0–1.25	0.001
Ca²⁺ total	2.12–2.65	
Mg²⁺	1.0	40
Anions		
Bicarbonate	25	10
Cl⁻	95–105	15
Phosphate	1.1	100
Organic anions	3.0	0
Protein	1.1	8

Intracellular fluid (ICF): K^+ and Mg^{2+} are the main **cations**. Phosphate, proteins and organic ions are the main **anions.**

Extracellular fluid (ECF): Na^+ is the main **cation**. Chloride and bicarbonate are the major **anions.**

In each compartment the total positive charges are balanced by an equivalent number of negative charges, therefore maintaining electrical neutrality.

8.3 Starling hypothesis

The distribution of ECF between plasma and the interstitial space is regulated at the capillaries and lymphatics.

Starling equation

Movement of fluid = K ⎡capillary hydrostatic pressure – tissue hydrostatic pressure⎤
⎣+ tissue oncotic pressure   + capillary oncotic pressure⎦

        Outward pressure   **Inward pressure**

K = filtration constant for the capillary membrane

The capillary membrane

This barrier between the plasma and interstitium allows the free passage of water and electrolytes, but restricts the passage of larger molecules (such as proteins), thus enabling oncotic and hydrostatic forces to control the flux of water across the membrane. There tends to be a net flow of water out of the capillary into the interstium at the arteriolar end of the capillary, and a net flow back into the capillary at the venular end of the capillary.

Oedema

This describes the clinical observation of excess tissue fluid (i.e. interstitial fluid).

Causes

- Increased capillary hydrostatic pressure (e.g. venous obstruction, fluid overload)
- Decreased capillary oncotic pressure (e.g. causes of hypoproteinaemia – nephrotic syndrome, cirrhosis)
- Increased tissue oncotic pressure (e.g. resulting from increased capillary permeability due to burns or inflammation)
- Decreased tissue hydrostatic pressure

The cell membrane

This is freely permeable to water but not to sodium ions, which are actively pumped out of the cells. Hence sodium is mainly an extracellular ion, whereas potassium is mainly an intracellular ion. Water will move freely across the cell membrane if there is any difference in osmolality between the two sides.

Movement of water between compartments

If water is given to a patient, it will rapidly distribute throughout the ECF with a resultant fall in ECF osmolality. Since osmolality must be the same inside and outside the cells, water will move from ECF to ICF until the osmolalities are the same. Thus water distributes throughout the whole body water. Since the intravascular space only comprises about 7.5% of the total body space, only 7.5% of infused water will stay in the intravascular compartment, and a large amount of fluid will need to be given to increase significantly the plasma volume.

If normal saline (0.9%, containing 150 mmol/l sodium ions) is infused, it will stay in the ECF. There is no change in osmolality inside or outside the cells, and there is no net flow of water into the cells. The saline will distribute throughout the extracellular space. The extracellular fluid makes up about 35% of the body water, and less saline will need to be given than water to lead to a corresponding increase in plasma volume.

Colloid solutions (albumin, starch solutions, gelatins) stay in the plasma compartment since the capillary membrane is impermeable to colloid. Consequently less colloid will need to be given than both water and saline to lead to a corresponding increase in plasma volume.

8.4 Daily fluid and electrolyte maintenance requirements

Daily maintenance requirements of H_2O + electrolytes

	Per kg body weight (mmol)	Total average male adult (mmol)
Na^+	1–1.5	70–100
K^+	1	70
Cl^-	1	70
$PO4^{2-}$	0.2	14
Ca^{2+}	0.1	7
Mg^{2+}	0.1	7
H_2O	35 ml	2500 ml

Average Daily Water Balance for Sedentary Adult in Temperate Conditions

Intake (ml)		Output (ml)	
Drink	1500	Urine	1500
Food	750	Faeces	100
Metabolic	350	Lungs	400
		Skin	600
Total	**2600**	**Total**	**2600**

Fever increases maintenance fluid requirement by 20% of the daily insensible loss for each °C rise. Most clinicians give an extra 1 litre per 24 hrs for each °C rise.

In general, fluid maintenance needs can be gauged by maintaining an adequate urine output (>0.5 ml/kg/hr). Patient's daily weight is also essential for adequate assessment.

(NB. Mechanical ventilation also increases insensible fluid loss.)

Fluid administration

Enteral
Oral fluid replacement is suitable if the GI tract is functioning and the deficiency is not excessive (i.e. post-obstructive diuresis). However, this is not always possible (e.g. paralytic ileus following surgery).

Parenteral
Intravenous fluid replacement is needed if the GI tract is not functioning properly or if rapid fluid replacement is required.

Parenteral fluid can broadly be divided into **crystalloid/colloid/blood**:

- **Crystalloid**: this is an electrolyte solution in water; crystalloids form a true solution and can pass through a semipermeable membrane; they diffuse out quickly into the interstitial space
- **Colloid**: these are regarded as plasma substitutes; colloids do not dissolve into a true solution and cannot pass through a semipermeable membrane; they contain high molecular weight molecules and remain in the intravascular compartment longer than crystalloids; they provide oncotic pressure
- **Blood**: (see Section 3.3).

8.5 Common fluid preparations

Crystalloid solutions (all are **isotonic** with body fluid)

- **Normal saline** (0.9%) contains 154 mmol/l Na^+; 154 mmol/l Cl^-
- **5% Dextrose** (calorific content is negligible) contains 278 mmol/l dextrose
- **Dextrose saline** (0.18% saline, 4% dextrose) contains 30 mmol/l Na^+; 30 mmol/l Cl^-; 222 mmol/l dextrose
- **Hartmann's solution** contains 131 mmol/l Na^+; 5 mmol/l K^+; 29 mmol/l, HCO_3^-; 111 mmol/l Cl^-; 2 mmol/l Ca_2^+
- **Ringer's solution** contains 147 mmol/l Na^+; 4 mmol/l K^+; 156 mmol/l Cl^-; 2.2 mmol/l Ca^{2+}

Colloid solutions

Albumin (4.5%)

- Natural blood product
- MR 45–70,000 (natural, therefore broad range MR)
- No clotting factors
- Small risk of anaphylaxis
- Limited availability/expensive

Gelatins (Haemaccel/gelofusin)

- Modified gelatins (hydrolysis of bovine collagen)
- Half-life 8–10 hours
- Low incidence allergic reaction

NB. Haemaccel contains K^+ and Ca^{2+} therefore if mixed with citrated blood in a giving set, leads to coagulation.

Dextrans

- Glucose polymers: Dextran 40 – average MR = 40,000; Dextran 70 – average MR = 70,000
- Half-life 16 hours

- Dextran 40 is filtered by the kidney but Dextran 70 is not, therefore Dextran 70 stays in circulation longer
- Dextran interferes with cross-matching blood and coagulation (forms red blood cell rouleaux) – nephrotoxic – allergic reaction

Hetastarch

- 6% Hetastarch in saline
- Half-life 16–24 hours
- MR 120,000
- Must limit dose to 1500 ml/kg – excess leads to coagulation problems
- Low incidence anaphylaxis/no interference with cross-matching
- Expensive

Fluid replacement

When prescribing fluid regimes for patients, we need to take three things into account:

- Basal requirements
- Continuing abnormal losses over and above basal requirements
- Pre-existing dehydration and electrolyte loss

Common daily maintenance regimes for 70 kg adult in temperate environment

- **Regimen A**
  1l normal saline + 20 mmol KCl over 8 hours
  1l 5% Dextrose + 20 mmol KCl over 8 hours
  1l 5% Dextrose + 20 mmol KCl over 8 hours

This provides: 3l water; 60 mmol K^+; 150 mmol Na^+

- **Regimen B**
  1l Dextrose saline + 20 mmol KCl over 8 hours
  1l Dextrose saline + 20 mmol KCl over 8 hours
  1l Dextrose saline + 20 mmol KCl over 8 hours

This provides: 3l water; 60 mmol K^+; 90 mmol Na^+

NB. Metabolism of dextrose may lead to effectively administering hypotonic saline. Therefore, Regimen B is only suitable in the short-term.

Fluid regimes and K^+

In the first 24 hours after non-cardiac surgery, potassium is often omitted from the IV fluid regime. There is a tendency for K^+ to rise during and after surgery because of

- Cell injury (high intracellular K^+ concentration released into plasma)
- Blood transfusions
- Decreased renal K^+ clearance due to transient renal impairment in the immediate post-operative period
- Opposed action of insulin by 'stress hormones' tend to cause K^+ release from the cells

Fluid regime and surgical trauma

Surgical trauma
- ADH release   – water conservation
- Aldosterone from   – Na^+ retention
  adrenals   – K^+ excretion

Therefore peri-operative fluid balance must be carefully monitored in relation to electrolytes and volume.

Sources of excess loss in surgical patients:

- Blood loss (e.g. trauma, surgery)
- Plasma loss (e.g. burns)
- GI fluid loss (e.g. vomiting, diarrhoea, ileostomy, bowel obstruction)
- Intra-abdominal inflammatory fluid loss (e.g. pancreatitis)
- Sepsis
- Abnormal insensible loss (e.g. fever, mechanical ventilation with no humidification)

It is essential for an accurate fluid chart to be kept. This records all fluid intake (oral and intravenous) and all output (urine, drain fluid, GI contents etc), and provides a balance for each 24 hours, once insensible loss has been estimated.

Correction of pre-existing dehydration

Patients who are dehydrated will need to be resuscitated with fluid over and above their basal requirements. The important issues are:

- To identify which compartment or compartments the fluid has been lost from
- To assess the extent of the dehydration

The fluid used to resuscitate the patient should be similar to that which has been lost. It is usually easy to decide where the losses are coming from. Bowel losses come from the ECF, pure water losses come from the total body water, and protein-containing fluid is lost from the plasma. There is frequently a combination of these.

Daily GI secretions and electrolyte composition

	Volume (ml/24 h)	Na$^+$ (mmol/l)	K$^+$ (mmol/l)	Cl$^-$ (mmol/l)	HCO$_3^-$ (mmol/l)
Saliva	1500 (1000–15,000)	10	26	10	30
Stomach	1500 (1000–2500)	60	10	130	–
Duodenum	Variable (100–2000)	140	5	80	–
Ileum	3000 (100–9000)	140	5	104	–
Colon	Minimal	60	30	40	–
Pancreas	500 (100–800)	140	5	75	115
Bile	800 (50–800)	145	5	100	35

8.6 Assessing fluid depletion

History

- Thirst/obvious fluid loss
- Fluid intake/output
- If patient on ward/ITU, check charts for fluid balance

Examination

- Dry mucous membranes
- Sunken eyes
- Low skin elasticity
- Low urine output
- Increase in heart rate
- Low pulse pressure/low BP
- Confusion
- Low capillary refilling

Central venous pressure (CVP)

- Normal = 3–8 cm H$_2$O
- Single values are not as useful as looking at the trend
- CVP measurement is best used as a guide to adequacy of treatment, i.e. it can be used to monitor response to a fluid challenge
- Consider a fluid challenge of 200 ml of colloid

- If dehydrated, the patient's CVP will rise in response to the challenge and then fall to the original value
- In a well-filled patient there will be a substantial rise (2–4 cm H_2O for 5 min) in the CVP
- If there is no overfilling, the CVP will rise >4 cm H_2O and will not fall again.

NB. CVP may be artificially elevated if rapid filling has occurred prior to measurement (due to venoconstriction), e.g. following rapid filling in 'shocked' patients.

Pulmonary arterial occlusion pressure (PAOP)

CVP reflects the function of the right ventricle which usually parallels left ventricular function. In cardiac disease, however, there may be a disparity between the function of the two ventricles. The Swan-Ganz catheter has a balloon on the tip with a pressure transducer beyond the balloon. The catheter is placed so that the balloon lies in a branch of the pulmonary artery, and when the balloon is inflated, the pressure beyond the balloon gives a good guide to the left atrial pressure – the pulmonary arterial occlusion pressure. This gives a better indication of the state of filling of the systemic circulation than the central venous pressure, although usually measurement of CVP will suffice (see Chapter 4).

Simple investigations

Simple indicators of dehydration are a rising haematocrit and albumin, and a raised urea, particularly in the presence of low volume concentrated urine.

Summary of fluid balance consideration

- Patient size and age
- Abnormal ongoing losses, pre-existing deficits or excesses, fluid shifts
- Renal and cardiovascular function
- Look at fluid balance charts over preceding 24 hours, and more
- Check serum electrolytes

9. SURGICAL COMPLICATIONS

No surgical procedure is without risk. A large percentage of complications can be minimised or avoided by early recognition, management and appropriate prophylaxis.

Many pre-existing conditions lead to increased risks of surgery – these are covered in detail in Chapter 1.

9.1 Risk factors (see Chapter 1)

- Extremes of age
- Obesity
- Cardiovascular disease
- Respiratory disease
- Diabetes mellitus
- Liver disease
- Renal disorders
- Steroids, immunosuppressant drugs

9.2 Post-operative complications

These may be **immediate**, **early** or **late** *and also* **specific** to the operation or **general** to any operation.

- **Immediate** complication is within 24 hours of surgery
- **Early** complication is within the 30–day period after the operation or during the period of hospital stay
- **Late** complication is after the patient has been discharged from hospital or more than 30 days after the operation.

Haemorrhage

- **Primary haemorrhage** occurs during the operation. It should be controlled before the end of the operation.
- **Reactionary haemorrhage** occurs usually in the first few hours after surgery, as a result of the patient warming up (vasodilating) and the blood pressure coming up after anaesthesia.
- **Secondary haemorrhage** occurs a number of days after the operation. The cause is usually infection-related, but can also be related to sloughing of a clot, or erosion of a ligature.

Predisposing factors

- Obesity
- Steroid therapy
- Jaundice
- Recent transfusion of stored blood
- Disorders of coagulation
- Platelet deficiencies
- Anticoagulation therapy
- Old age
- Severe sepsis with DIC

Prevention

- Recognise patients at risk
- Reverse risk factors if possible
- Liaise with haematologist re. managing disorders of coagulation
- Control of infection
- Meticulous surgical technique

Management

- Resuscitate
- Correct coagulopathy
- Surgical haemostasis if necessary
- Packing may be necessary

Infective complications

Risk factors

- Type of operation
  - Clean surgery
  - Potentially contaminated operations (e.g. elective operations on GI tract)
  - Contaminated operations (e.g. perforated duodenal ulcer)
  - Dirty operations (e.g. faecal peritonitis)
- Obesity
- Haematoma
- Diabetes
- Steroids
- Immunosuppression
- Malnutrition
- Obstructive jaundice
- Foreign material
  - Vascular grafts
  - Joint replacements
  - Heart valve
  - Mesh for hernia

NB Effects of infection in these cases can be devastating.

Prophylaxis

- Identify patients at risk
- Reduce/control risk factors
- Meticulous surgical technique
- Antibiotic prophylaxis
- Bowel preparation

Treatment

Wound infection

- Ensure adequate drainage
- Send pus for culture and sensitivity
- Debride if necessary
- Appropriate dressings
- Antibiotics only if acute infection (cellulitis, septic)

Abscess

- Drain – radiological, surgical
- Treat underlying cause e.g. anastomotic leak

Septicaemia/septic shock

- Early recognition
- Treat source of sepsis
- Organ support as required on Intensive Care Unit

Anastomotic leakage

Any anastomosis at risk, particularly oesophageal and rectal.

Predisposing factors

General

- Poor tissue perfusion
- Old age
- Malnutrition
- Obesity
- Steroids

Local

- Tension on anastomosis
- Local ischaemia
- Poor technique
- Local sepsis

Presentation

- Peritonitis
- Bowel contents in wound or drain
- Abscess
- Ileus
- Systemic signs of sepsis
- Fistula

Diagnosis

- Usually obvious
- Often made at laparotomy
- Contrast study/enema/swallow

Treatment

- Resuscitate
- Conservative (Nil by mouth, IV fluids, antibiotics, nutritional support)
- Surgery

Impaired wound healing – see Section 2, *skin and wounds*

Surgical injury

This can be **unavoidable** or **inadvertent**.

- **Unavoidable** (e.g. sacrifice of the facial nerve in total parotidectomy)
- **Inadvertent** (e.g. damage to the recurrent laryngeal nerve during thyroidectomy)

Post-operative deep vein thrombosis (DVT) and pulmonary embolism (PE)

DVT occurs in 50% of patients undergoing major abdominal or pelvic surgery if no pro-phylactic measures are taken. Twenty per cent of those with DVT are at risk of developing PE.

Predisposing factors

Patient factors

- Age
- Previous DVT or PE
- Immobility
- Obesity
- Pregnancy
- Thrombophilia (e.g. protein C and protein S deficiencies, lupus anticoagulant and factor V Leiden)
- Oral contraceptive pill

Factors involving the disease or surgical procedure

- Trauma or surgery, especially of the pelvis and lower limb
- Malignancy, especially pelvic and abdominal
- Myocardial infarction
- Congestive heart failure
- Polycythaemia
- Inflammatory bowel disease
- Nephrotic syndrome
- Length of operation

Risk of DVT

(THRIFT Study BMJ 1992; 305: 567–574.)

Low risk

- Minor surgery (<30 min); no risk factors other than age
- Major surgery (>30 min); age <40; no other risk factors
- Minor trauma or medical illness

Moderate risk

- Major general, urological, gynaecological, cardiothoracic, vascular or neurological surgery; age >40 or other risk factors
- Major medical illness; heart or lung disease; cancer; inflammatory bowel disease
- Major trauma or burns
- Minor surgery, trauma or illness in patients with previous DVT, PE or thrombophilia

High risk

- Fracture or major orthopaedic surgery of pelvis, hip or lower limb
- Major pelvic or abdominal surgery for cancer
- Minor surgery, trauma or illness in patients with previous DVT, PE or thrombophilia
- Lower limb paralysis
- Major lower limb amputation

Prevention of DVT (see Chapter 1)

General measures

- Early post-operative mobilisation
- Adequate hydration
- Avoid calf pressure
- Stop the oral contraceptive pill 6 weeks pre-operatively

Specific measures

Mechanical

- Graduated elastic compression stocking
- Intermittent pneumatic pressure device

Pharmacological

Anticoagulant drugs reduce thrombin formation.

- Low-dose subcutaneous heparin
- Low molecular weight heparins: the advantage of low molecular weight heparins over standard heparins is their longer half-life; there is also evidence that their use in high-risk patients is even more effective without increased risk of haemorrhage.

- Oral anticoagulants (e.g. warfarin) may be used after major gynaecological surgery and elective hip replacement in high-risk patients; however, there is increased bleeding risk and close laboratory monitoring of prothrombin time is essential.
- Dextran 70: found to be most effective in preventing thrombosis after hip fractures; it is given as a peri-operative intravenous infusion; antithrombotic effects include effects on blood flow, platelets, endothelium and lysability of fibrin. This is not used routinely in the UK.

General recommendations for prophylaxis for thromboembolism (THRIFT study, BMJ 1992; 305: 567–574).

Principles – the method used should be: simple to use; acceptable to patients; have minimal adverse effects.

- All hospital inpatients – need to be assessed for clinical risk factors and risk of thromboembolism; should have prophylaxis depending on the degree of risk
- Low-risk patients should be mobilised early
- Moderate and high-risk patients should be mobilised early AND receive specific prophylaxis

In practice, the methods used vary between clinicians and units but it is important that each centre has specific policies regarding prophylaxis.

Diagnosis of DVT

- Doppler ultrasound
- Venography – gold standard
- [^{125}I] fibrinogen scanning – research only

Complications of DVT

- Pulmonary embolus
- Post-phlebitic limb

Diagnosis of pulmonary embolus

- Ventilation-perfusion scan
- CT pulmonary angiography
- Pulmonary angiogram
- ECG

Treatment of DVT/PE

- Below knee – analgesia, graduated compression stocking
- Anticoagulation with heparin initially, then warfarin

Respiratory complications

Very common following surgery

Risk factors

- Age
- Pre-existing respiratory disease
- Smoking
- Obesity
- Pre-existing cardiac disease
- Excessive sedation
- Immobility
- Post-operative pain
- Upper abdominal/thoracic wounds
- One lung ventilation

Pathology

- Atelectasis – commonest
- Bronchopneumonia
- Pulmonary embolus
- Pleural effusion
- Pneumothorax
- ARDS/acute lung injury

Management

- Correct risk factors before surgery
- Adequate post-operative analgesia
- Minimise sedation
- Regular physiotherapy
- Antibiotics if evidence of infection
- Drain effusion/pneumothorax
- Ventilatory support if necessary

10. SUGGESTED FURTHER READING

Clinical Surgery in General, 3rd Edition, Kirk RM, Mansfield AO, Cochrane JPS, 1999, Churchill Livingstone, London
Pathology, Basic and Systemic, Woolf N, 1998, WB Saunders and Co, London

Chapter 3

Trauma

CONTENTS

Trauma

1. INITIAL ASSESSMENT AND RESUSCITATION AFTER TRAUMA

1.1 Historical perspective

Trauma care and Surgery have been inextricably entwined since the beginnings of uncivilised society. Battlefield surgeons such as Ambrose Pare (1510–1590) used empiric observation, common sense and 'hands-on' personal experience to improve the treatment of battle wounds during the Napoleonic wars. The plastic surgeon Archibald Hector McIndoe improved the treatment of burns in RAF pilots during World War II. He noted that those who ditched in the sea had less scarring and infection of their burn sites, leading to the use of saline soaks instead of tannins. Both men found that conventional practice was inadequate and sought to improve care and techniques for the sake of their patients and for the common good. In 1976, an orthopaedic surgeon crashed his light aircraft in Nebraska, resulting in the death of his wife and injuring his children. The emergency care that he and his family received was inadequate and this became the impetus to the development of the Advanced Trauma Life Support (ATLS) training course.

The Royal College of Surgeons of England was one of the first bodies outside of the USA to implement ATLS training (November 1988). This system has provided a framework and approach to acute trauma care so that the trauma team personnel can communicate and prioritise in a similar way, allowing parallel or simultaneous treatment in the multiply-injured patient, by a co-ordinated team approach. This has increased the speed with which injuries are identified and treated, making the most use of the 'Golden Hour', in order to improve survival and patient outcome.

1.2 'Trimodal' distribution of death

- Mortality from trauma can be considered in three phases – immediate, early and late. Immediate deaths are almost always unpreventable. They include massive brain injuries, or great vessel injuries (e.g. aortic avulsion associated with a fall from a height).

- 'Early' phase is within the first few minutes to hours when the opportunity for prompt and appropriate diagnosis and intervention can prevent loss of life or limb (the so-called 'Golden Hour'). The ATLS system mainly addresses this phase of care, and emphasises the need for rapid assessment and resuscitation.
- 'Late' phase occurs days to weeks after the injury, during which time deaths can occur due to sepsis and multiple organ system failure, or complications arising as a consequence of the initial injury or surgery. The quality of care in phases 1 and 2 will obviously have an impact on mortality in phase 3, and on overall outcome.

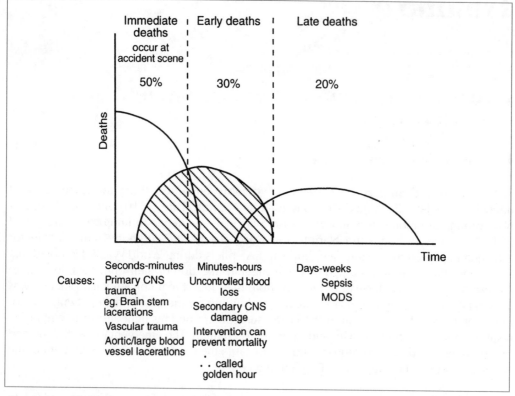

Mortality from trauma – trimodal distribution

Prehospital care

Information obtained from the emergency agencies in the field cannot be underestimated. Detailed and early information allows mobilisation of the Trauma team, including laboratory services, porters and the X-ray Department. Forward knowledge of the number of casualties and the type and extent of injuries allows the preparation of appropriate equipment such as chest drains, thoracotomy sets and O-negative blood to be ready and available as soon as the patient arrives. Ideally, continual updates should be provided by the emergency services so that the receiving team can be appropriately prepared both mentally and in terms of equipment.

Inhospital phase

Most Accident and Emergency Departments in the UK that deal with trauma cases have a designated area for receiving trauma cases and this is obviously essential for rapid access to specialist equipment and services.

The following should be readily available:

Airway management	Circulatory support	Infrastructure
• Laryngoscope	• Large bore cannulae	• Rapid communication-links
• Endotracheal tubes	• Warmed crystalloid solutions	• Laboratory support
• Fully stocked anaesthetic-trolley	• O-negative blood	• Radiology – immediate access
• Suction	• Giving sets	
• Oxygen	• Blood sampling equipment	

Multiple casualties

Dealing with large numbers of casualties is, fortunately, a rare occurrence in civilian practice in the UK. However, bombings such as Old Compton Street and Omagh, and rail disasters such as Selby, occur from time to time and may stretch resources to the limit. The best preparation is rehearsal, with a 'disaster plan' which is practised every few months.

1.3 Primary survey

'The ABCs'

The aim of this system is to save 'life before limb' i.e. preserve heart, brain and lung oxygenation and circulation. It is based on the ATLS format and involves continuous reassessment and adjustment in response to changing needs.

- **A** Airway: check that the airway is patent and protect it. Ensure that the cervical spine is protected, especially in the unconscious patient.
- **B** Breathing: check that there is adequate bilateral air entry and that there are no clinical signs of life-threatening chest conditions.
- **C** Circulation: detect shock and treat if present. Appropriate access is essential.
- **D** Disability: briefly assess the neurological status using the 'AVPU' mnemonic:

A = **A**lert
V = responds to **V**erbal stimuli
P = responds to **P**ain
U = **U**nresponsive

- **E** EXPOSURE: completely undress the patient. Inspect the entire body, including the spine, with a 'log-roll'. Keep the patient warm.

Check pupils:

- Size
- Symmetry
- Response to light

1.4 Secondary survey

To be carried out whilst continually reassessing ABC. Immediately life-threatening conditions should already have been detected and treated.

Objective

Re-examine patient thoroughly from head to toe:

- Obtain a complete medical history
- Obtain all necessary investigations: bloods, X-rays, cervical spine, chest and pelvis
- Perform any special procedures
- Monitor patient's response to treatment

'Fingers and tubes in every orifice':

- PR
- PV
- Check ENT
- NG tube insertion (if no skull fracture)
- Urinary catheter insertion if no evidence of genitourinary trauma

Head

- **Neurological state**
  Full GCS assessment
  Pupils
  Eyes

- **Face**
  Check facial bones for stability
  Teeth loose or absent

- **Scalp**
  Presence of soft tissue injuries/haematoma
  Signs of skull fracture
  Periorbital haematoma
  Scleral haematoma with no posterior margin
  Battle's sign
  CSF/blood from ears or nose

Neck

- **Risk factors for cervical spine injury**
  Any injury above the clavicle
  High speed RTA
  Falls from height

- **Examination**
  Thorough palpation of bony prominences
  Check for soft tissue swellings
  Check for muscle spasm

- **Exclude**
  Penetrating injuries of the neck
  Subcutaneous emphysema
  Elevated JVP

Thorax

- **Examination**
  Exclude pneumothorax
  Full respiratory system examination especially reassessing air entry
  Inspect chest wall – bony or soft tissue injury missed on primary survey?
  CXR
  ECG
  ABG should be obtained to monitor whether ventilation adequate

- **Abdomen**
  Examine thoroughly, abdominal wall injury suggests internal viscus injury
  NG tube insertion to decompress the stomach is suggested as long as there are no facial fractures or basal skull fractures
  Involve surgeons early if suspicious of internal injury
  After general resuscitation the main decision to be made in this area is whether a laparotomy is necessary

- **Pelvis**
  Check for bony instability which indicates significant blood loss
  Identify any genitourinary system injuries suggested by: high-riding prostate felt PR; blood found on PR examination; blood found on PV examination; blood at external urethral meatus; gross haematuria
  Urethral catheterization is only performed if there is no evidence of genitourinary injury

- **Extremities**
  Examine the full extent of each limb (remember hands and feet)

- Exclude soft tissue injury, bony injury, vascular injury, neurological injury
  Control haemorrhage; elevate limb; apply direct pressure (tourniquets are not favoured)
  Correct any obvious bony deformity as this will decrease: fat emboli; haemorrhage; soft tissue injury; requirement for analgesia; skin tension in dislocations
  Caution: check and document neurovascular supply to limb before and after any manipulation

Spine

- **Spinal column**
  Examine the peripheral and central nervous system
  Exclude sensory or motor deficits

Medical history

Minimum information required

A = **A**llergies
M = **M**edications
P = **P**ast medical history
L = **L**ast meal
E = **E**vents leading to injury environment

Check tetanus status.

Tetanus status and prophylaxis

Tetanus status	Minor injuries	Major injuries
Unknown or <3 doses	Tetanus toxoid only	Tetanus toxoid and Tetanus immune globulin
Full course received with last booster <10 years ago	No treatment necessary	No treatment needed

1.5 Maintenance of airway and ventilation

Hypoxia is the quickest killer of trauma patients, therefore maintenance of a patent airway and adequate oxygen delivery are essential.

SUPPLEMENTAL OXYGEN MUST BE DELIVERED TO ALL TRAUMA PATIENTS

Airway

Recognise a compromised airway

Airway obstruction can be gradual or sudden and the clinical signs (tachypnoea, cyanosis, and agitation) may be subtle. An altered level of consciousness due to head injury, drugs, alcohol or these factors combined makes airway compromise particularly likely especially from the risk of aspiration of stomach contents.

Vomiting or the presence of stomach contents in the oropharynx requires immediate suction and turning the patient into the lateral 'recovery' position.

Associated chest injuries may reduce ventilation/oxygenation and injuries of the neck may cause airway compromise by pressure from oedema or an expanding haematoma or tracheal perforation.

LOOK   Facial or airway trauma, agitation, cyanosis, use of accessory muscles
LISTEN   Stridor, gurgling, snoring or hoarseness
FEEL   Chest wall movement

Administer supplemental oxygen 15 l/min with reservoir bag.

Management of an obstructed airway

(The following must be achieved with simultaneous immobilisation of the cervical spine.) In the unconscious patient the airway may be obstructed by vomit, dentures, broken teeth or the tongue falling backwards. The mouth should be gently opened and inspected. A gloved finger may be used to remove debris and a Yankauer sucker used for secretions.

The 'chin lift' and 'jaw thrust'

Both of these manoeuvres are aimed at maintaining the patency of the upper airway (e.g. when the tongue has fallen backwards). The mandible is gripped and lifted forward whilst the neck is extended.

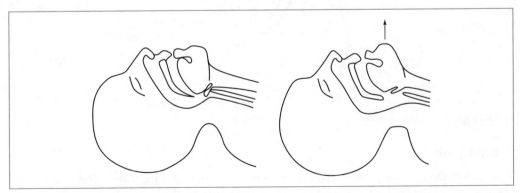

The 'chin lift' and 'jaw thrust'

The Guedel airway

Uses: for temporary 'bag-and-mask' ventilation of the unconscious patient prior to intubation.

Advantages: easy to insert, widely available, multiple sizes.

Disadvantages: sited above vocal cords therefore does not prevent airway obstruction at this site. Can provoke gag reflex.

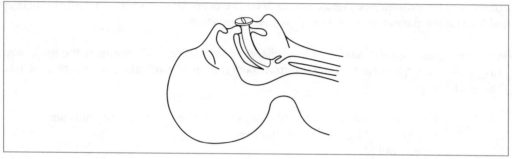

The Guedel airway

The nasopharyngeal airway

Uses: to prevent upper airway obstruction e.g. in a drowsy/still conscious patient.

Advantages: fairly easy to insert. Unlikely to stimulate gag reflex in comparison with oropharyngeal (Guedel) airway.

Disadvantages: less widely available, uncomfortable for the patient, sited above the vocal cords, insertion dangerous if facial trauma present.

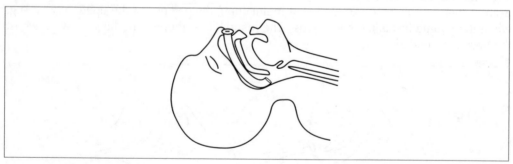

The nasopharyngeal airway

Definitive airway

If the above measures are insufficient then a definitive airway is indicated. This will ensure free passage of oxygen to the trachea, distal to the vocal cords.

Indications for a definitive airway

- Apnoea
- Hypoxia refractory to oxygen therapy
- Protection from aspiration pneumonitis
- Protection of the airway from impending obstruction due to burns/oedema/facial trauma/seizures
- Inability to maintain an airway by the above simpler measures
- Head injury with a risk of raised intracranial pressure
- Vocal cord paralysis

Types of definitive airway

- Orotracheal intubation
- Nasotracheal intubation
- Laryngeal mask
- Surgical airway (e.g. tracheostomy or cricothyroidotomy)

Orotracheal intubation

- Familiarise yourself with the technique and check all equipment before starting (laryngoscope, suction, ET tube (size 7–8 for females, size 8–9 for males), Ambu bag, oxygen supply, assistant, muscle relaxant, sedation, IV access)

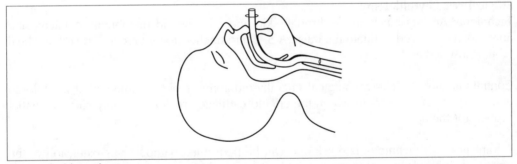

Orotracheal intubation

- Allow a maximum of 30 seconds for each attempt at insertion (hold your own breath!)
- Perform with direct visualisation of the vocal cords
- Check position of tube by auscultation of both lungs and the epigastrium. End tidal CO_2 monitors help verify correct position.
- Secure tube by tying in place (average length is 21–23 cm to teeth for females, and 23–25 for males)

Nasotracheal intubation

This technique is contraindicated in the apnoeic patient and in patients in whom mid-face or basal skull fractures are suspected.

Guiding the tip of the tube into the trachea is achieved blindly by auscultation for the point of maximum breath sounds, which is not as reliable as visualisation of the cords using the orotracheal route. An alternative method is fibreoptic guided insertion of the nasotracheal tube, but these endoscopes are costly and not widely available. This technique would seldom be advised in the acute trauma situation where speed and reliability are paramount.

Surgical airways

Indications: failed orotracheal intubation due to severe oedema of the glottis, fracture of the larynx, or severe oropharyngeal haemorrhage obstructing passage of a tube past the vocal cords.

Jet insufflation

Uses: temporary ventilation (30–40 minutes) until a definitive airway can be established.

Method: insert 14 gauge cannula through cricothyroid membrane. Cut side-hole in oxygen tubing. attach oxygen tubing with 15 l/min O_2 to cannula and cover side-hole intermittently with thumb to deliver inspired breath (1 second on, 4 seconds off).

Limitations: CO_2 gradually accumulates due to inadequate exhalation
Cannot be used with chest trauma
Not recommended for children

Surgical cricothyroidotomy

Technique: An incision is made through skin and cricothyroid membrane. A haemostat/artery forceps is used to dilate the track. A 5–7 mm tracheostomy tube (or an endotracheal tube) is inserted and secured.

Contraindications: (Relative) surgical cricothyroidotomy is not recommended in children under the age of 12 years in whom the cricoid cartilage provides the only circumferential support for the upper trachea.

Advantages: this technique is quick and can be performed without hyperextension of the potentially injured cervical spine. It provides a large calibre airway that can be secured, and it is therefore the technique of choice for a surgical airway in the early management of trauma patients.

Tracheostomy

An open surgical tracheostomy is slow, technically more complex, with potential for bleeding and requires formal operating facilities. It is not appropriate in the acute trauma situation, but is better suited to the long-term management of a ventilated patient.

Percutaneous tracheostomy is also time-consuming and requires hyperextension of the neck. In addition the use of a guidewire and multiple dilators make it an unsuitable technique in the acute trauma situation.

Complications of tracheostomy

Early
- Asphyxia
- Aspiration
- Creation of a false track
- Subcutaneous/mediastinal emphysema
- Haemorrhage/haematoma
- Laceration of the oesophagus or trachea

Late
- Vocal cord paralysis/hoarseness
- Cellulitis
- Laryngeal stenosis
- Tracheomalacia

1.6 Shock and haemorrhage

Shock

Definition: *tissue perfusion insufficient to meet metabolic requirements leading to disordered physiology.*

Types of shock

- Hypovolaemic
- Septic
- Anaphylactic
- Cardiogenic
- Neurogenic
- Vasovagal

In trauma cases, hypotension is always assumed to be hypovolaemia due to haemorrhage, until proven otherwise. This leads to a typical picture of a patient who is cold, pale, clammy, anxious or confused and peripherally 'shut-down'.

Pathophysiology of hypovolaemic shock

In hypovolaemic shock the reduction in blood flow leads to decreased tissue perfusion, causing hypoxia and lactic acidosis, both of which lead to further circulatory collapse and the result may be multiple organ dysfunction (MODS).

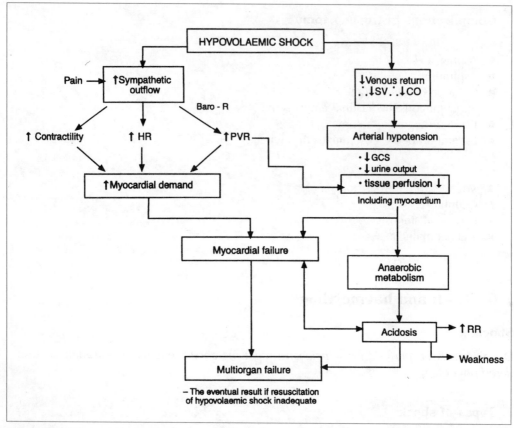

Pathophysiology of hypovolaemic shock

This model hinges on the fact that **acidosis leads to actual cellular destruction.** This is caused by dysfunction of the cell membrane Na^+/K^+ pump in the acidotic environment. Normally, intracellular Na^+ is exchanged for extracellular K^+. When this system fails Na^+ accumulates intracellularly taking water with it, causing the cell to swell. The intercellular spaces enlarge as the cells pull away from each other, allowing fluid to escape into the interstitium and disrupting the integrity of the individual organs.

In situations where there is inadequate cardiac output despite fluid replacement, inotropes (such as dopamine, dobutamine or adrenaline) may be considered.

Remember

CO = SV × HR (normal value = 6 l/min)
SBP = DBP + PP
CO = cardiac output; SV = stroke volume; HR = heart rate; SBP = systolic blood pressure; DBP = diastolic blood pressure; PP = pulse pressure; PVR = peripheral vascular resistance.

This demonstrates that PP, a major determinant of SBP, is governed in part by the PVR which will be raised due to peripheral vasoconstriction following hypovolaemic insult. Therefore the SBP will appear normal in a situation where the cardiac output may be much reduced. This is especially true in the young fit patient, compensating for the blood loss.

Haemorrhage

Definition: *acute loss of circulating blood volume.*

The direct systemic effects of haemorrhage are detailed in the table below. These values refer to the 'average' 70 kg male with a blood volume of 5 litres.

PHYSIOLOGICAL RESPONSES TO HYPOVOLAEMIA

	Class I	Class II	Class III	Class IV
Volume loss (ml)	0–750	750–1500	1500–2000	>2000
Loss (%)	0–15	15–30	30–40	>40
Pulse (bpm)	<100	>100	>120	>140
Blood pressure	Unchanged	Unchanged	Decreased	Decreased
Pulse pressure	Unchanged	Decreased	Decreased	Decreased
Urine output (ml/h)	>30	20–30	5–15	Anuric
Respiratory rate (breaths/min)	14–20	20–30	30–40	>40
Mental state	Restless	Anxious	Anxious/ confused	Confused/ lethargic
Fluid replacement	Crystalloid	Colloid and crystalloid	Colloid and blood	Colloid and blood

Values are irrespective of body fat proportions. Calculate fluid replacement in an obese patient to be the same as the expected weight, to avoid overfilling.

Management of hypovolaemic shock

- Control any obvious haemorrhage
  Direct pressure
  Elevation of injured limb
  Head-down tilt

- Establish IV access
  2 × 16 gauge cannulae

- Access options
  Forearm antecubital veins
  Cutdown to great saphenous vein
  Intra-osseous access in children (<6 years) if initial IV access fails
  Central access only after the patient more stable; this is useful as a guide to fluid replacement after the initial resuscitation.

Remember

- CVP may be falsely raised in tension pneumothorax, pericardial effusion, air embolus, pericardial effusion, MI.
- Physiological responses may be distorted by beta blockers, coronary heart disease, pacemakers, age, narcotics, anatomical location of injury, prehospital fluid replacement, pneumatic antishock garment, spinal injury, head injury.

Fluid replacement

Crystalloid versus colloid

Use initial bolus of 1–2 litres of Ringer's lactate (equivalent to Hartmann's solution). Titrate fluid resuscitation thereafter to response following initial bolus.

- Normal saline
  25% remains in the intravascular compartment; excess may lead to hyperchloraemic acidosis and sodium overload.

- Haemaccel/Gelofusine
  Exert greater oncotic pressure than isotonic crystalloid solutions therefore fluid tends to remain in the intravascular compartment longer.

- Blood

The patient's response to fluid resuscitation is indicated by improvement of the following signs and evidence of organ perfusion:

- Pulse (see graphs)
- Blood pressure
- Skin colour
- CNS state

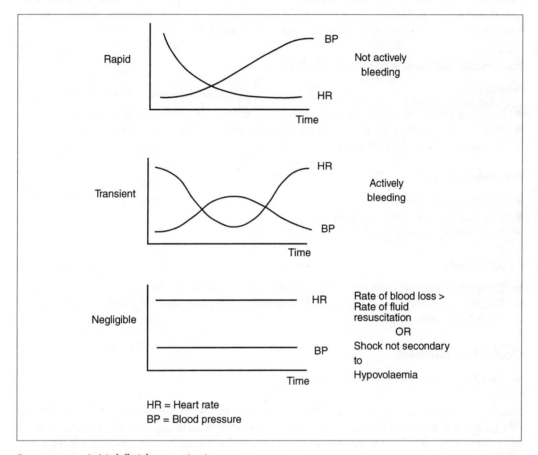

Response to initial fluid resuscitation

Urine output

This is a sensitive and quantitative indication of progress of resuscitation and reflects end-organ perfusion. A normal urine output reflects that resuscitation has been sufficient to reach the renal autoregulatory threshold, and achieve normal renal blood flow. A urinary catheter can be placed quickly and safely in the trauma patient, in the absence of a urethral injury.

Adult   0.5 ml/kg/hr
Child   1.0 ml/kg/hr
Infant   2.0 ml/kg/hr

Acid/base balance in shock

Initial respiratory alkalosis occurs due to increased respiratory rate. Later, metabolic acidosis ensues if there is uncompensated tissue hypoperfusion or insufficient fluid replacement leading to anaerobic metabolism. This will be reflected by a lowered pH, a progressive base deficit and low bicarbonate. Adequate fluid resuscitation, oxygen administration and transfusion to maintain adequate oxygen delivery can correct this process.

Pneumatic antishock garment (PASG)

Indications

- Splinting pelvic fractures with concomitant haemorrhage and hypotension
- Interim support for a shocked patient with abdominal trauma en route to theatre
- Support for lower limb fractures

Contraindications

- Pulmonary oedema
- Suspected diaphragmatic rupture
- Haemorrhage above the PASG

Complications

- Compartment syndrome and skin problems associated with prolonged use
- Deflation accompanied by sudden hypotension, therefore deflate gradually and resuscitate accordingly

Occult haemorrhage

'In the chest, in the belly, or on the road'

Possible locations of significant 'hidden haemorrhage' are in the thorax, in the abdomen, including the retroperitoneal space and pelvic fractures. If there are multiple long bone fractures there may be enough soft tissue haemorrhage to cause hypotensive shock. In compound fractures expect double the blood loss. This illustrates the importance of adequate prehospital information and the clinical history.

2. CHEST, ABDOMINAL AND PELVIC TRAUMA

2.1 Life threatening thoracic trauma

- Causes 25% of trauma deaths in the UK
- <15% will require surgery

Blunt chest trauma as a result of road traffic accidents predominates in the UK. Penetrating trauma of the chest has a greater incidence in countries such as South Africa and the United States.

Tension pneumothorax

Signs

- Respiratory distress
- Tracheal deviation AWAY from the side of injury
- Unilaterally decreased breath sounds
- Raised JVP
- EMD arrest

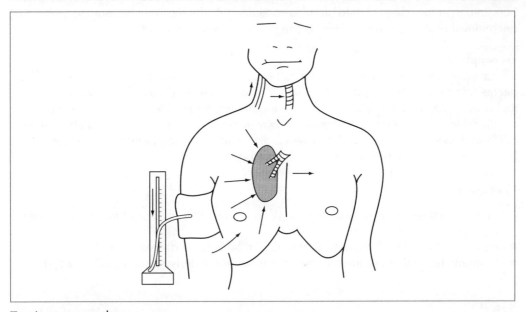

Tension pneumothorax

Treatment

- Immediate decompression
- Aspiration with a 14G venflon in the second intercostal space, mid-clavicular line
- IV access
- Formal chest drain insertion

NB. Chest X-ray must not delay treatment.

Cardiac tamponade

This condition has certain similarities to tension pneumothorax, which may also be present. A suggestive history of penetrating trauma plus failure to respond to thoracostomy tube drainage should lead to the diagnosis of pericardial tamponade being considered.

Cardinal signs

- Raised JVP, low BP, muffled heart sounds (Beck's triad)
- Kussmaul's sign: (JVP raised on inspiration)
- EMD arrest

Treatment

- Pericardiocentesis

This is both a diagnostic and therapeutic manoeuvre, which can decompress the pericardial space until formal cardiac surgery can be performed. A plastic cannula can be left in situ for repeated aspirations until thoracotomy is feasible. There is however a high false negative diagnostic rate (50%) and a high rate of perforation of previously uninjured cardiac chambers. In one in four cases clotted blood is encountered which cannot be aspirated, however the removal of just 15–20 ml of blood can provide temporary relief.

Technique

Under strict aseptic technique and with full resuscitative measures in progress, an 18gauge needle (plastic sheathed, Seldinger catheter or spinal needle) is advanced from the left sub-xiphoid approach, aiming toward the left shoulder tip. An ECG lead can be attached to the needle which will demonstrate increased T-wave voltage when the needle touches the epicardium. Blood is aspirated from the pericardial space and the plastic sheath or catheter is left in situ until urgent thoracotomy can be performed.

Flail chest

Definition: *segment of chest wall loses bony continuity with the rest of the thoracic cage.*

- Paradoxical chest wall movement, therefore tidal volume decreases
- Dramatic hypoxia is commonly seen due to severe underlying pulmonary contusion

Signs

- Respiratory distress
- Paradoxical chest wall movement
- Crepitus of ribs
- Hypoxia
- Hypovolaemia if associated with significant blood loss

Treatment

- Main aim of treatment is respiratory support
- IPPV indicated if there is failure to maintain adequate oxygenation
- Drain any haemopneumothorax
- Adequate analgesia (epidural often helpful; intercostal block may be adequate)
- Careful fluid management essential as patients are prone to pulmonary oedema
- Operative intervention for stabilization rarely indicated

Massive haemothorax

Definition: *1500 ml or more blood drained from chest cavity on insertion of chest drain.*

Signs

- Hypovolaemic shock: ↓ blood pressure, tachycardia; peripheral vasoconstriction
- Absent breath sounds
- Dull percussion note
- Signs of penetrating wound
- ↑ JVP if concomitant tension pneumothorax
- ↓ JPV if hypovolaemic shock prevails

Causes

- Usually penetrating injury

Treatment

Simultaneous drainage of haemothorax and fluid resuscitation. Chest drain must be wide bore (>32 French) AAL fifth intercostal space. Thoracotomy indicated if immediate loss >2000 ml or continuing loss >200 ml/h.

> **Any signs of penetrating injury medial to the nipples/scapula posteriorly –
> assume damage to great vessels or hilar structures.**

Open pneumothorax

Definition: *chest wound which is associated with air in the pleural space.*

Signs

- Respiratory distress
- Sucking chest wound: ↓ air entry; ↑ percussion note over affected side

Treatment

- Occlude wound with sterile dressing: fix three sides only (flutter valve)
- Using different site, insert chest drain
- Surgical closure usually indicated

Pulmonary contusion

- Bruising of lung tissue
- Usually blunt trauma
- Insidious onset of symptoms and signs
- Respiratory distress
- Increased airway resistance
- Decreased lung compliance
- Increased shunting leading to hypoxia
- Atelectasis

Treatment
Support the respiratory system, including intubation and IPPV if necessary.

Myocardial contusion

- Most common undiagnosed fatal injury
- Blunt trauma/deceleration injury
- Area injured: RV>LV
- Damaged heart tissue behaves similarly to infarcted myocardium

Cardiogenic shock possible

- Treat early
- Aberrant conduction may need treatment with a pacemaker
- ECG changes: premature ventricular ectopics or complexes ("PVCs"); sinus tachycardia; atrial fibrillation.

ST changes; T wave abnormalities; RBBB

Aortic disruption

- 90% immediately fatal
- Deceleration injury mechanism most common
- Site of rupture usually ligamentum arteriosum
- Early diagnosis essential for survival

Signs

- Hypovolaemia
- CXR widened mediastinum the only consistent finding
- Treatment involves fluid resuscitation whilst maintaining blood pressure >100 mmHg systolic
- Definitive treatment is surgical or stenting

Diaphragmatic rupture

- Blunt trauma: large defects in the diaphragm – allow herniation of abdominal viscera
- Penetrating injuries: small and rarely life-threatening
- Side affected L>R; R protected by liver; L more easily diagnosed
- Bilateral rupture rare
- Differential diagnoses: acute gastric dilatation; raised hemidiaphragm; loculated pneumothorax
- If CXR ambiguous consider contrast radiography, or CT
- Treatment is by surgical repair

Oesophageal trauma

- Usually penetrating
- Can follow blunt trauma to upper abdomen; oesophagus distends with gastric contents producing a linear tear

Clinical picture

- Mediastinitis
- Empyema

Confirmation

- Contrast studies/endoscopy/CT

Treatment

- Surgical repair
- Drainage of the empyema
- Drainage of the pleural space

2.2 Abdominal injuries

Often missed and frequently under-estimated therefore management should be aggressive.

Blunt

RTAs are the most common cause of blunt trauma and are usually associated with simultaneous head, chest or pelvic trauma.

Penetrating

- Low velocity: knives – 3% cause visceral injury
- High velocity: bullets – 80% cause visceral injury

Abdominal viscera

Spleen

This is the most commonly injured abdominal organ. Management is conservative unless there are signs of continuing haemorrhage, where laparotomy with splenectomy is indicated. Currently, there is a trend towards conservative management to avoid subsequent complications of overwhelming sepsis. This injury is tolerated better in children. Long-term prophylaxis against encapsulated organisms is essential to prevent postsplenectomy sepsis syndrome. Vaccination with Pneumovax, *Haemophilus Influenzae B* vaccine and Meningovax should be administered in the post-operative period. Long-term penicillin prophylaxis may also be advisable in susceptible individuals.

Liver

Managed conservatively if patient haemodynamically stable. In the case of penetrating trauma, assess with CT/USS/laparoscope.

Surgery – haemostasis by:

- Suture
- Packing
- Lobectomy (rarely needed)

Pancreas

- Usually compressive injury against vertebral column
- Difficult diagnosis
- Helping diagnosis: increased amylase level; CT scan

Intestine and mesentery

Blunt injury leads to shearing, compression or laceration injuries. Injuries can be direct, or secondary to devitalization when mesenteric blood supply is compromised. Damage occurs at points where viscera are tethered (i.e. become intraperitoneal from retroperitoneal or vice versa).

- Peritonism slow to develop
- Treatment (surgical): end-to-end anastomosis; defunctioning colostomy – usually due to contamination.

Blunt abdominal trauma

A careful history of the mechanism of injury, combined impact speed, whether a seat belt was worn or an air-bag inflated, whether a pedestrian or motorcyclist, combined with a modicum of imagination, will enable the trauma surgeon to develop an idea of which viscera are at risk. Investigations are useful but should not delay an essential laparotomy, which is necessary in approximately 10% of blunt trauma patients, 40% of stab wound victims and 95% of patients with gun shot wounds.

The physical examination should include:

- Inspection: bruising, seat belt marks, entry and exit wounds, distension may all denote underlying injury
- Palpation: signs of peritonism may be elicited
- Percussion: a crude indicator of the presence of free fluid
- Auscultation: of little practical value in abdominal trauma, but essential in evaluating the chest

Special investigations

- Baseline blood tests, including amylase
  The full blood count may be normal in the acute phase even with significant haemorrhage when dilution and equilibration has not yet occurred. Arterial blood gas estimation may provide evidence of shock in terms of acidosis or a significant base deficit.

- Erect CXR and AXR
  These may reveal a haemo or pneumothorax, diaphragmatic rupture, rib fractures associated with splenic or hepatic trauma, gas under the diaphragm associated with visceral perforation and pelvic fractures associated with massive blood loss.

- Ultrasound scan
  A portable scanner may provide a rapid, inexpensive way of detecting free fluid in the abdomen with a sensitivity of 86–97%.

- CT scan
  This is suitable for patients who are haemodynamically stable, but is slow to complete; involves moving the patient into the scanner, and relies on specialist interpretation. It provides good imaging of the retroperitoneum and is 92–98% accurate in guiding the decision to operate.

- Diagnostic peritoneal lavage
  This provides a rapid way of determining whether an unstable patient with abdominal trauma requires a laparotomy. It does not reveal retroperitoneal blood loss however and carries a 1% complication rate, even in experienced hands. It is made more difficult by obesity, but can be up to 98% sensitive.

Diagnostic Peritoneal lavage

Indications for DPL

- Multiply injured patient with equivocal abdominal examination
- Suspicion of injury with difficult examination
- Refractory hypotension with no other obvious sites of haemorrhage

Contraindications

- Absolute: decision already made for laparotomy
- Relative: previous abdominal surgery, obesity, advanced cirrhosis, coagulopathy, pregnancy

Technique of Diagnostic Peritoneal Lavage

Empty the stomach and bladder with a nasogastric tube and a Foley catheter respectively. Prep and drape the lower abdomen. Infiltrate local anaesthetic with adrenaline at the site of incision, in the midline, one third of the distance from umbilicus to pubic symphysis. Make a 2–3 cm vertical incision (long enough to expose the linea alba and peritoneum under direct vision) and dissect down in the midline. Elevate the peritoneum between haemostats and carefully incise. Thread DPL catheter gently into the pelvis and aspirate gently. If blood is found, proceed to laparotomy. Otherwise, instil 1 litre of warm saline, and then allow this to drain back into the bag under gravity. If macroscopic blood or contamination is seen, proceed to laparotomy. If macroscopically clear, send sample to the lab for analysis.

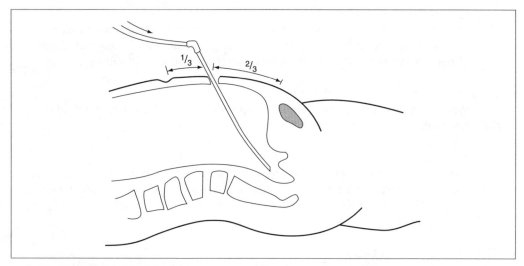

Diagnostic peritoneal lavage

Positive results of DPL

- >100,000 RBC/mm³
- Gram stain showing organisms
- Peritoneal lavage fluid found in urinary catheter or chest drain
- >500 WBC/mm³
- GIT contents aspirated on DPL

2.3 Renal and genitourinary injuries

Kidney

Ninety per cent of renal injuries in the UK are blunt. There is a higher frequency of renal trauma in children as there is less perinephric fat for support.

- Direct: usually crush injuries; between 12th rib and lumbar spine
- Indirect: deceleration injuries; pedicle and PUJ vulnerable

---

Renal injuries

- 85% 'minor' injuries (i.e. contusions)
- 10% 'major' injures (i.e. deep lacerations, parenchymal damage with capsular tears)
- 5% 'critical' injuries (i.e. pedicle injury (classically following a fall from a height and renal fragmentation)

Presentation

- Overlying evidence of trauma
- Loin mass and tenderness
- Loss of the loin contour
- Gross/microscopic haematuria
- +/− paralytic ileus

Investigations

- Baseline bloods
- MSU and dipstix
- USS if stable
- IVU
- Arteriography
- CT is NOT very helpful in this situation

Management

- Resuscitate where injury necessitates
- Bed rest
- Analgesia
- Antibiotics
- Serial MSU and USS

Surgery – intervention necessary for critical injuries of aortic aneurysm.

Complications of renal trauma

- Hypertension
- AV fistula
- Hydronephrosis　　　　} therefore follow-up is essential
- Chronic pyelonephritis
- Renal failure

Urethral injuries

The most common mechanism is via direct trauma e.g. falling onto crossbar of bike.

Can be recognized by:

- History
- Difficulty passing urine
- Blood at urethral meatus
- Perineal bruising
- Free floating prostate

Management
No urethral catheter.

If able to pass urine:

- Antibiotics
- Discharge
- Follow-up clinic appointment

If unable to pass urine:

- Antibiotics
- Urethography

Follow-up is essential to exclude stricture formation.

Scrotal injury

- Unusual
- Healing potential good
- Repair erectile mechanism if damaged
- Drain tense haemotocoeles

2.4 Pelvic fractures

- Severe injury; potential for large blood loss; rarely isolated injury
- Mortality rate 50% if 'open'

- 97% diagnosed on AP film
- Found in 90% of patients with bladder or posterior urethral injuries
- The latter is vulnerable through attachment to the puboprostatic ligaments

Investigations

- Pelvic X-ray (as part of three initial radiological investigations used to determine the degree of bone disruption)
- CT scan
- Angiography

Management

- Aggressive fluid replacement
- Stabilize pelvis early – PASG useful, external fixators used most commonly
- Antibiotics
- Treatment for bladder rupture is repair, suprapubic catheter insertion and broad-spectrum antibiotics
- May cause loss of up to six litres of blood

3. CENTRAL NERVOUS SYSTEM TRAUMA

Head injuries account for approximately 10% of A&E attendance in the UK. Approximately 50% of trauma deaths are associated with head injury.

3.1 Anatomy

Layers of the scalp

S	=	**S**kin
C	=	**C**onnective tissue
A	=	**A**poneurosis (galia aponeurotica)
L	=	**L**oose connective tissue
P	=	**P**eriosteum

Scalping injuries divide the aponeurosis and periosteal layers.

Bones of the skull

Important to revise basic osteology.

Danger area – pterion; middle meningeal artery is located immediately inside this thin layer of bone.

NB. External carotid → Maxillary artery → Middle meningeal.

Meninges

Dura, arachnoid and pia mater.

Neuroanatomy

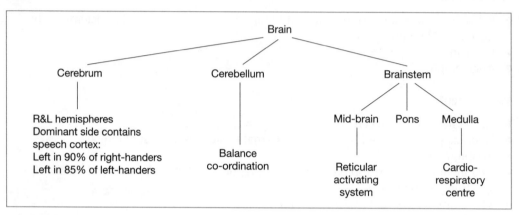

Schematic of neuroanatomy

Lobes of the brain

- **Frontal lobe**
  Emotions
  Personality
  Primary motor
  Motor speech (Broca's area: expressive)

- **Parietal lobe**
  Primary sensory
  Spatial orientation
  Sensory speech (Wernicke's area: receptive)

- **Temporal lobe**
  Memory
  Olfaction

- **Occipital lobe**
  Vision

Blood supply to the brain

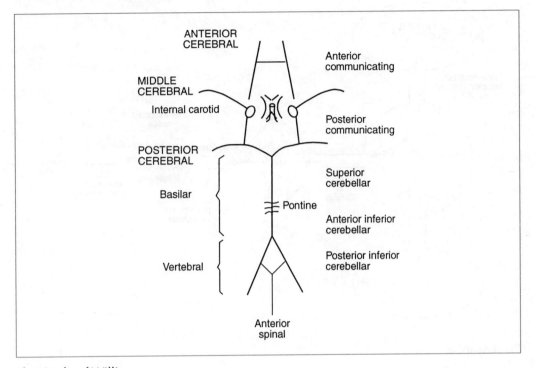

The Circle of Willis

3.2 Physiology

CSF production

- Total volume 130–150 ml
- Production rate – 30 ml/hr by choroid plexus
- CSF reabsorption occurs at arachnoid villi (projections into the sagittal venous sinus)

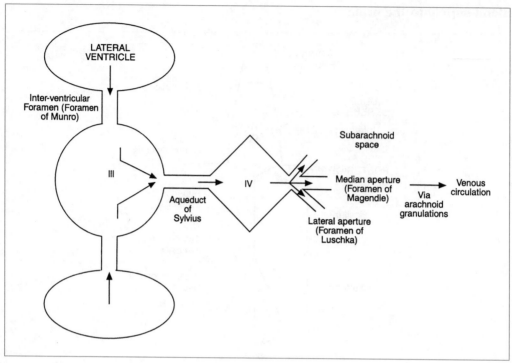

Cerebro-spinal flow

Blood can block the arachnoid villi thereby ↓ CSF reabsorption and ↑ ICP (communicating hydrocephalus).

Intracranial pressure (ICP)

- Normal – 10 mmHg
- Abnormal – >20 mmHg

The Monroe-Kellie doctrine explains intracranial compensation for an expanding intracranial mass.

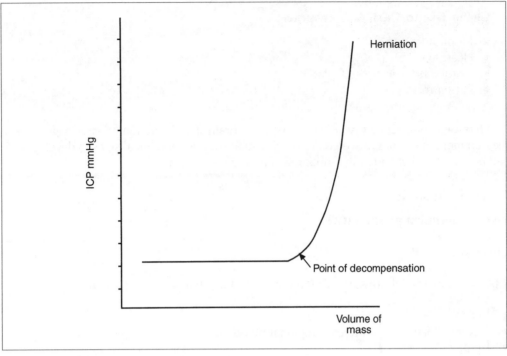

Volume pressure curve

The addition of a mass (e.g. haematoma) within the constant intracranial volume results in an extrusion of an equal volume of CSF and venous blood so that ICP remains normal. However, when this compensatory mechanism reaches its limit the ICP will increase exponentially with increased volume. Normal ICP does not exclude a mass lesion.

Causes of ↑ ICP

- Haematoma
- Focal oedema secondary to contusion/haematoma
- Diffuse cerebral oedema secondary to ischaemia
- Obstruction of CSF flow (rare)

Effects of ↑ ICP

- Tentorial herniation
- Pupillary dilatation as a result of third cranial nerve compression
- Motor weakness as a result of corticospinal tract compression
- Coning resulting in vital cardiorespiratory centres compression

Giving rise to Cushing's response

- Respiratory rate ↓
- Heart rate ↓
- Systolic BP ↑
- Pulse pressure ↑

Death results from respiratory arrest secondary to brain stem infarction/haemorrhage. Direct measurement of ICP has proved more reliable than waiting for clinical signs to develop. ICP can be monitored extradurally, subdurally and intraventricularly.

Cerebral blood flow

Cerebral perfusion pressure (CPP)

CPP = MAP – ICP

(MAP = mean arterial pressure). CPP has a control mechanism called autoregulation:

- ↑ pCO_2
- ↑ extracellular K^+ } increase regional blood flow
- ↓ pO_2

Autoregulation is severely disturbed in head injury and CPP <70 mmHg is associated with poor outcome. Therefore the priority with a head injury is to maintain cerebral perfusion.

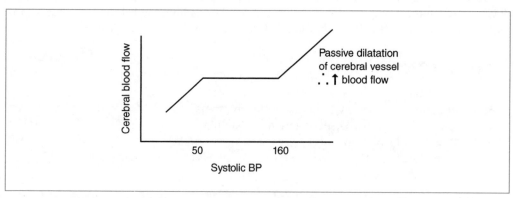

Control of cerebral blood flow

3.3 Assessment of conscious level

Consciousness is controlled by the reticular activating system.

Causes of altered conscious level

- Trauma
- Poisons
- Shock
- Epilepsy
- Opiates
- Infection
- Psychiatric
- Alcohol
- ↑ ICP
- Metabolic (e.g. uraemia)

The Glasgow Coma Scale offers a reproducible, quantitative measure of the patient's level of consciousness.

GLASGOW COMA SCALE

Best motor response	6	Obeys commands
	5	Localizes to pain
	4	Withdraws from pain
	3	Abnormal flexion
	2	Extension
	1	None
Best verbal response	5	Orientated
	4	Confused
	3	Inappropriate
	2	Incomprehensible sounds
	1	None
Best eye opening response	4	Open spontaneously
	3	Open to speech
	2	Open to pain
	1	None

Classification system for head injuries

Patients with head injuries are a very diverse group and their injuries may be classified in a number of ways:

- Severity
  minor GCS 8–15
  major GCS <8
- Mechanism
  blunt
  penetrating injuries
- Pathology
  focal/diffuse
  primary/secondary
  skull/intracranial lesions

Patients after a head injury ± LOC who are able to talk and appear to have made a complete recovery would have a GCS of 15.

Therefore the management aim is to detect those at risk of developing an intracranial haematoma.

- Primary brain injury: neurological damage produced by causative event
- Secondary brain injury: neurological damage produced by subsequent insults (e.g. hypoxia, hypovolaemia, ischaemia, increased ICP, metabolic imbalance or infection)

The main direction of treatment is:

- To diagnose a primary brain injury and provide the optimum conditions for recovery
- To minimize/prevent secondary brain injury by maintaining brain tissue oxygenation

3.4 Mechanisms of brain injury

Hypoxia/ischaemia

Permanent damage within 3–4 min.

Contusion

The brain has a soft consistency and is poorly anchored within the cranial cavity, it therefore moves with acceleration/deceleration. Contact with the skull can cause bruising (contusions). The frontal and temporal lobes are particularly vulnerable.

Diffuse axonal injury

Axonal tracts may be torn by the shearing forces involved, resulting in a spectrum of damage from reversible to irreversible. The transient LOC known as concussion is due to this mild stretch injury. Microscopically this causes 'retraction balls'.

3.5 Intracranial haemorrhage

Focal injuries

- Extradural haematoma
- Subdural haematoma
- Intracerebral haematoma
- Large contusion

Diffuse axonal injury

Mild:	Coma lasting 6–12 hours – 'concussion'
Moderate:	Coma >24 hours – no brainstem dysfunction, mortality = 20%
Severe:	Coma >24 hours with brainstem dysfunction, mortality = 57%

Extradural haematoma

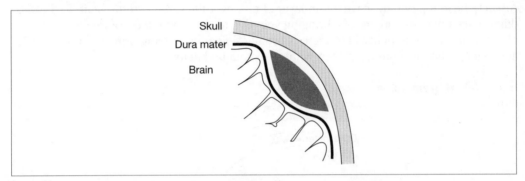

Extradural haematoma

Trauma (often trivial) e.g. a blow to the temporal or parietal bone causing rupture of the underlying middle meningeal artery. Children and young adults are more susceptible as the dura becomes more adherent to the skull with advancing age. Initial concussion is typically followed by a 'lucid interval' as the expanding haematoma is accommodated. Rapid decompensation may then follow as intracranial pressure rises as the inner edge of the temporal lobe descends into the tentorial opening (mid-brain cone).

Acute subdural haematoma

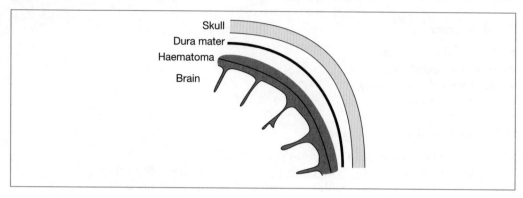

Acute subdural haematoma

A severe head injury may leave a thin layer of clot over the surface of the brain in the sub-dural space either by rupture of a bridging vein due to shearing forces, or due to laceration of brain substance. In either case there is usually severe underlying primary brain damage and deterioration is more rapid than with an extradural haematoma.

Intracerebral haematoma

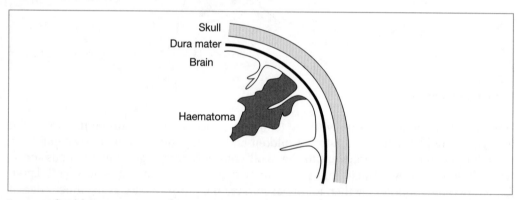

Intracerebral haematoma

These injuries are the least remediable compressing intracranial haematomas. They are usually associated with cerebral laceration, contusion, oedema and necrosis, all of which contribute to their compressive effects. Removal of such a clot has unpredictable and often disappointing results.

3.6 Management of head injuries

Treatment priorities and management decisions depend on whether the head injury is minor or major.

Minor head injuries

The management aim is to detect those at risk of developing an intracranial haematoma.

RISK OF HAEMATOMA

	Skull fracture	No skull fracture
Fully conscious	1:45	1:7900
Confused	1:5	1:180
Coma	1:4	1:27

Criteria for skull X-ray after recent head injury

- Loss of consciousness or amnesia at any time
- Suspected penetrating injury
- Large scalp haematoma/laceration
- Difficulty in assessing the patient (e.g. alcohol intoxication, the young, epilepsy)
- Neurological symptoms or signs
- Cerebrospinal fluid or blood from the nose or ear
- History of high velocity injury

The skull X-ray is a useful adjunct to clinical examination. (NB. Simple scalp laceration is not a criterion for skull X-ray.)

Criteria for admission

- Loss of consciousness >5 min (or amnesia)
- Confusion or decreased GCS
- Skull fracture
- Neurological symptoms and signs
- Worsening headache, nausea or vomiting
- Extensive laceration
- Difficult to assess (alcohol intoxication)
- No responsible adult at home
- Other medical conditions (e.g. clotting abnormalities)

Note:

- Post-traumatic amnesia with full recovery is not an indication for admission
- Patients sent home should be given written instructions about possible complications and appropriate action

Major head injury

Aim of management – prevention of secondary cerebral damage.

NB. Major head injury will often have concomitant cervical spine injury.

Management of major head injury

- **Maintain ventilation with PaO$_2$ >13 and PaCO$_2$ <5.3**
  Intubation is appropriate when absent gag reflux, PaO$_2$ <9, PaCO$_2$ >5.3
  Use rapid sequence intubation
  Exclude any pneumothoraces before ventilation
  Remember, a talking patient indicates a reduced risk of complications

- **Maintain adequate mean arterial pressure**
  NB. CPP = MAP – ICP

- **Mannitol 0.5–1 g/kg over 10–30 mins to help reduce ICP**

- **Antibiotics**
  Penicillin V six-hourly if any signs of open fracture of the skull

- **Analgesia**

Criteria for consultation with a neurosurgical unit

- Fractured skull in combination with any abnormal neurology
- Confusion or other neurological disturbance persisting for more than 12 hours
- Coma continuing after resuscitation
- Suspected open injury of the vault or the base of the skull
- Depressed fracture of the skull
- Deterioration of patient's GCS

Note:

- Before assuming that the deterioration is due to CNS, exclude possible hypoxia and metabolic causes (e.g. hypoglycaemia).

3.7 Spinal injuries

The overriding concern with spinal injuries is the risk of either causing or completing an injury to the spinal cord, which can result in devastating and permanent neurological injury. This causes tragedy at a personal level, and has a long-term economic impact on medical resources. The utmost caution and vigilance should therefore be exercised when dealing with trauma victims at risk of having a spinal injury. In the British Isles these injuries are most commonly seen in victims of road traffic accidents, and are frequently associated with blunt injuries to head, chest and abdomen, and also with long bone fractures. If such a life-threatening injury co-exists with a suspected or proven spinal injury, then it must be dealt with, whilst maintaining strict immobilisation of the spine. This may not be achieved satisfactorily with a hard collar alone, but sand-bags, tape, a spinal board or in-line traction with skull tongs may be necessary until definitive treatment of the spinal injury can be safely addressed.

Trauma patients at risk of a spinal injury

- Unconscious/head injury (10% risk of associated C-spine injury)
- High speed road traffic accident
- Injury above the clavicle
- Sensory or motor deficit
- Brachial plexus injury
- Falls from >3× the patient's height

Clinical findings that suggest a C-spine injury in an unconscious patient

- Flaccid areflexia
- Abdominal breathing/use of accessory muscles of respiration
- Elbow flexion without extension
- Grimaces to pain above, but not below the clavicle
- Hypotension with bradycardia (and euvolaemia)
- Priapism

NB. Accurate and repeated documentation of clinical findings is essential in order to establish a baseline with which to compare trends of improvement or deterioration.

Assessment of the cervical spine

If a cervical spine injury is suspected then strict immobilisation must be maintained until accurate assessment can be performed by an adequately qualified individual. Assessment should include an accurate history with careful consideration to the mechanism of injury and energy of impact.

Clinical symptoms in a conscious patient may include pain and neurological deficit. Clinical signs may include deformity (a palpable 'step-off'), bruising, crepitus and muscle spasm. A full radiological assessment (PA and lateral C-spine, visualisation of C7 with an effective pull-down, or a swimmer's view, additional CT scanning if necessary). Only when there is an absence of clinical and radiological evidence of a C-spine injury, should spinal precautions be dispensed with. The cervical spine, if injured, is at particular risk during endotracheal intubation, 'log-rolling', and transfer onto the operating table. During these manoeuvres, extreme caution must be exercised, for example, fibreoptic intubation to avoid extending the neck from the neutral position, and log-rolling should be the minimum necessary to complete the secondary survey, and only performed with an adequate number (4) of trained assistants.

Neurological assessment

Sensory function

Pain and temperature perception are conveyed by the spinothalamic tract which supplies the contralateral side of the body. Deep and superficial pain should be tested separately (pinch test and pricking with a broken tongue depressor, respectively). Superficial pain and light touch must be carefully distinguished as light touch is widely conveyed in the spinal cord and may be preserved when superficial pain sensation has been lost, enabling the diagnosis of a partial, as opposed to complete, spinal cord injury. The former have some potential for recovery whereas the latter carry a dismal prognosis. In extreme cases the peri-anal and scrotal areas may be the only region preserved (sacral sparing) and this should be carefully tested for sensation and anal contraction.

NB. Loss of sensation below the level of spinal injury may obscure the diagnosis of other life-threatening injury.

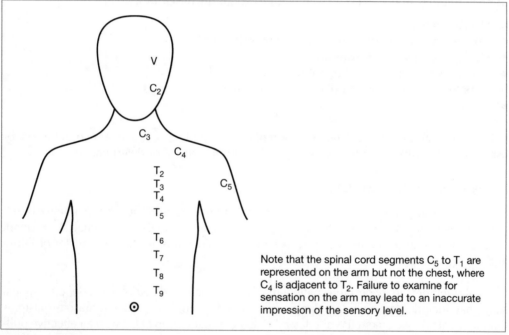

Note that the spinal cord segments C_5 to T_1 are represented on the arm but not the chest, where C_4 is adjacent to T_2. Failure to examine for sensation on the arm may lead to an inaccurate impression of the sensory level.

Sensory levels

Motor function

This is transmitted via the corticospinal tracts which run on the ipsilateral side. Voluntary movement and involuntary response to painful stimuli can be assessed.

Proprioception

This is subserved by the posterior columns on the ipsilateral side and can be tested by joint position sense, and vibration sense using a tuning fork.

Reflexes

These should be assessed in the standard fashion using a reflex hammer and carefully documented for serial evaluation.

Autonomic function

Evidence of damage to the autonomic nervous system can manifest as priapism and/or incontinence.

Neurogenic shock

Injury to the descending sympathetic pathways can lead to loss of vasomotor tone with pooling in capacitance vessels and failure to generate a tachycardic response. This results in profound hypotension which in the trauma setting may be mistakenly attributed to hypovolaemia. Appropriate treatment requires the selective use of inotropic agents, rather than aggressive and inappropriate volume replacement which may result in pulmonary oedema. Atropine may be necessary to counteract an associated bradycardia.

Spinal shock

In the immediate post-injury phase, the injured spinal cord may appear completely functionless with resulting flaccidity and loss of reflexes. Several days or weeks later, characteristic spasticity, hyperactive reflexes and upgoing plantar response supersede the flaccid state.

Radiological assessment of the cervical spine

Patients requiring radiographs of the cervical spine:

- Any injury above the clavicle
- Head injuries
- Unconscious trauma patients
- Multiply injured patients
- Brachial plexus injuries

In the first hour

Lateral cervical spine radiographs are obtained as part of the standard trauma series (C-spine, chest , pelvis). Adequate views from the base of the skull to T1 must be obtained and the region of C7/T1 requires either a 'pull-down' technique, or a swimmer's view for proper assessment. The area of the atlas and axis can be rapidly assessed during CT scanning for a head injury. It must be noted that portable films taken in the emergency setting miss up to 15% of fractures, therefore if a spinal injury is suspected on clinical grounds, then such an injury should be assumed to be present until proven otherwise. If a C-spine injury is present, then the rest of the spine needs to undergo radiological assessment.

Secondary evaluation

After the acute phase of the patient's assessment and resuscitation, if a C-spine injury is suspected or proven, then specialist evaluation by the Orthopaedic or Neurosurgical team will follow. This will include A-P and oblique views of the C-spine, odontoid views and a chest

X-ray. Bony fragments within the spinal canal can be revealed by CT or MRI scanning. Flexion/extension views of the C-spine may also be deemed necessary and should only be performed under the strict supervision of an experienced specialist.

Specific types of cervical spine fracture

C-1 Atlas fracture

Axial loading can cause a blow-out of the ring of C1 (Jefferson fracture) best seen on the open mouth view. One third of these are associated with a fracture of C2, but cord injuries are uncommon. These fractures are unstable and require specialist referral and management.

C-1 Rotary subluxation

Usually presents in a child as torticollis. Odontoid views show the peg to be asymmetric with respect to the lateral masses of C-1. No attempt should be made to overcome the rotated position of the head and specialist referral and management is required.

C-2 Odontoid dislocation

Bony injury may be absent and dislocation may be due solely to disruption of the transverse ligament on C-1. Suspect when space between anterior arch of C-1 and the odontoid is greater than 3 mm. (Steel's rule of three: adjacent to the atlas, one third of the spinal canal is occupied by the odontoid, one third intervening space, one third spinal cord.) This condition is unstable with high risk of cord injury. Strict immobilisation and specialist management are mandatory.

C-2 Odontoid fractures

- Type 1 Above the base
- Type 2 Across the base (NB. childhood epiphysis may resemble this on X-ray)
- Type 3 Fracture extends onto the vertebral body

All require strict immobilisation and specialist referral.

'Hangman's fracture'

This results from an extension-distraction injury, plus axial compression, and involves the posterior elements of C-2. (In judicial hanging the slip knot was placed under the chin.) This is a highly unstable injury and traction is strictly contraindicated. Strict immobilisation and specialist referral are essential.

C-3 to C-7 injuries

These can arise through a variety of mechanisms, and apart from obvious bony injury and clinical signs, may be revealed by a haematoma reducing the space between the anterior border of C-3 and the pharynx (normally less than 5 mm.) In children this distance is normally 2/3 the width of C-2 and increases on Valsalva. These require strict immobilisation, followed by specialist referral and management.

Facet dislocations

These may be unilateral (suspect if displacement between adjacent vertebral bodies = 25%) or bilateral (displacement = 50%). May also see displacement of spinous processes on A-P views with unilateral dislocation.

Cervical cord injuries

At risk are injuries associated with a bone fragment from the anterior/inferior vertebral body giving the classic 'tear drop' appearance on X-ray. The posterior vertebral fragment may displace into the canal and cause cord damage.

Thoracic spine injuries

These usually result in wedge fractures from hyperflexion injuries. Cord injury is uncommon but as the canal is narrow in this region, is frequently complete when present. This more commonly occurs with a rotational injury. Wedge fractures of thoracic vertebrae are splinted by the rib cage and only require internal fixation if kyphosis exceeds 30° or neurological deficit is present.

Thoracolumbar injuries

Usually result from hyperflexion and rotation and are commonly unstable. The cauda equina is at risk and will produce bladder and bowel signs, and deficits in the lower limbs. These patients are at high risk during log-rolling and this may need to be minimised or deferred until X-ray studies obtained.

4. PRINCIPLES OF LIMB INJURIES

4.1 Peripheral nervous system: anatomy and physiology

Nervous system

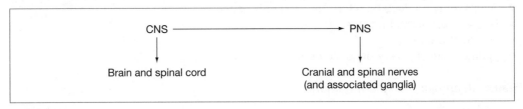

Nervous system

Acute injury to peripheral nerves is usually the result of direct mechanical trauma:

- Blunt: pressure
- Penetrative: laceration
- Traction: RTA and fracture

Nerve damage is commonly missed therefore assume injury present until proven otherwise. Chronic nerve injuries are more common. Leprosy is the most common cause of chronic loss of sensation worldwide, but diabetes is more common in developed countries.

Most common causes of sensation loss

- **UK**
  Diabetes mellitus (DM)
  Peripheral vascular disease (PVD)
  Radiotherapy

- **World-wide**
  Leprosy

Structure of peripheral nerve

Endoneurium
Connective tissue around individual axons, containing collagen, capillaries and lymphatics. Protects from stretching forces.

Perineurium
Dense connective tissue surrounding fascicle. Strong mechanical barrier. Diffusion barrier protecting fibre from large ionic flux.

Epineurium
Outermost layer of connective tissue. Binds fascicles together and forms thick protective coat. Forms 25–75% cross-sectional area of nerve. Thicker over joints.

Classification of nerve lesions

Neuropraxia

- Conduction ceases due to segmental demyelination
- Axons remain intact, therefore Tinel's sign is negative
- Nerve looks normal macroscopically
- Transient lesion
- Spontaneous recovery occurs over days or weeks

Causes: tourniquet palsy, crush injuries

Axonotmesis

- 'Axonal separation'
- Axons damaged, therefore distal portions degenerate
- Endoneurium intact, therefore recovery is possible by axonal regrowth along the endoneural tube at 1 mm/day
- Recovery delayed but likely

Causes: closed stretch injury

Neurotmesis

- Nerve completely divided and spontaneous recovery unlikely
- Motor recovery is usually better than sensory following surgical repair

Nerve recovery

- Stump oedema occurs after 1 hour
- Axons start to sprout filopodia from the proximal to last node of Ranvier and rely on the myelin sheath to guide them to the end organ; Day 3
- Chromatolysis: this is the cell body regenerative response, where the cell body enlarges; days 14–20 in response to the increased metabolism
- Distal axon undergoes Wallerian degradation; complete in 6 weeks
- Muscle innervated by the injured nerve wastes

Tinel's sign – painful paraesthesia on percussion over the area of regeneration.

4.2 Diagnosis and investigation of nerve injuries

Arterial bleeds suggest possibility of nerve injury. Check individual peripheral nerves. (See the table below.)

PERIPHERAL NERVE CHECKS

Upper limb	Sensory	Motor
Axillary	Regimental badge area – lateral upper arm	Abduction of shoulder
Musculocutaneous	Lateral area of forearm	Flexion of elbow
Median	Palmar aspect index finger	Abductor pollicis brevis
Radial	Dorsal web space between thumb and index finger	Wrist extension
Ulnar	Little finger	Index finger abduction
Lower limb		
Femoral	Anterior aspect of knee	Knee extension
Obturator	Medial aspect of thigh	Hip adduction
Superficial peroneal	Lateral aspect of foot dorsum	Ankle eversion
Deep peroneal	Dorsal aspect of first web space	Ankle and toe dorsiflexion

Sensation can be maintained for 72 hours therefore look for sensation distortion.

Nerve comparison

- Hypersensitivity
- Reduced two-point discrimination
- Test with light touch
- Vasomotor function: reduced sweat production; disturbance of sympathetic function is an important early sign of nerve damage.

Electromyography

Objective investigation which is time-consuming and unpleasant. It is the electrical assessment of nerve injury and extent of injury.

Approaches used are:

- **Direct nerve stimulation:** the nerve is stimulated above and below the injury and the threshold of muscular response is compared with that of the opposite side.
- **Detection of potentials within the motor unit:** either surface or needle electrodes are used to establish close muscle contact; abnormal or reduced/absent action potentials indicate nerve injuries.
- **Nerve conduction velocity determination:** this determines the interval between stimulation of nerve and detection of muscle action potential at distal sites; very useful for chronic lesions (e.g. normal velocity median nerve – 57 m/s; in carpal tunnel syndrome – 49 m/s).

None of the above are very effective immediately after injury as muscle stimulation continues before Wallerian degeneration is complete. When denervation is complete, fibrillation occurs.

NB. Nerve conduction is affected by age and temperature.

4.3 Treatment of nerve injuries

Aim to maximize the chance of recovery. Primary repair is always favourable as the outcome is better.

Open injuries

- Always surgically explore and debride the wound thoroughly
- Clean cuts should be repaired or marked with 6.0 nylon
- Crushed/torn nerves are lightly opposed and re-operated upon at 2–3 weeks

NB. Vascular and orthopaedic injuries take priority over nerve injuries.

Closed injuries

- Mostly axonotmesis/neuropraxia
- Late surgery scar tissue should be excised; clean-cut ends anastomosed
- Use of nerve grafts
- Limb splints to decrease tension

Techniques for repairing nerves

- Epineural
- Fascicular
- Grouped fascicular
- Mixed repair

All wounds should be free of foreign bodies and nerves aligned with no tension.

4.4 Brachial plexus injuries (BPI)

There are a number of classification systems for brachial plexus injury:

- Birth versus traction injuries in later life
- Pre- versus post-ganglionic injuries

Most injuries caused at birth are post-ganglionic and recovery spontaneously. The cause of injury is the traction applied to the head, away from the shoulder during birth. These can be divided anatomically into upper (Erb's palsy) and lower (Klumpke's palsy) plexus injuries.

Injuries in later life may be pre- or post-ganglionic depending on mechanism of injury, which may be penetrating (e.g. stab injury) or blunt (e.g. traction). Pre-ganglionic injuries are less likely to recovery as they usually indicate spinal root avulsion.

Clinical features (i.e. pattern of paralysis and sensory loss) will indicate the type of lesion.

The following suggest a pre-ganglionic injury:

- Severe pain
- Paralysis of diaphragm or scapular muscles
- Spinal cord injury
- Cervical spine injury
- Vascular impairment
- Horner's syndrome

If the whole of the brachial plexus is non-functional, the limb will be completely numb and paralysed and may necessitate amputation if there is no recovery.

4.5 Reflex sympathetic dystrophy (Sudeck's atrophy)

Causes

- Trauma to region
- Peripheral nerve lesion
- Medical (e.g. MI or CVA)

Due to sympathetic overactivity. Most often affects hands and feet, knees, hips and shoulders.

Signs and symptoms

- Persistent regional pain
- Trophic skin changes
- Swelling
- Stiffness of neighbouring joints
- Skin often blotchy, blue and cold
- LATER skin becomes smooth and shiny
- Nails become atrophic and brittle

4.6 Skeletal system: anatomy and physiology

Bone

- Dense connective tissue
- Very vascular
- Blood supply runs in canals – canaliculi
- Haversian canals
- Volkmann's canals (at 90° to Haversian canals) } (both contain blood vessels)

Bone types

- Compact: 80% of appendiceal skeleton; very dense
- Cancellous: spongework of trabeculae

Significant in calcium metabolism. No microscopic difference between the types. Bone marrow – functionally independent of the bone.

Periosteum

- Layer of thick fibrous tissue
- Deepest cell layer contains osteoblasts therefore osteogenic
- Sharpey's fibres attach the periosteum to the bone

Endosteum

- Single layer of cells
- Lines the marrow cavity and channels
- Also osteogenic

Bone development

Intramembranous: osteoblasts lay down bone in fibrous tissue (e.g. clavicles)
Endochondral: pre-existing hyaline cartilage model is destroyed and replaced with bone

Sites of primary ossification

- Diaphysis: midshaft of a long bone
- Epiphysis: growing ends of long bone

Calcium

Normal range in plasma: $2.15–2.65 \times 10^3$ m

Functions:

- Constituent of hormones
- Neurotransmitter
- Mitosis
- Fertilization
- Clotting
- Teeth and bone structure

Intracellular – mostly bound to albumin; main 'store' of calcium

Extracellular – mostly free; free portion is active

Total body plasma calcium:

- 50% free
- 40% albumin bound
- 10% complexed

NB. Reduced pH $\rightarrow$ decreased protein binding $\rightarrow$ increased fraction of free calcium

Calcium irregularities

- **Symptoms of hypocalcaemia**
  Paraesthesia
  Tetanus – carpopedal or laryngeal spasm
  Fitting
  ECG changes

- **Symptoms of hypercalcaemia**
  Abdominal pain
  Decreased GI motility
  Muscle weakness
  Polydipsia
  Sudden cardiac arrest
  Renal failure with or without calculi
  ECG changes

NB. Trousseau's sign or Chvosteck's sign

Calcium metabolism

- Absorption of Ca^{2+} from gut is proportional to total body quantity
- Excretion is via gut and renal system
- Fine tuning of body Ca is mainly under endocrine control

Phosphate

Normal plasma range $0.81–1.45 \times 10^3$ m. Mainly an intracellular anion.

Needed for:

- Glucose metabolism intermediate
- All energy compounds
- Cofactors
- Lipids
- Enzymes

Absorption

- Directly proportional to intake; not related to total body calcium

Storage

- Soft tissue
- Bone

Symptoms of phosphate deficiency

- Skeletal dysfunction
- Cardiac dysfunction
- Abnormal bone growth

Magnesium

Normal range in plasma – 0.75–1.0×10^3 m. Major intracellular cation.

Needed for:

- Neuromuscular transmission
- Cofactors, especially ATP
- Protein synthesis

Storage

- 1/3 is protein bound
- 65% in bone
- 35% in cells

Magnesium deficiency

- **Deficiency seen in**
  Inflammatory bowel disease
  Alcohol excess
  Diuretics use
  TPN

- **Deficiency leads to**
  Cardiac arrhythmias
  Paraesthesia
  Fits and tetani

Vitamin D

Main modulator of Ca^{2+} and phosphate. Action via gut to alter these substrates' absorption.

Needed for:

- Normal bone formation

Metabolism
Dietary source (D2) Skin + UV (D3).

- Milk 7–dehydroxy cholesterol
- Fish
- Liver

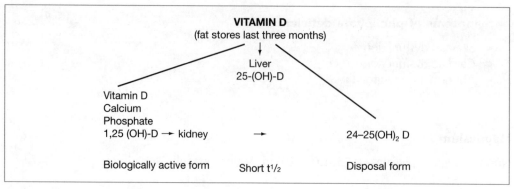

Vitamin D

1,25 Dihydroxycholecalciferol actions

- Absorption of Ca^{2+} from gut against concentration gradient
- Bone reabsorption via osteoclast
- Calcium and phosphate uptake into sarcoplasmic reticulum of muscle cells
- Mineralizes bone – otherwise unmineralized bone assimilates (rickets)
- Decreased lymphokines
- Decreased lymphocyte proliferation

Parathyroid hormone (PTH)

Parathyroid glands

- Posterior to thyroid gland
- Within or outside thyroid capsule
- Usually × 4
- Superior glands fairly constant position
- Inferior glands position varies
- Blood supply – inferior thyroid artery
- Superior glands originate from IV pharyngeal pouch
- Inferior glands originate from III pharyngeal pouch

Chief/principal cell – PTH; main bulk of gland.

Oxyphil cells – function unknown; scattered throughout gland.

PTH

- Maintains or increases plasma calcium level
- Facilitates metastasizing Ca^{2+} from bone renal system intestinal tract

PTH prevents build-up by stimulating urinary excretion of phosphate. Concentration of plasma PTH is regulated by plasma $[Ca^{2+}]$ via a negative feedback mechanism.

Other integrated feedback systems

- Increased phosphate $\rightarrow$ decreased free Ca^{2+} (phosphate binds Ca^{2+}) therefore increased PTH
- Increased 1,25 $(OH)_2$ D $\rightarrow$ decreased PTH
- Decreased Mg $\rightarrow$ decreased PTH

PTH stimulates Ca^{2+} uptake by target cells therefore there is an initial decreased Ca^{2+} and later increased Ca^{2+}.

Summary of effects of PTH

- **Renal**
  Increased Ca^{2+} – reabsorption from ascending loop of Henle
  Decreased PO_4^{2-} – increased renal excretion
  Decreased Na^+ – decreased bicarbonate; due to increased renal excretion

- **Gut**
  Stimulates formation of 1,25 $(OH)_2$ D therefore increased Ca^{2+} absorption from gut
  (NB. Indirect effect via 1,24 $(OH)_2$ D.)

- **Skeletal**
  Stimulates osteocytic osteolysis: increased Ca^{2+} release from bone
  Simultaneous osteoclastic reabsorption
  Inhibition of collagen synthesis

- **PTH excess**
  Primary hyperparathyroidism (e.g. parathyroidadenoma)
  Parathyroid-related protein (e.g. tumours with ectopic hormone product)
  Secondary hyperparathyroidism (e.g. CRF)

- **Symptoms**
  Non-specific abdominal pain
  Duodenal ulceration
  Pancreatitis
  Depression

Remember
'Bone, stones, abdominal groans, psychic moans'

Calcitonin

Antagonizes action of PTH on bone therefore decreased $[Ca^{2+}]$. Origin of hormone: C cells (parafollicular cells) in thyroid gland. Embryological origin – neural crest cells. Release of hormone governed by $[Ca^{2+}]$ in plasma.

Action

- Decreased plasma [Ca^{2+}] inhibits bone reabsorption, inhibits osteolysis. Extent of effect of hormone dependent on baseline turnover of calcium of individual.
- Decreased [PO_4^{2-}] via increased urinary excretion.

NB. No clinical picture for deficient state. PTH and Vitamin D compensate for any abnormal calcitonin level.

4.7 Fractures: aetiology and healing

Aetiology

- Traumatic: direct, indirect (i.e. via pull from ligament or tendon)
- Repetitive stress (e.g. March fracture of the metatarsals)
- Pathological (e.g. malignant bone involvement, metabolic disease)

Anatomical description

Complete fracture

- Stable fracture: transverse, impacted
- Unstable fracture: oblique, comminuted

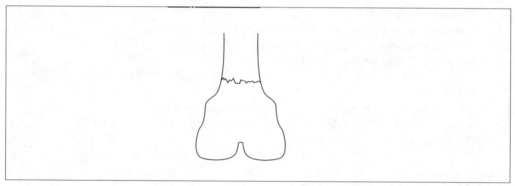

Stable fracture – Transverse Impacted

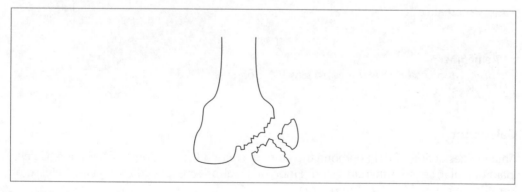

Unstable fracture – Oblique/Comminuted

Incomplete fracture

- Greenstick fracture: periosteum remains intact; quick healing
- Compression fracture: cancellous bone crumples (e.g. crush fracture of vertebrae), unreducible

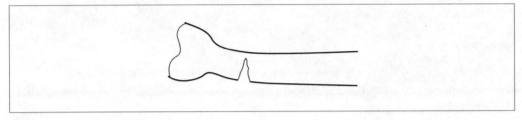

Greenstick fracture

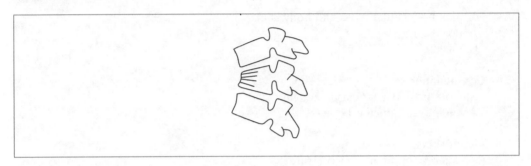

Compression fracture

Displacement

After a fracture the amount of displacement is reliant on:

- Force of injury
- Gravitational pull
- Muscle attachment and its pull

Description

Rotation
Opposition
Angulation
Displacement
Site

Stages of fracture healing

- **Immediate**
  Tissue death and haematoma formation
  Torn vessels bleed
  Avascular necrosis of fracture ends

- **8 hours**
  Inflammation and cellular proliferation
  Acute inflammation
  Cellular tissue attempts to bridge the fracture site
  Haematoma absorbs
  Angiogenesis

- **Formation – cellular mass and bony islets**
  Chondrogenic
  Osteogenic

- **Consolidation**
  Osteoblastic and osteoclastic activity
  Woven bone – lamellar bone

- **Remodelling**
  Restoration of normal bone density
  Repair complete

The speed of repair varies with:

- Bone type: cancellous >cortical
- Type of injury: transverse fracture heals slower than a spiral fracture
- Site of injury
- Poor circulation
- Amount of movement at the fracture site

4.8 Complications of fractures

Complications of fractures

- **Immediate**
  Internal or external bleeding
  Organ injury (e.g. brain, lung)
  Skin or soft tissues
  Neurovascular damage

- **Later**
  Local
  Skin necrosis
  Gangrene
  Pressure sores
  Infection

- **General**
  Venous thrombi
  Pulmonary emboli
  Pneumonia
  Renal stones
  Fat embolism (see notes)

Crush syndrome: this may be a feature of any severe injury, which results in ischaemia of large amounts of soft tissue; fluid loss, DIC and release of toxins lead to acute tubular necrosis; temporary dialysis may be needed; watch urine output and plasma K^+.

Late complications

- Wound sepsis (early wound toilet is vital)
- Failure of fixation (e.g. plates or nails break or dislodge)
- Joint stiffness, contractures, malalignments (malunions)
- Sudeck's atrophy (joint stiffness and patchy osteoporosis)
- Psychological problems immobilizing ('compensation neurosis')
- Non-union

Non-union

The signs of fracture (pain, mobility and tenderness, swelling) persist for longer than expected (e.g. >3 months, in the case of a long bone in an adult) (true union, with trabeculae crossing the fracture site may take much longer).

If X-rays then show the absence of callus (new unremodelled bone) at the fracture site diagnose **delayed union**.

If X-rays shows that the medullary cavity has closed off, diagnose **non-union**.

Non-union is more common in cortical bone than in cancellous bone, where there is often impaction.

Factors delaying union

- Where there is an avascular fragment (scaphoid, femoral neck)
- Comminuted fractures, particularly if there has been infection
- Generalized disease (e.g. malignancy, infection)
- Distraction of the bone ends by soft tissue (open reduction ± internal fixation attempts to prevent this)
- Osteoporosis and elderly patients (more common)

Management of non-union

- Rigid immobilization will help (e.g. internal fixation). If there is no callus, a cortical bone graft may help by providing both fixation and an osteogenic stimulus.
- If realignment is not necessary a cancellous graft (using marrow-rich chips) may be used (± internal fixation).
- If infection is present, it will be necessary to remove dead bone. Bone chips then fill in the space, which is held open by external fixation (Steinmann pins).

Fat embolism

Most commonly seen after long bone fractures, especially proximal femoral shafts, although may follow all traumatic conditions. Classic presentation occurs after a 12–48 hour asymptomatic period, with pulmonary and neurological features coinciding with a petechial haemorrhagic picture.

Biphasic course

- Initial systemic symptoms caused by a mechanical occlusion of the vasculature by fat globules. These symptoms may fluctuate reflecting the flexibility of the fat within the vessels.
- Later presentation resulting from the eventual degradation of the fat particles into irritant constituents. These migrate systemically causing a later phase systemic upset.

Risk factors

- Age – young men have an increased risk
- Closed fracture has an increased incidence of fat embolism
- Unstable fracture
- Reaming of the marrow cavity for internal bone fixation

> **Clinical presentation of fat embolism**
>
> - Increased heart rate and respiratory rate
> - Pyrexia
> - Hypoxia and hypocapnia
> - Thrombocytopenia
> - Mild CNS symptoms (confusion, anxiety)
> - Petechial rash (especially over the upper anterior portion of the body – due to occlusion of dermal capillaries by fat)

Laboratory tests

- Arterial blood gases
- Cytology – Sudan black staining
- Free or macrophage-consumed fat globules
- Reduced haematocrit (due to intra-alveolar haemorrhage)
- Altered coagulation, including thrombocytopenia

Treatment

- Reduce fractures early
- Maintain intravascular volume
- Mechanical ventilation and PEEP
- Use of high-dose steroids is controversial but sometimes used

5. SPECIAL PROBLEMS

5.1 Post-traumatic stress disorder (PTSD)

This occurs when a person has experienced a traumatic event involving actual or threatened death or injury to themselves or others. The individual will have felt fear, helplessness or horror.

There are three classic symptoms which usually cluster:

- **Intrusions:** re-experiencing the event via flashbacks or nightmares
- **Avoidance:** the person attempts to reduce exposure to people, places or things that exacerbate the intrusions
- **Hyperarousal:** physiological signs of increased arousal, including hypervigilance and increased startle response.

These symptoms must persist for more than 1 month after the event to qualify as PTSD, causing significant distress or impairment of social or occupational situations.

Lifetime prevalence in the USA is 5–10% (Kessler et al., 1996). This value increases to >20% in inner city populations.

Other symptoms include:

- Insomnia
- Anorexia
- Depression with low energy
- Difficulty in focusing
- Withdrawal

5.2 Paediatric trauma

Accidents are the most common cause of death in children aged >1 year. They account for 150,000 paediatric admissions and 600 deaths per year in the UK. The most common form of accidents resulting in death from head injuries are road traffic accident (RTAs).

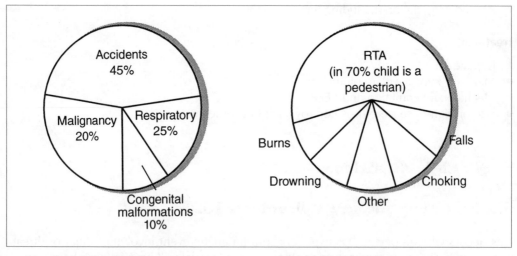

Causes of death 1–14 years   Causes of accidents 1–14 years

The assessment and resuscitation of the injured child is the same as for the adult, but taking note of the anatomical and physiological differences.

Anatomical

- Children frequently have multisystem trauma due to their small size and shape
- Increased force per body area
- Decreased fat layer
- Closer proximity of organs
- Rapid thermal losses
- Elastic skeleton often conceals underlying organ damage without fractures

Physiological
Tend to compensate well and therefore serious pathology goes unnoticed until decompensation occurs.

Psychological
Long-term effects can be social or affective resulting in learning disabilities. Communication difficulties can give rise to increased fear. Parents should always be allowed maximal contact.

Airway management

- Relatively large occiput causes relative increased flexion of cervical spine
- Soft tissues such as the tongue and tonsils are relatively large compared to the oral cavity and therefore obstruct the airway easily
- Short trachea often results in right bronchus intubation
- Narrow nasal passages
- Under 6 months are obligate nose breathers

Breathing

- Small airways more easily obstructed (NB. Resistance is proportional to $\dfrac{1}{R^4}$)
- Muscles more likely to fatigue
- Chest wall more compliant – can have pulmonary contusions without rib fracture therefore actively seek injury
- Mobility of the mediastinal structures makes the child more sensitive to tension pneumothorax and flail segments

Intubation

- Use straight blade laryngoscope
- Uncuffed ET tube used to avoid subglottic oedema
- Tube size is equivalent to child's little finger girth or use formula: age/4 + 4
- Use of nasopharyngeal tube is debatable but is often safer for transport

Circulation
Recognition of early shock may be difficult due to their great physiological reserve.

Remember

$CO = SV \times HR$

In infants the SV is small and relatively fixed, therefore CO varies with HR. Thus the primary response to hypovolaemia is tachycardia and their response to fluid resuscitation is blunted.

Caution: $\uparrow$ HR compounded by pain and fear

NORMAL VALUES IN CHILDREN

Age (years)	Heart rate (bpm)	Blood pressure (mmHg)	Respiratory rate (breaths/min)
<1	110–160	70–90	30–40
2–5	95–140	80–100	25–30
5–12	80–120	90–110	20–25

>12 years: values very similar to those of adults.

Other useful features in assessing paediatric circulation are:

- Pulse volume
- End organ perfusion: (i) skin perfusion; (ii) respiratory rate; (iii) urine output; (iv) mental status
- Temperature: toe-core gap

PHYSIOLOGICAL RESPONSE TO HAEMORRHAGE

Blood volume loss (%)	<25	24–45	>45
Cardiac	↑ Heart rate Weak thready	↑ Heart rate Bradycardia	Hypotension Pulse
CNS	Lethargic Irritable Confused	↓ Consciousness Dulled response	Coma
Skin	Cool Clammy	↓ Capillary refill, Cold extremities, Cyanotic	Pale and cold
Kidneys	↓ Urine output	Minimal output	No urine output

Intravenous access

After two attempts at percutaneous access, consider:

- Under 6 years old: intra-osseous needle (anterior surface tibia 2 cm below tuberosity)
- Over 6 years old: venous cutdown

Fluid resuscitation

Initial bolus 20 ml/kg crystalloid (warmed whenever possible).

Reassess, looking continually for response to bolus:

- Slowing of the HR
- Increased BP
- Increased pulse pressure
- Increased urine output
- Warm extremities
- Improved mental status

If there is no improvement to the bolus give 20 ml/kg colloid (usually haemaccel).

Head trauma

The Glasgow Coma Scale is still useful in children aged >4. If under 4 then the verbal response score must be modified.

Exposure

Remember that due to their relatively large surface area:weight ratio children lose heat quickly. Overhead heaters and blankets are essential.

NB. Remember that all drug dosages should be worked out per kg body weight.

Weight estimate in kg for those <10: (age + 4) × 2.

Non-accidental injury

Always be aware of the possibility. A number of features raise suspicion.

In the history:

- Late presentation
- Inconsistent story
- Injury not compatible with history (e.g. long bone fracture in children under walking age)

In the examination:

- Abnormal interaction between child and parents
- Bizarre injuries: bites, burns, shape of injury (e.g. finger tip bruising)
- Perioral injuries
- Perianal/genital injuries
- Previous injuries: old scars, healing fracture

5.3 Trauma in pregnancy

Treatment priorities are the same as for the non-pregnant patient, treating mother first as the fetus is reliant on her condition. Resuscitation and stabilization need modification to account for the anatomical and physiological changes which occur in pregnancy.

Anatomical changes in pregnancy

- **1st trimester:** uterus is relatively protected by bony pelvis and thick-walled uterus
- **2nd trimester:** uterus becomes intra-abdominal and more vulnerable to injury; amniotic fluid cushions fetus
- **3rd trimester:** relative decrease in amniotic fluid and thickness of uterus, therefore fetus more vulnerable to blunt and penetrative trauma.

The placenta contains no elastic tissue and is vulnerable to shearing forces, resulting in incidences of placental abruption and damage to dilated pelvic veins.

Physiological changes in pregnancy

Due to the effect of oestrogen and progesterone:

- ↓ Smooth muscle tone: ↓ gastric emptying with LOS reflux therefore risk of aspiration
- ↓ $PaCO_2$ to 30 mmHg: this is the 'physiological hyperventilation of pregnancy' secondary to the respiratory stimulant effect of progesterone. FEV_1/FVC remains the same, whereas TV increases by 40%
- ↑ Pulse rate
- ↓ Blood pressure (10–15 mmHg in the second trimester); normalizes near term
- ↑ Plasma volume by 50%
- ↑ Cardiac output by 1.0–1.5 l/min; CVP is usually normal despite the increased total volume.

This means that pregnant women have to lose more of their total circulating volume before signs of hypovolaemia develop. Blood is shunted away from the utero-fetal circulation to maintain the mother's vital signs. Therefore the fetus may be shocked before maternal tachycardia, tachypnoea or hypotension develop. For these reasons, vigorous replacement is required.

Aorto-caval compression

The enlarged uterus can compress the IVC and impair venous return, reducing cardiac output by up to 40%. This can cause a drop in blood pressure unless the pressure is minimized by placing patients in the left lateral position.

Secondary survey in pregnancy

Urgent X-rays (C-spine etc.) are still taken as the priority is to detect life-threatening injuries.

Special considerations
Search for conditions unique to the pregnant patient:

- Blunt/penetrating uterine trauma
- Placental abruption
- Amniotic fluid embolism
- DIC
- Eclampsia
- Uterine rupture
- Premature rupture of membranes in labour
- Isoimmunization: prophylactic anti-D should be given to Rhesus-negative mothers within 72 hours; the Kleihauer-Betke test (maternal-blood smear looking for fetal RBCS) is specific, but not very sensitive and is therefore of little use.

5.4 Burns

Comprises 6% of Accident and Emergency presentations.

Types of burn

- Thermal: the most common
- Chemical: alkali burns are more severe than acidic burns as the latter limit their own extent of damage by producing a coagulated barrier
- Electrical
- Radiation

Physiology of burns

There is coagulative necrosis of tissues exposed. Capillary beds are disrupted, which then leak plasma into the surrounding interstitium. Damage equates to the time of exposure to the injurious element, in the case of thermal burns, the actual temperature. Thus lower temperatures with longer exposure, may cause the same amount of damage as higher temperatures.

Major burn

- 15% total body surface area (TBSA) in adults
- 10% TBSA in children

At this point the body's response is generalised with global oedema and profound hypovolaemic shock.

Results of burns

- **Hypovolaemic shock**
  Consequent reduction in cardiac output
  Increased peripheral vascular resistance

- **Increased haematocrit**
  Due to loss of plasma

- **Increased metabolism**
  Increased oxygen demand
  Increased nitrogen loss

- **Increased levels of cortisol**
  Increased catabolism
  Increased gluconeogenesis

Depth of burn

Burns should be clinically judged by their depth. Ultimate classification may not be until operative assessment.

BURNS: A HELPFUL GUIDE

	Superficial	Deep dermal	Full thickness
Appearance	Pink and painful Often blistered	Pink-white with reduced blanching Dull to pinprick	Black/white No sensation

Repair	Takes 14 days
	  to repair 100%
		Takes 3–4 weeks
		  to heal
			Minimal healing
			  from wound edges only

	± Pigment
	  changes
		Heals from adnexa
		Scarring
			Usually needs grafts to
			  cover the site

Initial resuscitation

Follow the ABCDE protocol. Beware impending airway compromise with inhalational injury.

- Facial or oropharynx burns
- Hoarseness or stridor
- Soot in the nostrils or sputum
- Expiratory bronchi
- Dysphagia
- Epiglottic swelling with drooling

Intravenous fluid resuscitation is essential when the burn exceeds 15% (consider oral rehydration if less than this). Wallace's Rule of Nines is used to estimate area of significant burn. Do not include areas of simple erythema.

Wallace's Rule of Nines

- Head 9%
- Arms (each) 9%
- Legs (each) 18%: (9% anterior surface, 9% posterior surface)
- Trunk 36%
- Perineum 1%
- Palm of hand 1.25%

Intravenous fluid replacement formulae

There are many available formulae.

The Brooke Army Hospital Formula is used commonly, but requirements should be tailored to each patient. In the first 24 hours:

- Colloid (plasma, plasma substitutes, dextran). Give 0.5 ml/Kg/% TBSA of burn IV
- Electrolytes (Ringer's lactate). Give 1.5 ml/kg/% TBSA of burn IV
- Water (5% dextrose in water). Give 2000 ml IV (less for children)

Half the above volumes are given in the second 24 hours, after which most patients can drink normally.

Like all other formulae, the physiological response of the patient needs to be taken into account (i.e. urine output, blood pressure and pulse, respiratory rate and peripheral perfusion) and the volume replacement should be adjusted to these values. Hb and HCT measured regularly can be a helpful guide to rate of resuscitation.

Consider blood transfusion: 1 unit for each 10% of deep burns.

Remember analgesia (pain increases catecholamine release which increases catabolism).

Continual reassessment essential.

Transfer to burns unit only when:

- FT burns >10% total body surface (children 5%)
- Burns involving hands, feet or perineum
- Involvement of respiratory system
- Circumferential burns
- Significant electrical or chemical burns

Transfer is safe only when:

- Airway stable
- Fluid resuscitation instigated
- Escharotomies performed in any areas of FT circumferential burns (otherwise asphyxia (due to trunk burns) and compartment syndrome (due to limb burns) are inevitable).

Local treatment of burns

Partial thickness
Expose to allow wound to dry, thus reducing access by organisms and the subsequent risk of infection. Silver sulphadiazine dressing reduces the number of Gram-negative organisms.

Deep dermal
Clean and dress and leave undisturbed for two weeks. Then shave the wound down to healthy tissues in areas which have not healed and graft if necessary.

Full thickness
Immediate excision and grafting is the aim (if the patient is elderly, grafting is kept to an absolute minimum), allowing the wound a delay to see if it will heal unaided.

NB. Allo/xeno-grafts are useful in the short-term, for coverage which reduces the need for analgesia and the risk of infection.

Complications of burns

- **Infection**
  Usually endogenous organisms; can lead to MODS
  Damaged local circulation: ↓ immune defences; compromised phagocytosis; ↓ chemotaxis.
- **Electrolyte disturbances**
  ↑ K^+
  ↑ Na^+ – inadequate fluid resuscitation
  ↓ Na^+ – dilutional, over-enthusiastic resuscitation
- **Respiratory failure**
  Upper respiratory tract damage as direct result of heat
  Lower respiratory tract damage – oedema
  ↓ surfactant
  reduced lung compliance
  ↓ macrophages
  Lung parenchyma damage – by toxic products

- **Myonecrosis**
  Commonly seen with electrical burns and some deep burns.
- **RBC breakdown**
  Results in haemoglobinuria and consequent renal failure. Causes increase in plasma K^+. May exacerbate DIC.
- **Massive increase in catabolism**
  Resultant huge N_2 losses. Stress ulcers common. Therefore feed patients early with high energy diet.
- **Pancreatitis**
- **Acalculus cholecytitis**
- **Increased risk of pulmonary embolism**
- **Septic thrombophlebitis**
  Often exacerbated by IV access, therefore limit this access to essential access. CVP lines discouraged.

5.5 Traumatic wounds

Key issue is contamination.

Micro: bacteria
Macro: foreign bodies

Needs extensive debridement to remove foreign bodies and all necrotic tissue. Clostridium enjoy the anaerobic environment of traumatic wounds. Full tetanus and antibiotic coverage is essential. These wounds should never be closed primarily.

5.6 Orbital trauma

Examination

- Acuity
- Eyelids
- Eyeball:
  Assess early bleeding
  Look for anterior chamber haemorrhage
  Look for conjunctival haemorrhage
  Look for foreign body
- Orbital: clinical evidence includes reduced eye movements; check with OM views on XR.

5.7 Facial injuries

- Facial lacerations: clean meticulously; alignment of the tissues must be exact to produce a good cosmetic result.
- Complex lacerations: is there a plastic surgeon available?
- Dog bites: give antibiotic cover
- Rugby player's ear: aspirate haematoma (repeat every few days) and then strap orthopaedic felt pressure pads against the head
- Ruptured ear drum: advise against letting water into the external auditory meatus
- Avulsed teeth may be replaced; if inhaled, arrange expiratory CXR
- Bleeding socket: bite on an adrenaline-soaked dressing or use sutures

Bony injury classification

- **Le Fort I:** severs the tooth-bearing portion of the maxilla from the upper maxilla. Signs: crepitus on manipulation. It causes epistaxis but rarely threatens the airway.
- **Le Fort II:** the middle third of the facial skeleton is driven back and downwards. If the bite is open, airway is at risk.
- **Le Fort III:** the fracture extends into the anterior fossa via the superior orbital margins. There may be CSF rhinorrhoea.

6. PRE-HOSPITAL CARE

Trauma is the leading cause of death in the first four decades of life.

Aims of pre-hospital care

- Stabilize the patient's condition
- Extract patient from incident situation
- Transfer patient safely: full primary survey; secure airway and C-spine; × 2 IV access; monitor set-up; appropriate analgesia (inc. splinting).

> **Remember**
>
> 'First do no harm'
>
> Approach with **horizontal organization** (i.e. each member of team doing their own task concomitantly).

6.1 National pre-hospital services

- All members of service should have the same accepted routine of approach
- Communication between all the services should be maintained
- There should be close connection with a trauma centre

6.2 Major incidents

'Number or severity of live casualties needs special arrangements of emergency services'

Requires triage system ('Triager' = to sort).

To be of use, needs to be **Quick, Efficient** and **Reproducible**. It should involve continual re-assessment of patients by appropriate medical staff, with regular readjustment of patient priorities.

Identify major groups:

- Those needing immediate resuscitation (e.g. airway compromise, life-threatening chest condition, immediately life-threatening haemorrhage, massive burns (airway often in danger here too)).
- Those needing early resuscitation, but can survive a delay of a few hours (e.g. torso injuries, including non-life-threatening chest injuries, major fractures, major burns)
- Delayed treatment (i.e. those able to withstand delayed treatment with no risk of life-threatening injuries)
- Dead

6.3 Trauma scoring systems

- **Injury severity score** (ISS): anatomical description. A score of 0–6 is given to each body region depending on severity of injury. The three highest scores are then squared and added together to produce the ISS score. Disadvantages are static score. Needs absolute diagnosis before score can be calculated. Subjective.
- **Revised trauma score** (RTS): physiological description. Score calculated using the GCS, respiratory rate and systolic BP. This system is flexible, varying with patient's progress. It is objective with little inter-observer variability.
- **Trauma score–injury severity score** (TRISS): combined ISS and RTS scoring, as well as including age of patient and mechanism of injury (i.e. penetrating or blunt). Indicator of patient's prognosis.

7. SUGGESTED FURTHER READING

Advanced Trauma Life Support Course for Physicians, Committee on Trauma, American College of Surgeons Student Manual

Bailey and Love's Short Practice of Surgery (Twenty second edition), Mann CV, Russell RCG, Williams NS, Chapman and Hall Medical

Current Therapy of Trauma (Fourth edition), Trunkey DD, Lewis FR jr, B.C. Decker

Chapter 4

Intensive Care

CONTENTS

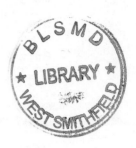

Intensive Care

1. CARDIOVASCULAR ANATOMY

1.1 Thoracic cavity

Lungs (in pleural cavities)

The **mediastinum** (the space between the pleural cavities) contains the heart and great vessels, the oesophagus, the trachea and bifurcation, the thoracic duct, and the phrenic and vagus nerves. An anatomical plane passing through the sternal angle and the lower border T4 divides it.

Divisions of the mediastinum

- **Superior**
  Above this plane

- **Middle**
  Containing fibrous pericardium and heart

- **Anterior**
  In front of fibrous pericardium

- **Posterior**
  Behind fibrous pericardium

The pre-vertebral and pre-tracheal fascia from the neck extends into the superior mediastinum. Neck infection will therefore

- Pass into the anterior mediastinum if in front of pre-tracheal fascia in neck
- Be confined to the superior mediastinum in front of vertebral bodies if behind pre-vertebral fascia in neck.

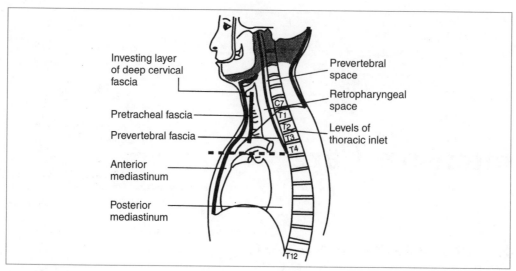

Investing layer of deep cervical fascia

Pretracheal fascia

Prevertebral fascia

Anterior mediastinum

Posterior mediastinum

Prevertebral space

Retropharyngeal space

Levels of thoracic inlet

C7
T1
T2
T3
T4

T12

Divisions of the mediastinum demonstrating the continuity with the tissue spaces of the neck

1.2 Superior mediastinum

Boundaries of the superior mediastinum

- **Anterior**
  Manubrium

- **Superior**
  Thoracic inlet (often clinically referred to as thoracic outlet)

- **Posterior**
  Bodies of T1 to T4

- **Inferior**
  Plane through T4

The great vessels are contained within the superior mediastinum (veins on right, arteries on left). There is more 'dead space' on the right side (to accommodate venous distension), therefore fluid in the mediastinum may collect there. Its contents are listed below.

Arterial

The arch of the aorta lies wholly in the superior mediastinum, behind the manubrium.

Arterial branches in the superior mediastinum

- **Brachiocephalic trunk**
  Arises behind the manubrium; termination of the left brachiocephalic vein lies in front of the artery; it divides behind the right sterno-clavicular joint into the right subclavian artery and the right common carotid artery

- **Left common carotid artery**
  Passes up next to the trachea into the neck; there are no branches in the mediastinum

- **Left subclavian artery**
  Supplies the head and neck, the upper limb and some thoracic wall structures; there are no branches in the mediastinum

Ligamentum arteriosum

The fibrous remnant of fetal ductus arteriosum (between pulmonary artery and aortic arch). The left recurrent laryngeal nerve (from vagus) hooks around it.

Venous

- **Brachiocephalic veins** are formed behind the sternoclavicular joints, from internal jugular and subclavian veins: **right** passes vertically downwards; **left** passes nearly horizontally through the superior mediastinum behind the manubrium, meets the right brachiocephalic vein at the lower border of the first costal cartilage on the right.
- **Superior vena cava** (SVC) is formed by the two brachiocephalic veins and passes vertically downwards behind the right sternal border, through the pericardium and joins the right atrium at the lower border of the third right costal cartilage; the azygous vein drains into the SVC behind the sternal angle, opposite the second right costal cartilage.

Nerves

Phrenic

- Supplied by C3 to C5 (mainly C4) – 'keeps diaphragm alive'
- Passes in front of the lung root on each side
- Adjacent to the mediastinal pleura throughout its mediastinal course, i.e. lies as far medial as possible in the thorax.

Medial relations are different on each side:

> **Medial relations**
>
> - **Right phrenic nerve medial relations**
>   (= venous structures throughout its course)
>   Right brachiocephalic vein
>   Superior vena cava
>   Right atrium
>   Inferior vena cava
>
>   Passes through the vena caval
>   foramen in central *tendon* of
>   diaphragm
>
> - **Left phrenic nerve medial relations**
>   Left common carotid artery
>   Left subclavian artery
>   Arch of aorta (lateral to superior
>   intercostal vein)
>   Pericardium over left ventricle
>
>   Passes through *muscular* part of
>   diaphragm to left of pericardium

Vagus

As medial in their course as structures permit.

- **Right nerve**
  Lateral to trachea
  Passes behind lung root
  Enters oesophageal plexus in midline (with left vagus)
  Right recurrent laryngeal branch given off in root of neck
  Hooks around the right subclavian artery (non-recurrent in 1–2% of cases)

- **Left nerve**
  Separated from trachea by left common carotid and subclavian arteries and passes
  over the aortic arch
  Passes behind lung root
  Enters oesophageal plexus

Left recurrent laryngeal branch

- Given off on the aortic arch
- Hooks around the ligamentum arteriosum and passes up on the right side of the
  aortic arch

Recurrent laryngeal nerves

- Supply trachea and adjacent oesophagus

They are extremely important due to their innervation of the muscles of the larynx and their
potential for injury in thyroid surgery.

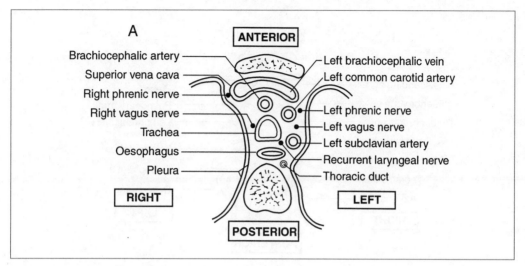

Transverse section through T3

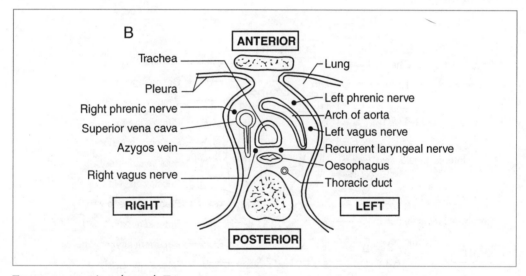

Transverse section through T4

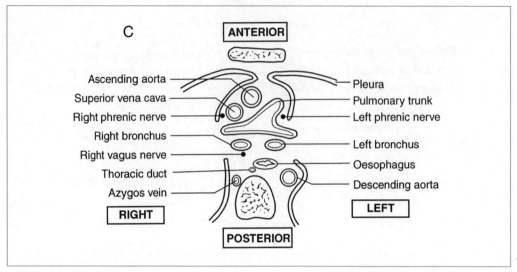

Transverse section through T5

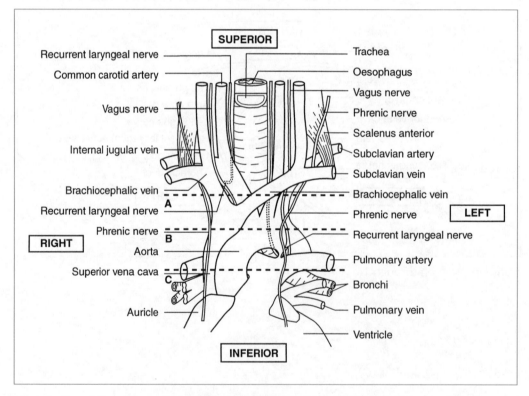

Lines A, B and C correspond to diagrams A, B and C (horizontal sections) on previous pages

Cardiac plexus

- Sympathetic and parasympathetic afferent fibres
- Supply SA node, AV node and bundle, ventricular myocardium
- Also contain afferent pain fibres

Trachea

- Continuation of larynx
- Commences in neck at level of C6
- Bifurcates just below manubrium
- Thoracic part descends in superior mediastinum in front of oesophagus to upper part of posterior mediastinum

Oesophagus

- Crossed by arch of the aorta on the left and azygous vein on the right

1.3 Anterior mediastinum

Contains the thymus (although the thymus may only be present in the anterior part of the superior mediastinum).

- Surgical approach is via median sternotomy
- Continuous through superior mediastinum with pre-tracheal space of the neck

1.4 Middle mediastinum

- Pericardium and heart
- Adjoining parts of the great vessels
- Lung roots
- Phrenic nerves

Pericardium

Fibrous (outer part):

- Fuses with all vessels except inferior vena cava
- Blends with central tendon of the diaphragm
- Also attached to the sternum (sternopericardial ligaments)
- Supplied by the phrenic nerve

Serous (inner part):

- Parietal (outer layer) phrenic nerve supply
- Visceral (inner layer) no sensation
- Transverse and oblique sinuses = folds of pericardium between parietal and visceral layers

NB. *Pericardiocentesis* = needle aspiration of fluid (e.g. blood) in pericardial cavity. (See Chapter 3, *Trauma*, for details.)

1.5 Posterior mediastinum

Boundaries of the posterior mediastinum

- **Anteriorly**
  Pericardium (upper part), posterior part of the diaphragm (lower part)

- **Posteriorly**
  T4 to T12

Contents

- Descending aorta: commences at lower border of T4; exits posterior mediastinum at midline at level of T12 by passing behind the crura of the diaphragm
- Oesophagus: commences at C6 and ends at cardia of the stomach at level of T10; exits posterior mediastinum at level of T10
- Thoracic lymph nodes
- Thoracic duct
- Azygos veins
- Thoracic sympathetic trunk

1.6 The heart

Borders of the heart

- **Left border**
  Mostly left ventricle
  Auricle of left atrium (upper part)
  Surface marking = apex to lower
    border left 2nd costal cartilage,
    2 cm lateral to the sternum

- **Right border**
  Right atrium
  Surface marking = level of 3rd–6th
    right costal cartilage,
    right margin of the sternum

- **Inferior border**
  Mostly right ventricle
  Small amount of left ventricle (which forms the apex)
  Surface marking = right 6th costal cartilage to apex (usually left 5th intercostal space, in mid-clavicular line)

Surfaces of the heart

Anterior/sternocostal surface

- Right atrium and ventricle, small amount of left ventricle, forming left border

Diaphragmatic surface

- Right atrium, receiving inferior vena cava; anteroposterior AV groove
- Part of both ventricles (1/3 right, 2/3 left)

Posterior surface/base of heart

- Left atrium, receiving pulmonary veins

Tissues of the heart

- Epicardium (outer part)
- Myocardium (muscle layer, makes up the bulk of the heart)
- Endocardium (inner part of the chambers of the heart)

Valves of the heart

Tricuspid

- Three cusps (anterior, posterior and septal)
- Surface marking: behind sternum, level of 5th and 6th costal cartilages
- Auscultation area: 5th intercostal space, right sternal edge

Pulmonary

- Three semilunar cusps (anterior, left and right)
- Surface marking: left of midline behind sternum, level of 3rd costal cartilage
- Auscultation area: 3rd costal cartilage, left sternal edge

Mitral

- Cusps (large anterior and small posterior)
- Surface marking: left of midline behind sternum, level of 4th intercostal space
- Auscultation area: at the apex beat

Aortic

- Three cusps (right, left and posterior)
- Surface marking: left of midline behind sternum, level of 3rd intercostal space
- Auscultation area: 2nd intercostal space, right sternal edge

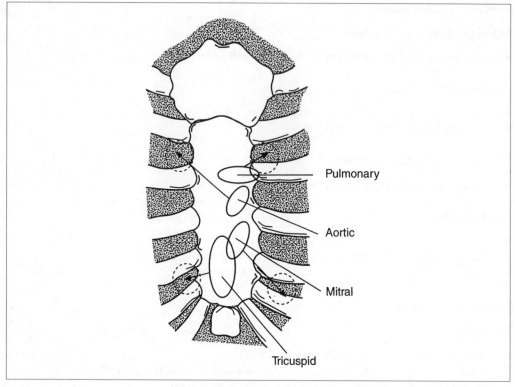

Surface markings of the heart valves. The arrows indicate the directions in which sounds of the closing valves are propagated and the circles indicate the generally preferred sites for auscultation

Conducting system

This is formed by specialized cardiac muscle cells and initiates, co-ordinates and controls the rhythm of cardiac muscle contraction.

Main elements:

- **Sinoatrial node (SA node)**: acts as a pacemaker for the heart; situated in the wall of the right atrium, just below the superior vena cava
- **Atrioventricular node (AV node)**: situated in the wall of the interatrial septum (above and to the left of the opening of the coronary sinus); electrical impulses which have been conducted from the SA node through the atria are conducted through the AV node to the Bundle of His
- **'Bundle of His'**: arises from the AV node; passes through the membranous part of the interventricular septum; divided into right and left branches. **Right branch**: initially runs in the muscle of the septum then becomes subendocardial on the right side of the septum; reaches the anterior wall of the ventricle then divides into multiple subendocardial branches, supplying the right ventricle (branches are made up of

Purkinje fibres); **Left branch**: this reaches the endocardium of the septum then divides into multiple subendocardial branches (Purkinje fibres); Purkinje fibres make up the terminal subendocardial plexus.

Blood supply

By region

- Right ventricle – right coronary artery
- Left ventricle – left coronary artery
- Atria: arterial supply – variable
- Interventricular septum – right and left coronary arteries

NB. There can be considerable variation from this general scheme.

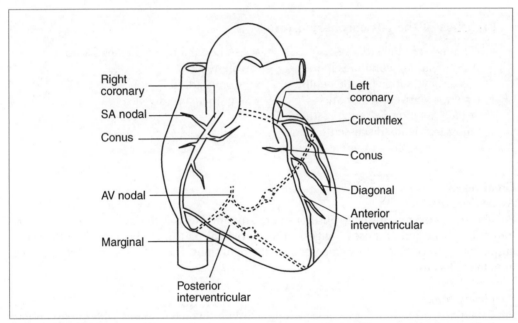

Coronary arteries and their main branches, viewed anteriorly. Interrupted lines show the vessels on the posterior surface

By vessel
Right coronary artery
Arises from the right aortic sinus branches (passes between the right auricle and infundibulum of the right ventricle; downwards in AV groove and backwards at inferior surface of the heart).

Branches of the right coronary artery

- Conus artery
- SA nodal artery
- Right marginal artery
- AV nodal artery
- Posterior interventricular artery
- Atrial and ventricular branches

Left coronary artery
Arises from the left aortic sinus (behind the pulmonary trunk – passes between the left auricle and infundibulum of right ventricle).

Branches of the left coronary artery

- Circumflex branch (direct continuation); continues in the AV groove supplying the ventricle
- Anterior interventricular artery (= left anterior descending artery); most frequently discussed
- SA nodal artery (supplies SA node in 40%)
- Conus artery
- Ventricular branches

Great vessels

Ascending aorta
Proximal part covered in sleeve of serous pericardium (which it shares with the pulmonary trunk). There are three sinuses (bulges) in the proximal part (one above each aortic valve cusp). The right coronary artery emerges from the right sinus. The left coronary artery emerges from the left sinus.

Pulmonary trunk
Proximal part covered in sleeve of serous pericardium (which it shares with the ascending aorta), passes backwards, divides into the right and left pulmonary arteries in the concavity of the aortic arch (in front of the left main bronchus).

2. CARDIOVASCULAR PHYSIOLOGY

2.1 Basic concepts

- Cardiac output is intermittent – continuous capillary flow is due to the elasticity of the aorta and branches. During diastole, continuous flow is maintained in the capillary bed, by relaxation of the arterial elastic wall, previously stretched during systole. This 'capacitance' mechanism maintains the diastolic pressure and permits continuous flow into the capillaries.
- Peripheral vessels more muscular, less elastic than great vessels
- Greatest resistance (and therefore the greatest pressure drop) in arterial circulation is across small arteries and arterioles; the flow changes from pulsatile to continuous while passing through arterioles; the greatest total cross-sectional area is at the level of the capillaries and this causes the blood velocity to slow considerably at this level; slow flow + thin walled vessels = ideal conditions for transfer of substances between blood and tissues.
- The total cross-sectional area and the number of vessels decreases on passing from the venules to small veins to large veins and therefore increases velocity
- The majority of the blood volume of the systemic circulation is in the venous vessels

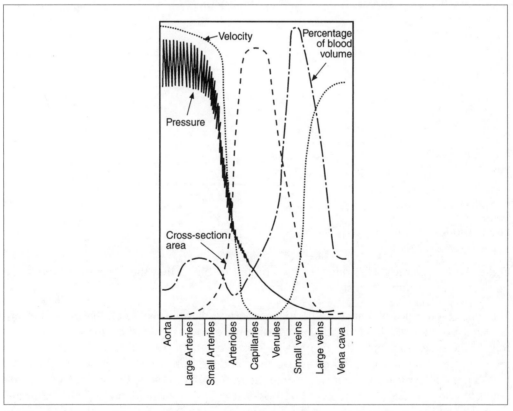

Pressure, velocity of flow, cross-sectional area and capacity of the blood vessels of the systemic circulation

2.2 Physiology of heart muscle function and Starling's law

Cardiac muscle cells (like skeletal muscle cells) are made up of **sarcomeres**. Sarcomeres contain thick filaments (**myosin**) and thin filaments (**actin**).

The filaments slide over each other (expending energy) and so shorten the sarcomere (and therefore shortening of several sarcomeres is the mechanism by which the muscle cell contracts). The force that the muscle sarcomere can exert is in part dependent on the sarcomere length, which, in turn, is a reflection of the degree of overlap of the thick and thin filaments.

- When the sarcomere is very short, the high degree of overlap interferes with contraction, and the force is therefore reduced
- When the sarcomere is very long, the relative lack of overlap means that less force can be exerted in between these two extremes
- A length of sarcomere exists where the overlap is high enough to produce maximum force, but not so high as to interfere with force production

This has implications for the force that the heart can exert to pump blood (known as the Frank–Starling mechanism or 'Starling's law of the heart').

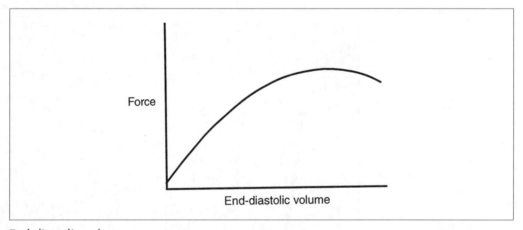

End-diastolic volume

End-diastolic volume (EDV) refers to the amount of blood that the ventricle of the heart holds at its maximum, i.e. just before it contracts.

The more blood in the heart (i.e. the higher the end-diastolic volume), the more the sarcomeres are stretched. Up to a point, increasing the amount of blood (by increasing venous return) increases the force the heart muscle can exert. Beyond a critical point, further increasing the amount of blood decreases the force the heart muscle can exert. Clinically EDV is difficult to measure but it can be inferred from CVP or Wedge Pressures. CVP is analogous to end-diastolic pressure of the right ventricle, which is analogous to EDV, assuming normal compliance and valve function. On the Starling curve force is analogous to measured values of Cardiac Output or Stroke Volume.

Functionally, the heart acts as a **syncytium** (a single multi-nucleated cell formed from a number of fused cells (although this is not anatomically the case). This means that when one part of the heart depolarises, the wave of depolarisation passes throughout the entire heart muscle.

The heart has a large number of **mitochondria**. This means that energy for heart muscle function can be continuously generated via aerobic metabolism.

Heart muscle contraction relies heavily on optimal concentrations of calcium, potassium, and sodium.

Excitation-contraction coupling – the mechanism by which the action potential causes the myofibrils of muscle to contract. Heart muscle differs from skeletal muscle. Therefore, in addition to the release of Ca^{2+} ions into the sarcoplasm, large quantities of extra Ca^{2+} ions also diffuse into the tubules (tubules of cardiac muscle have a **diameter five times larger** than skeletal muscle with **twenty-five times** the volume).

Free intracellular calcium ions are the most important factor in regulating the contractility of the myocardium.

- **Increased intracellular calcium will increase the force of myocardial contraction**
- **Decreased intracellular calcium will decrease the force of myocardial contraction**

Many drugs that increase cardiac muscle contractile force involve increasing intracellular calcium.

2.3 Pressure, flow and volume changes in the heart

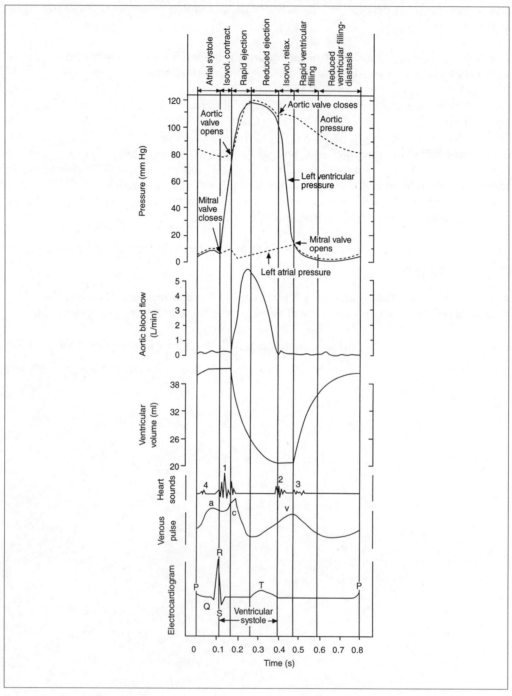

Events in the cardiac cycle

Main features

When left atrial pressure (LAP) is >left ventricular pressure (LVP), the left ventricle fills.

Period of rapid filling:

- First 1/3: diastolic rapid filling
- Second 1/3: slow filling directly from venous system though atria
- Final 1/3: atrial contraction (responsible for 25% filling)

In fast atrial fibrillation, ventricular filling and cardiac output is compromised particularly on induction of anaesthesia, hence every effort must be made to reduce the rate to <100 prior to surgery.

When the left ventricle contracts, left ventricular pressure rises:

- When LVP >LAP, mitral valve closes
- When LVP >aortic pressure, aortic valve opens, allowing blood to flow from the ventricle to the aorta

When ventricle is relatively empty, and relaxing, LVP falls:

- When LVP <aortic pressure, aortic valve closes
- When LAP >LVP (again), left ventricle fills, and the cycle begins again

Normal values for aortic and intracardiac pressures

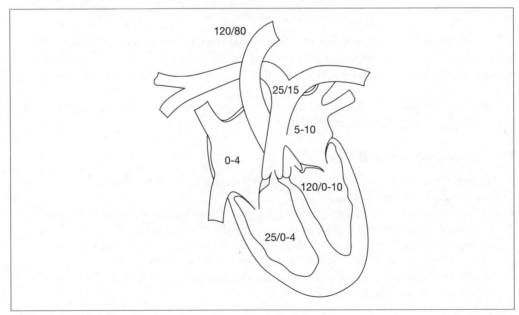

Cardiac catheter measurements (as mmHg)

2.4 Electrocardiography and cardiac conduction

All heart muscle cells can depolarise, but the shape of the action potential varies between cells.

Cells of the Sinoatrial (SA) and Atrioventricular (AV) nodes, as well as the cells of the Purkinje conducting system have the ability to depolarise themselves (*self-excitation*: a process causing automatic rhythmical contraction) at regular intervals, thereby initiating a wave of depolarisation which passes throughout the heart.

This slow spontaneous depolarisation of the membrane potential is due to slow inward calcium conductance. Repolarisation occurs following increased potassium conductance when the calcium channels close.

This ability is referred to as **automaticity** (pacemaking ability) and is due to the unusual shape of the action potential.

The cells of the SA node have the highest frequency of self-depolarisation, followed by the cells of the AV node, with the Purkinje system cells having the lowest frequency. The ventricular rate is around 40 bpm.

These cells have a long **refractory period** (a period following depolarisation during which any further depolarisation cannot take place). This means that the cells with the highest frequency of firing (the SA node) will therefore control the rate at which the entire heart depolarises (and hence controls the rate at which the heart beats). It follows that a denervated heart will continue to beat (e.g. this is seen after heart transplantation). Transplanted hearts increase rate via circulating adrenaline, but atropine (vagal block) has no effect on heart rate.

If the SA node cells fail to function, the cells with the next highest frequency (those in the AV node) will take over the pacemaking function of the heart. The SA node is normally slowed physiologically by vagal activity and accelerated by sympathetic hormones and innervation.

Conduction through the heart can be disturbed by disease processes (e.g. ischaemia, infarction) or by drugs (e.g. digoxin, adenosine).

The electrocardiogram (ECG)

- Records the sum of the electrical impulses generated by the heart during depolarisation and contraction
- Provides information on the rate and rhythm of heart contraction, as well as information on pathological processes (e.g. infarction, inflammation)
- A standard ECG consists of 12 'leads'; these are best thought of as extensions of the direction of electrical flow from the heart, which can be measured. A positive deflection on the ECG (upwards) shows that depolarisation is conducted towards that electrode and vice versa.

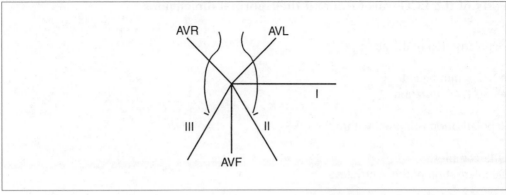

12–Lead ECG

6 V leads look at the heart in a horizontal plane from the front and left side

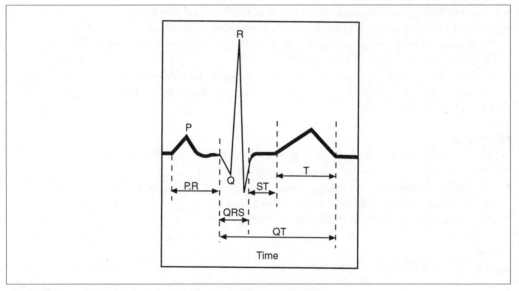

The important deflections and intervals of a typical ECG

The waveform produced by one (normal) heart contraction is shown. Different parts of the waveform have their own name and are related to different physiological actions occurring within the heart.

Parts of the ECG waveform and their normal dimensions

P wave

Depolarisation of the atria:

- <2.5 mm height
- >0.1 sec duration

Repolarisation is hidden within the QRS.

QRS complex

Depolarisation of the ventricles:

- If first deflection is downwards, is called a **Q wave**
- The first upward deflection (whether preceded by a Q wave or not) is called the **R wave**, and usually has increasing amplitude from V1 to V6
- The first downward deflection after the R wave is called the **S wave**
- The QRS should be <0.10 sec (three small squares) in duration
  An S wave in lead I suggests right axis deviation, an S wave in II suggests left axis deviation. Normal Axis is –30 to +90.
  A wide QRS (greater than 0.12) occurs when depolarisation does not pass down the Purkinje fibres as in bundle branch block and complexes of ventricular origin (ectopics and Third Degree Block).

PR interval

Represents the (normal) conduction delay between the atria and the ventricles.

- Should be between three and five small squares (0.12–0.20 sec)
  Greater than 0.2 seconds shows first degree block.
  A variable PR occurs in second degree blocks.

T wave

Represents repolarisation of the ventricles.

ST segment

The line between the S wave and the T wave.

- Usually isoelectric, i.e. level with the baseline of the ECG
- May be elevated acutely when myocardial infarction is present
- May be depressed when myocardial ischaemia is present

NB. May be normal, despite presence of either infarction or ischaemia.

Rhythm recognition

1. Rate	>100 Tachycardia	
	<60 Bradycardia	
2. QRS width	<0.12 secs Narrow complex (supraventricular origin)	
	>0.12 secs Broad complex	
3. Irregular	Regularly irregular	Ectopics
		Second-degree block
	Irregularly irregular	Atrial fibrillation
4. P wave activity	Absent in AF, Flutter, nodal, VT	
5. P relations to QRS	Not in ventricular ectopics or complete heart block	

2.5 Coronary circulation

The most important determinant of coronary blood flow and myocardial perfusion is aortic pressure. However, during systole, ventricular contraction causes compression of the coronary vessels, reducing or even briefly reversing the flow of blood to the myocardium. Most of the perfusion to the left ventricle therefore occurs in diastole, and so the diastolic aortic pressure is also important in coronary perfusion. The diastolic time is also important, hence at fast rates inadequate myocardial perfusion occurs. The direction of flow is from the outer surface inwards, therefore the sub-endocardial region is vulnerable to ischaemia.

Normally, autoregulation of coronary blood flow occurs by changes in the calibre of the coronary resistance vessels; this is in response to changes in myocardial activity and metabolic demand. It is thought to be mediated by the release of vasodilator metabolites. The coronary arteries are 'end-arteries' thus occlusion will lead to ischaemia or infarction of the myocardium.

If, however, there is a slowly developing partial occlusion (e.g. due to atherosclerosis) a collateral circulation can develop to a degree, but this can never compensate for reduced flow through 'main' vessels.

2.6 Cardiovascular variables and definitions

CARDIOVASCULAR VARIABLES*

Some variables such as CO, SV, and left ventricular stroke work are indexed to body surface area (BSA) to make different sized patients comparable.

Variables	Definition
Heart rate [60–80 beats/min]	Number of heart beats per minute
Blood pressure	Pressure in the arteries during blood flow
Systolic [100–120 mmHg]	Highest pressure recorded (peak systolic)
Diastolic [60–90 mmHg]	Lowest pressure recorded (diastolic)
Pulse pressure [40 mmHg]	Difference between the systolic and the diastolic
Mean pressure (MAP) [70 mmHg]	Calculated as approximately diastolic pressure + 1/3 of pulse pressure
Central venous pressure (CVP) [2–8 mmHg]	Pressure in the central venous system (e.g. superior or inferior vena cava) Equivalent to Right Atrial Pressure (RAP)
Stroke volume [60–130 ml] SV	Volume of blood ejected by the heart with each contraction CO/HR
Stroke volume index [41–51]	Indexed stroke volume CI/HR = SVI
Cardiac output [5 L/min] CO	Volume of blood ejected by the heart in one minute (= heart rate × stroke volume)
Cardiac Index [2.5–4.0] CI	CO/BSA
Systemic Vascular Resistance (SVR) [770–1500 dyne.sec.cm^{-5}]	Resistance to flow of blood through the systemic circulation $$= \frac{MAP - CVP}{CO \times 80} \qquad [80 = \text{correction factor}]$$
Pulmonary Artery Pressure(PAP) [25/15 mmHg]	Pressure in PA
Pulmonary Artery Occlusion pressure (PAOP) [10mmHg]	Wedge pressure, analogous to LA pressure
Left Atrial Pressure (LAP)	Preload of left atrium, indirectly inferred from PAOP
Left Ventricular Stroke Work Index	LVSWI [44–68 g-m/m^2] Measurement of ventricular performance. Increased in hypertension, decreased in shock, failure, aortic stenosis. Stroke work (g) = SVI × (MAP-PAOP) × 0.0136
Right Ventricular SWI [4–8g-m/m^2]	SVI × (MPAP-RAP) × 0.0136

*Normal values for adults are shown in square brackets [ ].

NB. Blood flow is essential to organs. Cardiac output is difficult to measure. Blood pressure is easy to measure. However, blood flow from the heart to the systemic circulation (cardiac output) may be impaired (e.g. due to myocardial dysfunction, or hypovolaemia), but blood pressure may change very little. This is because vasoconstriction (increased SVR) will occur in vessels to 'non-vital' organs and in the venous system, in order to maintain blood pressure and flow to more vital organs (heart, brain). It is therefore important to remember that circulating volume may have been lost (e.g. post-op or after trauma) without the blood pressure changing very much. This is discussed in more detail in Chapter 3, *Trauma*.

2.7 Regulation of cardiac output

Regulation of heart rate

As described earlier, the heart SA node has its own intrinsic rate (100 beats/min). This rate is influenced by the autonomic nervous system.

Sympathetic nerve fibres (from C8 to T5) cause noradrenaline release at nerve endings, which acts on cardiac beta-receptors, increasing heart rate and force. **Parasympathetic** nerve fibres (in vagus nerves) cause acetylcholine release at nerve endings, acting on muscarinic receptors, causing a slowing of heart rate.

Parasympathetic control predominates (therefore causing 'normal' heart rate to be 60–80, despite intrinsic rate of 100 beats/min).

Autoregulation reflexes:

- Baroreceptor reflexes
- Respiratory reflexes
- Bainbridge reflexes

Regulation of stroke volume

Preload
End-diastolic ventricular wall tension (initial fibre stretch as in **Starling's law**). This is a description of the volume of blood available to fill the heart during diastole. Preload is dependent upon

- Venous filling time
- Diastolic filling time
- Atrial systole (i.e. in fibrillation)
- Myocardial/pericardial distensibility (compliance)

As preload increases, so does the force of contraction up to a certain point, after which increased preload causes a *decrease* in the force of contraction.
Measured by CVP or PAOP.

Contractility
Force of myocardial contraction, determines CO, SV and myocardial O_2 demand.

Increased by

- Preload
- Nerves: sympathetic stimulation increases contractility as well as heart rate
- Hormones (the following all increase contractility): adrenaline, thyroxine, glucagon
- Drugs (i.e. inotropic)

The following all decrease contractility:

- Hypoxia
- Ischaemia and cardiac disease
- Acidosis and alkalosis
- Parasympathetic stimulation mainly by suppressing the SA node
- Electrolyte imbalance K, Ca
- Reduced filling (Starling's law)
- Drugs (i.e. anaesthetics)

Measured indirectly via;

- Stroke volume and CO
- Ejection fraction (echocardiography) [70%]

Afterload
Ventricular wall tension required to eject stroke volume in systole.

Increased by:

- Aortic stenosis
- Raised SVR as in shock
- Increased ventricular volume (greater tension to contract, Laplace Law)
- Increased afterload increases cardiac work and oxygen consumption

Decreased by:

- Vasodilator drugs
- Vasodilator mediators as in septic shock

2.8 Shock syndromes

Shock is defined as inadequate tissue perfusion and oxygenation.

Types of shock include:

- Hypovolaemic   See Trauma chapter 3
- Septic   See section 11.4
- Cardiogenic   Infarction or negative inotropes
- Anaphylactic   Vasodilatory and cardiac suppressing mediators
- Obstructive   Tamponade and tension pneumothorax
- Neurogenic   Vasodilatation, sympathetic innervation blocked

Early signs include tachycardia, decreased urine output and tachypnoea. Blood pressure may be maintained due to vasoconstriction, but as shock decompensates the BP will fall.

Monitored variables in types of shock

	HR	CVP/PAOP	CO	SV	SVR
Hypovolaemic	↑	↓	↓	↓	↑
Cardiogenic	↑	↑	↓	↓	↑
Septic	↑	↓ →	↑	↓	↓
Tamponade	↑	↑ ↑	↓	↓	↑
Neurogenic	↓	–	↓	–	↓

2.9 Cardiovascular monitoring

Clinical

The most important for the majority of patients are:

- Pulse
- Pulse character   Palpable radial pulse suggests BP of >90 mmHg
- Capillary refill time   Compress 5 secs, usually <2 secs
- Skin temperature   Warm or cold
- Skin colour
- Respiratory rate   Increased
- Urine output   (0.5 ml/kg minimum, aim 1 ml/kg)
- Mental state   Anxiety, aggression, obtunded, coma

Adjuncts

Blood pressure, cuff width should be 40% of circumference of limb. Systolic becomes inaccurate in shock, but MAP measured with automated devices is reliable.

ECG, 3 lead. Lead II is best as p wave optimal for rhythm assessment and easier to see ischaemia.

Pulse oximetry, measures oxygen saturation by absorption of light wavelengths in fingertip. Demonstrates heart rate, perfusion and arterial Hb saturation. Normal around 97%, below 90% risk of severe hypoxaemia as steep part of oxygen dissociation curve. Inaccurate when cold peripheries, severe shock, nail varnish and carbon monoxide poisoning.

Invasive

CVP monitoring
(See Chapter 2, *Peri-operative management 2*, for insertion of CVP lines and complications.)

Uses of central venous cannulation in the ICU include:

- Monitoring; CVP, passage of PA catheter
- Infusion of drugs; multilumen catheters usually used
- Haemofiltration; 8.5F double lumen

- Parenteral feeding; tunnelled lines are best to reduce sepsis
- Fluid challenge; assess the response to a bolus of fluid (e.g. 250 ml)

Fluid challenge

The CVP is more useful as a trend in response to the rapid administration of 250 ml of colloid rather than as an absolute number. The fluid challenge assesses the compliance of the vascular system. The end point is return of normal BP and urine output or a filled vascular system. Overfilling with poor BP usually requires inotropic or vasopressor support.

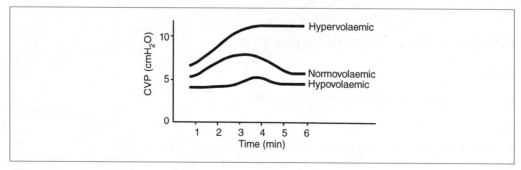

Changes in CVP in response to an IV fluid bolus

CVP lines are NOT normally used for initial resuscitation (e.g. in trauma) as placement of the line takes time, has complications and fluid infusion through the line is slow compared to a big peripheral cannula. However a large bore, short cannula inserted centrally such as a 12 or 14G or a 8.5Fr Swan introducer catheter allows very rapid infusion.

Infection control

Risk of infection least with subclavian, then internal jugular, and finally femoral. There is no evidence for routine changes of lines within 30 days unless there are local signs of infection. If systemic sepsis, then blood cultures should be taken from both the line and peripherally, if positive then remove line. PA catheters should be removed after 5 days. Peripheral lines after 72 hrs.

Transducer systems

CVP can be measured using a manometer but electromechanical transducer systems are easier and more accurate and allow continuous measurement. They convert the mechanical energy of a pressure into an electrical signal by the changing of the capacitance or resistance through a flexible conductor.

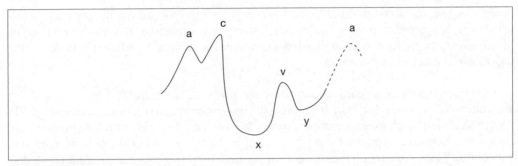

CVP waveform

a. Atrial systole		AV valve open
c. Contraction of ventricle	Carotid pulse	AV valve closed
v. Filling of atria		AV valve closed
x. Ventricles relax		AV valve closed
y. AV valve opens		

The CVP waveform swings with respiration. Inspiration dips if spontaneous breathing and increases if ventilated, and vice versa.

Pulmonary artery catheter ('Swan–Ganz catheter')

Generally, CVP (the preload of the right side of the heart) also fairly accurately reflects the preload of the left side of the heart. There are some situations where the CVP does not accurately reflect the left-sided filling pressures (e.g. pulmonary hypertension, right ventricular infarction, tricuspid valve disease).

In this situation, it is necessary to measure left atrial pressure. This is done by passing a pulmonary artery flotation catheter (a catheter with an air filled balloon near the end) into a central vein and feeding it in (guided by the characteristic pressure waveforms of different parts of the central circulation) until it is 'wedged' in a distal branch of the pulmonary artery.

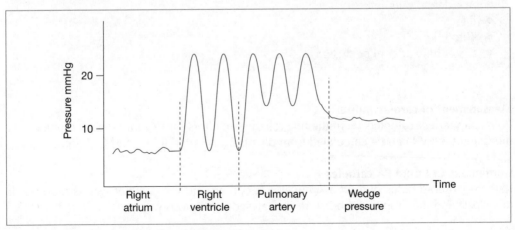

Pressure waves as catheter is passed through the heart.

When wedged, the pressure distal to the balloon is a close reflection of the pressure in the left atrium. This pressure reading (pulmonary artery wedge pressure, PAWP) can be used in the same way as the CVP to guide fluid replacement. The balloon is deflated between readings to avoid pulmonary infarction.

It can be used to measure cardiac output by the thermodilution method (Fick's principle) and, once this is known, it can be used with other cardiovascular measurements (CVP, PAWP, MAP, PAP (pulmonary artery pressure)) to calculate the SVR, PVR (pulmonary vascular resistance) and ventricle stroke work. A bolus (10 ml) of cold dextrose is injected and a thermistor at the catheter tip measures a temperature drop proportional to CO. Knowledge of the cardiac output and SVR is sometimes useful in helping to determine if a critically ill patient who is in shock has a myocardial, hypovolaemic or septic (vasodilatory) cause, and for guiding inotrope therapy. Other measurements include oxygen delivery and consumption (see section 5.3).

Fick's principle (classically using oxygen consumption VO_2)
$$CO = VO_2/CaO_2 - CvO_2$$

$$\text{Organ blood flow/time} = \frac{\text{Amount of marker substance taken up by organ/t}}{\text{Concentration difference between supply and drainage}}$$

Arterial line
A 20 G cannula within an artery (usually radial) allows optimal *continuous* measurement of arterial blood pressure. Also useful if multiple blood gas measurements are needed. Allen's test to assess collateral flow in the ulnar artery is unreliable.

Complications of insertion

- Haemorrhage/haematoma
- Ischaemia
- Aneurysm/AV fistula
- Accidental drug injection
- Infection
- Thrombosis
- Distal limb arterial occlusion

Measurement of cardiac output
Pulmonary artery catheters were the first reliable monitors for CO in the ICU. Once CO is measured the SVR can be calculated from data from an arterial line and CVP lines.

Continuous CO from PA catheter
Rather than cold bolus of fluid as indicator, a coil around the catheter warms blood as it flows past and the drop in temperature is analysed continuously.

PiCCO

Thermodilution from cold fluid injected via CVP line and analysed via a modified arterial line containing a thermistor. By a double indicator method it shows continuous CO, intrathoracic blood volume and pulmonary extravascular lung water. From the latter two values the requirement for fluids or inotropes can be judged.

Lithium dilution and pulse contour analysis

Similar to Fick's principle technique using small doses of lithium as the indicator with a lithium electrode attached to an arterial line. This calibrates the software, which calculates continuous cardiac output by pulse wave analysis.

Echo Doppler

Measures blood flow in the aorta via an oesophageal probe, hence gives indication of contractility and cardiac output. Patients need to have a patent oesophagus and be sedated to use this technique. From the Doppler waveform CO and contractility can be deduced.

Echocardiography

By visualization of the ventricle by a trained operator shows filling, myocardial wall motion and ejection fraction (EF). EF is normally 50–70%. May be used trans-thoracic or oesophageal.

2.10 Cardiovascular support

The principles of cardiovascular support in circulatory failure follow the VIP rule:

- Ventilate
- Infuse
- Pump

Ventilate

- ABC rule of resuscitation
- Improve oxygenation and gas exchange
- Reduce oxygen demand to respiratory muscles, up to 30% of cardiac output
- Control acidosis by CO_2 control

Infuse

- Always ensure adequate filling prior to vasoactive support (Starling)
- Fluid challenge using invasive monitoring
- Use of colloids as tighter dose response relationship

Pump

- First priority is to restore perfusion pressure, second to optimise cardiac output
- Blood pressure
- Aim MAP >60 or SBP >90 mmHg. (Elderly often require higher pressure)
- An adequate pressure should maintain urine flow

- If SVR is low then vasopressor such as noradrenaline is indicated to improve perfusion pressure
- Vasoconstriction may mask hypovolaemia, therefore closely monitor filling pressures and CO
- Cardiac output
- Sufficient organ blood flow
- Dobutamine in low output states increases CO. Risk of tachycardia in high dosage due to vasodilatation. If BP drops consider further fluid
- Adrenaline is sometimes used as acts as vasopressor and inotrope
- Monitor effect via DO_2, lactate, pHi, urine output, CO

Maximising blood flow to organs

Renal and mesenteric blood flow is increased by dopexamine infusion at rate of 0.5 to 1 microgram/kg/min. No evidence for prevention of renal failure.

Drugs

Inotropes	Increase force of ventricular contraction, usually beta effect
Lusiotropes	Enhance myocardial relaxation
Vasopressor	Vasoconstricts blood vessels, alpha effect
Vasodilator	Vasodilates blood vessels, arterial, venous or both
Chronotrope	Increase heart rate. Beta effect.

Usually infused in micrograms/kg/min. Dose ranges and individual effects are unpredictable in the critically ill patient.

Adrenaline: Inotrope, vasopressor, chronotrope. Activates beta-receptors increasing intracellular cAMP. Low dose beta effects mostly, becoming more alpha at high dose. Beta 2 effects cause vasodilatation in skeletal muscle beds lowering SVR.

Dobutamine: Inotrope, vasodilator. Synthetic. Predominant beta 1 effect increasing heart rate and force of contraction, hence cardiac output. Mild beta 2 and alpha effects overall causing vasodilatation.

Dopamine: Up to 5 μg/kg/min has dopamine receptor activity causing renal dilatation. Between 5 and 10 μg has mostly beta inotropic effect. Above 15 μg has mostly alpha vasoconstrictive effect. Unpredictable ranges in different patients.

Problems with dopamine include
- Gut ischaemia
- Growth hormone suppression, immunosuppression

Dopexamine: Mesenteric and renal vasodilatation via dopamine receptors, and also has beta 2 effects. Synthetic. Anti-inflammatory effect. May protect the gut against ischaemia in the presence of vasoconstrictors. Used at dose 0.5–0.9 μg/kg/min for mesenteric protection.

Noradrenaline: Vasopressor effect predominates, mild inotropic beta 1. Increases SVR to improve perfusion pressure but may suppress organ and skin perfusion due to capillary vasoconstriction. Used to increase perfusion pressure in septic shock.

Isoprenaline: Chronotrope used to increase heart rate in heart block while awaiting pacing. Beta 1 and beta 2 effects.

Phosphodiesterase inhibitors: Milrinone, Enoximone. Increase intracellular cAMP by decreasing its breakdown. Increase inotropic and vasodilatation, (inodilator and lusiotropic). Increased CO, lowered PAOP and SVR, but no significant rise in HR or myocardial oxygen consumption

Vasodilators
Hydralazine, mostly arterial vasodilatation, to control BP
Nitroprusside, arterial vasodilator with short half-life given as infusion
Nitrates, venodilators reducing pre-load

Fluids – the crystalloid colloid controversy
Crystalloids

- Salt ions in water. Volume infused, about one-third stays intravascular and two-thirds pass to ECF, hence risk of tissue oedema.
- E.g. normal saline, Hartmann's solution
- Advantage in that ECF fluid deficit in shock is replaced

Colloids

- Contain osmotically active particles in solution. Expand plasma volume by volume infused.
- May leak into interstitium in capillary leak syndrome.
- E.g. Gelofusine, Haemaccel. Gelatine based, half-life about 4 hours.
- Dextrans. Degraded dextrose. Interfere with cross-matching.
- Starches. Long half-life in some cases. 10% solutions hyperoncotic hence increase plasma volume more than volume infused. Some may have benefit in reducing capillary leak syndrome.
- Albumin. Pasteurised. Suppresses albumin synthesis. Normally some albumin leaks through the capillary membrane.
- Blood. Plasma reduced has haematocrit of about 70%.

A combination of crystalloids and colloids is probably the best approach.

Volume expanding fluids should be considered in separation to maintenance fluids.

Maintenance fluids

- Daily water requirement is 2–3 litres
- Daily sodium requirement is approximately 80 mmol day
- Daily potassium requirement is approximately 60–80 mmol
- Options for basic requirements include:
  - 3 litres of dextrose saline. 30 mmol sodium per litre hence total 90 mmol.
  - 2 litres of dextrose 5% with 500 ml of normal saline (150 mmol/l) hence 75 mmol.

Dextrose containing fluids are not useful for volume replacement as they only replace water which as the sugar is metabolised redistribute to intracellular and extracellular compartments. The dextrose allows water to be isotonic for IV infusion.

Potassium is replaced at a maximum of 20 mmol per hour in a monitored ICU environment. In hypokalaemic patients this reflects a large total intracellular deficit.

Magnesium replacement should be considered in this situation with the aim of a serum level of 1 mmol/l.

2.11 Cardiopulmonary bypass

Bypass is established prior to open-heart surgery and replaces the pumping of the heart and gas exchange of the lungs by a machine. Usually used for coronary bypass grafting (CABG) but new techniques for selected patients are available such as the use of suction retractors, which immobilises the myocardium around coronary arteries (Octopus).

Prior to establishing bypass full anticoagulation is required with 3 mg/kg heparin confirmed by regular ACT (activated clotting time) measurements. 1 mg heparin = 100u.

Bypass is established via placement of two catheters

● Venous – inserted into right atrium or femoral vein
● Arterial – inserted into ascending aorta or femoral artery

Parts of the bypass circuit
Venous blood drains into a **reservoir** primed with anticoagulated crystalloid.
Filter to remove bubbles and particles
Heat exchanger to cool or warm as appropriate. Blood is cooled during surgery to reduce tissue oxygen extraction. The blood is warmed when coming off bypass back to normal. However, afterdrop occurs due to delay in warming cold peripheries.
Pump Vortex or roller pump, provides non-pulsatile blood flow at rate of approximately 1.5–3.0 l/m^2. A mean blood pressure of 40 to 60 mmHg is achieved by the appropriate use of vasopressors and dilators.
Oxygenator either membrane (commonest) or bubble. Very efficient at removing CO_2, therefore CO_2 may need to be added.

During bypass the ventilator is stopped.

Anaesthesia during bypass is maintained via a volatile ether agent via the oxygenator or with an intravenous infusion.

During bypass the heart may need to be stopped. There are two methods.

● **Fibrillation** by AC current and reversed by direct DC shock via spoon paddles.
● **Cardioplegia**, an ice-cold solution including potassium and procaine, reversed by redistribution and warming.

Complications

- Anticoagulation. Heparin reversed with protamine sulphate 1mg:1mg heparin. Rapid injection may cause hypotension.
- Temperature. Hypothermia beneficial to myocardial oxygen consumption but post-op afterdrop can cause arrhythmias, fluctuations in peripheral resistance and awareness on rewarming.
- Prolonged bypass and complex surgery
- Poor ventricular function on coming off bypass may require inotropic agents
- Neurological. Confusion or stroke due to microaggregates, bubbles or hypocapnea.

Postoperative management

- Ventilation and continued rewarming on an ICU. Optimisation of analgesia with systemic opiates. Continued invasive monitoring to optimise cardiac function. Aim for Hb of 10 to 12 g/dl, normal acid base and urine output.
- Extubation is usually achieved within a few hours, after which facemask oxygen and physiotherapy is continued for a few days.

Postoperative complications

- Hypertension
- Acute bleeding, with tamponade due to bleeding point. Requires return to theatre and opening of sternotomy. For dilutional haemorrhage or DIC coagulation factors will be required.
- Renal impairment. Inadequate perfusion or haemolysis
- Pulmonary impairment. Excess fluid load, pneumothorax, manipulation of lungs or sternotomy pain.

ECMO, ECCO$_2$R

When lungs are so badly damaged that they cannot be adequately ventilated then in specialised centres Extra-Corporeal Membrane Oxygenation or Extra-Corporeal CO_2 Removal can be initiated. These devices are essentially cardiac bypass circuits and take over respiration while the lungs hopefully heal. There is evidence for benefit in paediatric patients but equivocal in adults.

2.12 Cardiopulmonary resuscitation

International guidelines are produced by the European Resuscitation Council and updated every few years. For latest guidelines liaise with your local Resuscitation Officer and obtain practical training. All hospital clinical staff must be proficient in basic life support (BLS).

Cardiac arrest is defined as absence of a palpable pulse. It is classified as shockable and non-shockable.

Shockable:	Ventricular fibrillation VF and pulseless ventricular tachycardia VT
Non-shockable:	Asystole, no electrical activity
	Pulseless electrical activity, (PEA), ECG rhythm compatible with a pulse but pulse is absent.

The commonest out of hospital cardiac arrest is VF due to ischaemic heart disease and myocardial infarction. This rhythm is treatable by defibrillation as rapidly as possible which stops the arrhythmia, puts the patient into asystole and hopefully a perfusing sinus rhythm ensues. The chance of recovery decreases rapidly in minutes.

The commonest in-hospital arrests are mostly asystole and PEA caused by continued cardio-respiratory deterioration. Recognition of the sick patient and early instigation of organ support such as oxygen, ventilatory and circulatory management can prevent arrest and death.

Main causes of cardiac arrest are the following (4H's and 4T's)

- Hypoxia
- Hypovolaemia
- Hypothermia
- Hypokalaemia, hyperkalaemia, hypocalcaemia

- Tension pneumothorax
- Tamponade
- Thromboembolism
- Toxicity

Important points in Advanced Life Support

Continue chest compressions at rate 100/min. Ratio of 15 compressions to 2 ventilations in single and two rescuer CPR. If intubated, chest compressions should be continuous.
Check pulse and give adrenaline 1 mg every 3 minutes if no pulse present to cause peripheral vasoconstriction to improve coronary and cerebral perfusion.
Intubate to improve oxygenation and prevent aspiration
Monitor ECG and defibrillate if VF or VT
During CPR check through 4H's and 4T's and treat as appropriate

Return of spontaneous circulation (ROSC); ventilate if required, 12 lead ECG, CXR, blood gases, U&Es and FBC. ICU support.

3. RESPIRATORY ANATOMY

3.1 Bony thorax

Sternum

This consists of three parts:

- **Manubrium**: jugular notch (upper concave margin); articulates with the clavicles, 1st costal cartilages and upper halves of 2nd costal cartilages; 1st costal cartilage joint is a primary cartilaginous joint (not synovial)
- **Body**: upper border is the manubriosternal symphysis, which is bridged by the 2nd costal cartilage; each lateral border has 5½ facets for articulation with costal cartilages 2–7
- **Xiphoid process**: posterior attachment of diaphragm; anterior attachment of rectus abdominus

Ribs

- **Head**: two facets for articulation with the two adjacent thoracic vertebrae (thoracic vertebra of the same number + the one above). (NB. The 1st rib's head has just one facet for articulation with T1 only.)
- **Neck**: tubercle – one facet for articulation with transverse process of vertebra; body – continues anteriorly as the costal cartilage

Costal cartilages

- 1–7 articulate directly with the sternum
- 8, 9 and 10 run into one another and then into 7
- 11 and 12 float free

3.2 Intercostal spaces

There are three muscle layers (as with the abdomen):

- **Outer**: external intercostal muscles (+ serratus posterior muscles and levator costae)
- **Middle**: internal intercostal muscles
- **Inner**: innermost intercostal muscles (+ transversus thoracis and subcostal muscles)

External intercostals

- Run obliquely downwards and forwards
- Replaced by the anterior intercostal membrane anteriorly

Internal intercostals

- Run downwards and backwards
- Complete anteriorly but replaced posteriorly by the posterior intercostal membrane

Innermost intercostals

- Cross more than one intercostal space
- Innermost layer includes transversus thoracis and subcostal muscles

Neurovascular bundle

- Between internal intercostals and innermost intercostals
- Under protection of the *lower* border of the ribs, hence drains or needles should always be sited *above* a rib

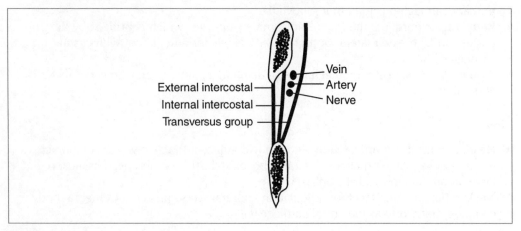

Vertical section through an intercostal space

Intercostal nerves

Derived from ventral primary rami of spinal nerves T1 to T11.

There are three branches:

- **Collateral** branch
- **Lateral cutaneous** branch – anterior and posterior branches
- **Anterior cutaneous** branch

NB. Skin above the 2nd rib is supplied by supraclavicular branches of cervical plexus, not by 1st intercostal nerve.

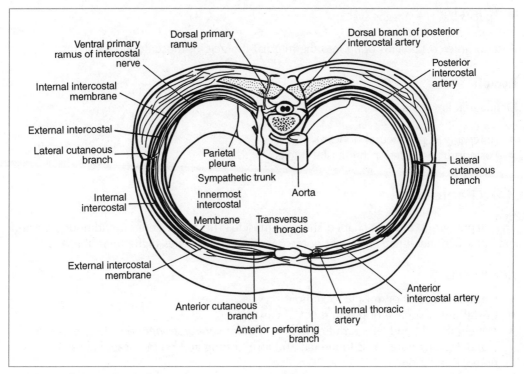

Contents of an intercostal space

Intercostal arteries

Posterior intercostal arteries

- Derived from the superior intercostal artery (from 2nd part of subclavian artery) in spaces 1 and 2
- Derived directly from the descending aorta in spaces 3–11

Anterior intercostal arteries

- Derived from internal thoracic artery in spaces 1–6
- From musculophrenic artery (continuation of above) in spaces 7, 8 and 9
- Spaces 11 and 12 do not have an anterior intercostal artery

Intercostal veins
There are one posterior and two anterior veins per space.

Posterior intercostal veins drain in various different ways:

- Space 1 → supreme intercostal vein
- Spaces 2 and 3 → superior intercostal vein
- Space 4 → either superior intercostal vein or azygos system

- Spaces 5–11 → azygos system

Anterior intercostal veins drain into the internal thoracic or musculophrenic veins.

Lymph

Drainage follows the arteries:

- Anteriorly → parasternal nodes
- Posteriorly → posterior intercostal nodes

3.3 Diaphragm

The diaphragm is a dome-shaped sheet of muscle. There is a central tendinous part and muscular peripheral part. The right dome (overlies the liver) lies higher than the left.

Attachments

- **Sternal**: two slips of muscle to xiphoid process
- **Costal**: inner surface of ribs and costal cartilages 6–12
- **Vertebral**: right and left *crura* from upper lumbar vertebrae; *right crus* larger, from L1, 2 and 3; some fibres pass to the left and form a sling around the oesophagus; *left crus* from L1 and 2 only.

Medial arcuate ligament: thickening of psoas fascia
Lateral arcuate ligament: thickening of lumbar fascia

Blood supply
Intercostal arteries 7–11 and the subcostal artery supply the periphery. The main body is supplied by the right and left phrenic arteries (direct from aortic branches).

Nerve supply
It is supplied by the right and left phrenic nerves (C3, 4 and 5) and the intercostal nerves (around the periphery).

Diaphragmatic openings

There are three main openings:

- **Aortic**: T12 level – behind the diaphragm and not actually in it
- **Oesophageal**: T10 level – site of sliding hiatus hernia
- **Vena cava**: T8 level – in the central tendon

Other structures penetrating the diaphragm

- Phrenic nerves: right with the inferior vena cava, left through left dome
- Splanchnic nerves: with corresponding crus

- Sympathetic trunk: behind medial arcuate ligament
- Hemiazygos vein: left crus
- Superior epigastric vessels
- Lymph vessels

3.4 Trachea

This commences at the level of C6. It is held open by C shaped 'rings' of cartilage. Trachealis muscle fills gap in the rings.

It is divided into two parts.

Cervical

5 cm in length (but stretches during respiration).

Related structures

- Oesophagus (directly behind the trachea)
- Recurrent laryngeal nerves (in the groove between the trachea and the oesophagus)
- Carotid sheath
- Thyroid (isthmus at 2nd, 3rd and 4th tracheal rings)
- Inferior thyroid veins
- Anterior jugular veins

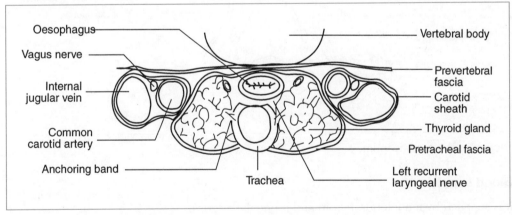

Relations of the thyroid gland

Thoracic trachea

5 cm in length (but stretches). Begins at jugular notch of manubrium. Bifurcates just below manubriosternal angle (position is dependent on respiratory cycle).

Related structures

- Oesophagus
- Vagus and recurrent laryngeal nerves
- Manubrium
- Thymus
- Brachiocephalic veins
- Brachiocephalic trunk and common carotid arteries
- Pulmonary trunk and bifurcation
- Superior vena cava
- Azygos vein
- Cardiac plexus
- Tracheobronchial lymph nodes

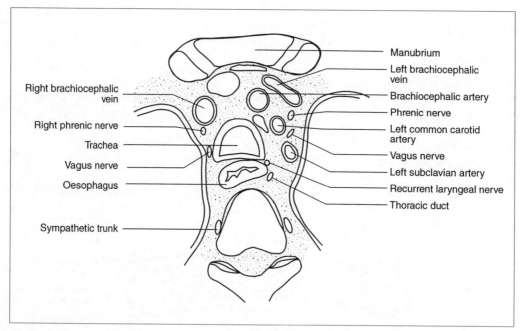

Section of the mediastinum

Blood supply

It is supplied by the inferior thyroid and bronchial arteries.

Nerve supply

The vagus and recurrent laryngeal nerves supply the mucous membrane. Parasympathetic (vagus) and sympathetic (upper ganglia of sympathetic trunk) supply the smooth muscle.

Lymph drainage

Deep cervical and paratracheal nodes.

3.5 Pleura

There are two layers separated by a small amount of fluid in a closed space. They couple the lungs and chest wall and allow the lungs to slide in the thorax during respiration.

Parietal pleura

- Outer layer covers the inside of the thoracic cavity
- Reflects around the root of the lung to be continuous with the visceral pleura

Visceral pleura

- Inner layer, firmly adherent to the surface of lungs.

Pulmonary ligament – loose fold of pleura that hangs from the lung root and allows movement during respiration.

Nerve supply

Parietal pleura

- Intercostal nerves
- Phrenic nerves

Visceral pleura

- Autonomic innervation only

3.6 Lungs

Left lung: two lobes separated by oblique fissure.
Right lung: three lobes separated by oblique and horizontal fissures.

Lung roots:

- Pulmonary artery lies superiorly
- Bronchus lies posteriorly
- Pulmonary veins lie inferiorly

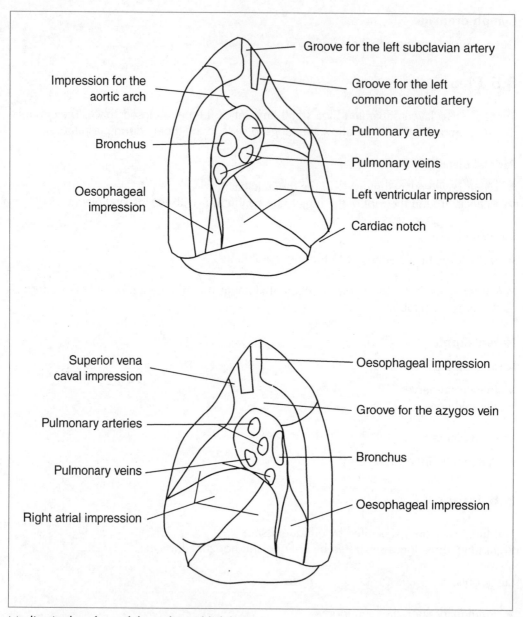

Mediastinal surface of the right and left lungs

Lobar and segmental bronchi

- Right (shorter and more vertical) and left main bronchi → lobar bronchi → segmental bronchi → bronchioles
- Each lung has 10 bronchopulmonary segments: 5 per lobe on the left and 3 (upper), 2 (middle) and 5 (lower) for right lobes
- Each branch of a bronchus is accompanied by a branch of the pulmonary artery
- Blood supply to the bronchial tree is from its own small bronchial arteries

Pulmonary plexus

- From cardiac plexus
- Lies at hilum of each lung
- Supplies lungs with sympathetic and parasympathetic innervation

3.7 Surface anatomy

Diaphragm (in full expiration): 4th intercostal space on the right – 5th rib on left.
Pleura and lungs: lung roots – costal cartilages 3 and 4 (or T5–7) at sternal edges.

Remember 2, 4, 6, 8, 10 and 12.

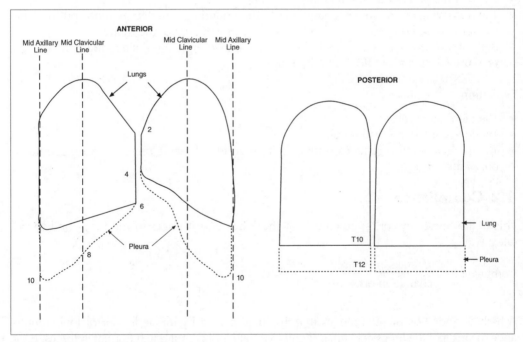

Surface anatomy of the lungs

4. MECHANICS OF BREATHING

4.1 Muscles of respiration

Inspiratory

- Diaphragm (main respiratory muscle)
- External intercostals

Accessory inspiratory muscles

- Scalenes
- Sternocleidomastoid
- Pectorals
- Latissimus dorsi

Expiratory

- Passive in quiet respiration
- Muscles of forced expiration: abdominal wall muscles; internal intercostals

Inspiration

- The diaphragm contracts, flattening its domes
- The ribs swing up in a bucket handle fashion, around their vertebral joints, pushing the sternum up and out, so increasing the cross-sectional area of the thorax
- Both of the above increase the thoracic volume leading to a reduced intrathoracic pressure causing air to flow into the lungs

Expiration

- The diaphragm relaxes
- The lungs and chest wall recoil
- The thoracic volume reduces leading to a raised intrathoracic pressure causing airflow out of the lungs

4.2 Compliance

This is the 'elasticity' or 'stretchiness' of the lungs and it refers to the lungs and/or the chest walls.

$$Compliance = \frac{change\ in\ volume}{change\ in\ pressure}$$

A high or good compliance means that the lungs are easily inflated. Poor or low compliance means that the lungs are stiff, difficult to inflate and do not reach normal volumes. Poor compliance is caused by lung disease (e.g. pulmonary fibrosis, sarcoidosis, ARDS) or by disease of the chest wall (e.g. thoracic scoliosis).

Dynamic lung compliance is visualized by flow volume loops. (See Section 6.3.)

4.3 Airway resistance

80% in upper airways.

$$Resistance = \frac{pressure}{flow}$$

(where pressure = atmospheric pressure – alveolar pressure).

- Under smooth muscle control
- Parasympathetic innervation increases smooth muscle tone and hence resistance. Thus ipratropium bromide (muscarinic antagonist) bronchodilates.
- Sympathetic innervation reduces it and sympathomimetics e.g. salbutamol
- Forced expiration increases airway resistance – due to increased intrathoracic pressure

5. CONTROL OF RESPIRATION

5.1 Outline

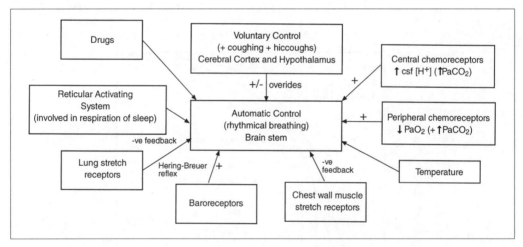

Hering–Breuer reflex = negative feedback from lung stretch receptors as the lung inflates

5.2 Chemoreceptors

Chemoreceptors

- **Central (medulla)**
  Detect changes in pH
  CO_2 crosses blood-brain barrier and dissolves in CSF releasing H^+ ions
  Receptors actually detect the increase in CSF H^+ concentration

- **Peripheral**
  Carotid bodies IX nerve
  (+ less important aortic bodies X nerve)
  Primarily detect changes in PaO_2
  Less important detector of changes in $PaCO_2$

Living at altitude means that there is a reduced inspired O_2 concentration causing:

- Initial hyperventilation
- Gradual acclimatization

5.3 Transport of oxygen

Haemoglobin

- Molecular weight 66,500 kDa
- Normal concentration 150 g/l
- Four O_2 binding haem molecules
- 1 g of haemoglobin binds 1.34 ml of O_2 when fully saturated
- O_2 saturation refers to the number of O_2-bound haem molecules expressed as a percentage of the total number available; it is measured by pulse oximetry
- Most O_2 is carried by haemoglobin
- A negligible amount of O_2 is dissolved in plasma (which gives PaO_2 value)

The relationship between O_2 saturation and PaO_2 is described by the O_2 dissociation curve.

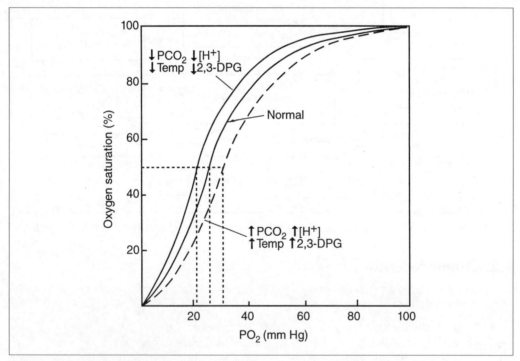

The O_2 dissociation curve

The sigmoid shape is because as each haem becomes O_2-bound it affects the O_2 binding of remaining haem molecules.

Factors that shift curve

- **To the left**
  Increased affinity for O_2
  Decreased: $PaCO_2$
  [H+]
  2,3 DPG
  Temperature decrease
  HbF, COHb

- **To the right**
  Reduced affinity for O_2
  Increased: $PaCO_2$
  [H+] (Bohr effect)
  2,3 DPG
  Temperature increase

Hb has a much greater affinity (×250) for carbon monoxide than O_2 (HbCO curve shifted far to the left). Myoglobin has only one haem molecule and its curve is again far to the left.

At the lungs, $PaCO_2$ and [H+] are low and so Hb has a high affinity for, and therefore binds, O_2. At the tissues, $PaCO_2$ and [H+] are high and therefore Hb gives up O_2 to the tissues. Anything that shifts the equilibrium curve to the left (e.g. ↓2,3 DPG, CO) will reduce the amount of O_2 given up to the tissues.

NB. Fetal Hb is not affected by 2,3 DPG and hence has a greater affinity for O_2.

5.4 Oxygen content, delivery and consumption

To calculate the content of oxygen in arterial blood the following equation is used:

$CaO_2 = (Hb \times 1.36 \times SpO2) + PaO_2 \times 0.0226$

0.0226 is ml of oxygen carried per kPa.

Using normal figures of Hb 15 g/dl, SpO_2 0.98, and PaO_2 of 13 kPa the content of oxygen can be seen to be 20 ml/dl or 200 ml/l.

The contribution carried by solution is trivial compared with carried on haemoglobin.

Global body oxygen delivery DO_2 can be calculated by:

Cardiac output × CaO_2 e.g. 5 l/min × 200 ml/l = 1000 ml/ min

Oxygen consumption can be calculated by subtracting the mixed venous content from the arterial content and multiplying the sum by cardiac output.

$(CaO_2 - CvO_2) \times CO$

CvO_2 is measured by substituting mixed venous saturations and PvO_2 into the equation for content. The values are measured directly via a blood gas analyser with blood obtained from the tip of a PA catheter. This provides true mixed venous blood. Some PA catheters have an oximeter at the tip to give continuous values.

CvO_2 is approximately 150 ml/l as SvO_2 is normally 0.75 (75%), hence Oxygen consumption is normally 250 ml/min.

It can be seen that there is more oxygen delivered than is consumed and consumption remains independent of delivery. In low delivery state and in critical illness oxygen consumption seems to become supply dependant.

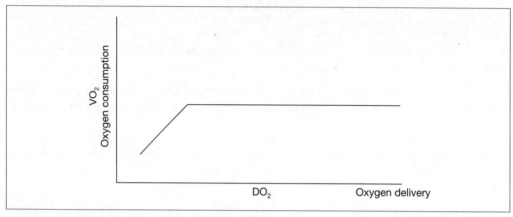

VO_2/DO_2

This was the basis for Goal Directed Therapy where DO_2, VO_2, and CI were increased to supra-normal levels with the intention of increasing VO_2. A flaw with this argument is that both equations contain common factors, which bias the result by mathematical coupling.

Goal values are:

CI >4.5 l/min per m^2
DO_2I >600 ml/min per m^2
VO_2I >168 ml/min per m^2

The results of studies showing this approach to be beneficial are countered by studies that have found deleterious effects from the high doses of inotropes and fluids required. It is likely that patients who respond to aggressive management will survive and non-responders are too ill to survive rather than a benefit of the management.

Current approaches to goal directed resuscitation are to maintain blood pressure to perfuse tissues hence urine output and correction of acidosis.

From the equation for DO_2 it can be seen that methods of increasing tissue oxygen delivery include

- Increasing cardiac output with fluids, inotropes
- Increasing SaO_2 with increased FiO_2, PEEP and other ventilatory strategies
- Increasing haemoglobin with transfusion

Optimal haemoglobin concentration in the critically ill is a compromise between oxygen carriage and perfusion. Perfusion is related to viscosity, which increases as the haematocrit increases. Usually when bleeding is not a risk then a Hb between 8 and 10 g/dl allows adequate oxygen delivery with good perfusion of narrow capillaries.

Oxygen extraction ratio (OER).

$$OER = CaO_2 - CvO_2/CaO_2 \times 100\% \; [25\%]$$

Shows adequacy of DO_2 especially in low flow states whereby the ratio increases and in septic shock the ratio decreases.

5.5 Transport of carbon dioxide

CO_2 is transported in three ways:

- Dissolved as CO_2 in plasma (10%)
- Reacts with amine side groups of deoxyHb to form carbaminohaemoglobin (30%)
- Reacts with H_2O of plasma to form $H^+ + HCO_3-$ catalysed within the red blood cells by *carbonic anhydrase* and transported as sodium bicarbonate (60%). The bicarbonate diffuses out of the red cells in exchange for chloride ions (**Chloride shift**).

Haldane effect: deoxyHb (venous) is a weaker acid than oxyHb and can hence carry more CO_2 in the carbaminoHb form.

6. LUNG FUNCTION TESTS

These tests measure for lung volumes, airway resistance and gas transfer.

6.1 Lung volumes

- A **volume** cannot be subdivided
- A **capacity** is the sum of two or more volumes
- Lung volumes vary with age/sex/height, but not weight

Spirometry

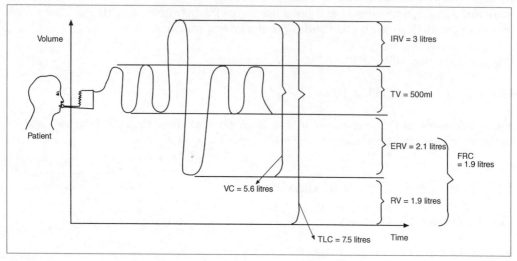

Predicted lung volumes for a 20-year-old male, height 1.8 m

Definitions

- **TV**: Tidal Volume (0.5 l) – volume of air moved in quiet respiration
- **IRV**: Inspiratory Reserve Volume (3 l) – maximum volume inspirable following TV inspiration
- **ERV**: Expiratory Reserve Volume (2.1 l) – maximum volume expirable following TV expiration
- **RV**: Residual Volume (1.9 l) – volume remaining in lungs after maximum expiration
- **FRC**: Functional Residual Capacity (1.9 l) – sum of ERV + RV – volume in which gas exchange takes place
- **VC**: Vital Capacity (5.6 l) – volume that can be expired after a maximal inspiratory effort
- **FVC**: Forced VC
- **FEV$_1$** : Volume expired in the 1st second of an FVC measurement
- **TLC**: Total Lung Capacity (6 L) – sum of VC + RV
- **PEFR**: Peak Expiratory Flow Rate – cheap and easy measure of airway resistance

All of the above except RV (and hence TLC) can be measured by spirometry. To measure RV (or TLC) requires helium dilution methods or whole body plethysmography.

NB. Above volumes are only meant as guides and relate to fit young adults.

- **Dead space**: total volume of parts of lung not taking part in gaseous exchange
  Anatomical: mouth, nose, pharynx, larynx, trachea and bronchi
  Functional: volumes of diseased parts of lung unable to perform gaseous exchange

- **Minute ventilation**: total volume entering/leaving the lungs per minute
- **Alveolar ventilation**: volume of new/fresh air entering the alveoli per minute

Ventilation = Alveolar ventilation – dead space

Dead space = VD/VT = $PaCO_2$– $EtCO_2$/$PaCO_2$ = 0.3 (normal value)

E +CO_2 = End tidal CO_2

6.2 Restrictive versus obstructive lung disease

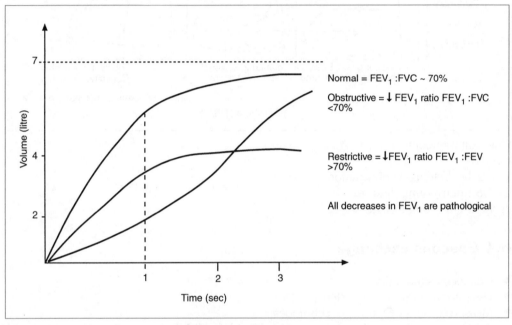

Simple spirometry in obstructive/restrictive disease

FEV$_1$:FVC ratio

- Normal value 0.7 (or 70%)
- Obstructive picture <70%
- Restrictive picture >70% or ratio stays the same

Peak Expiratory Flow measurement indicates airflow resistance but is patient effort and technique dependant. The PEFR 25–75 is less subjective for objective assessment.

6.3 Flow volume loops

These loops help to characterize airflow obstruction as extra- or intra-thoracic and measure severity – useful for work up of neck/mediastinal masses.

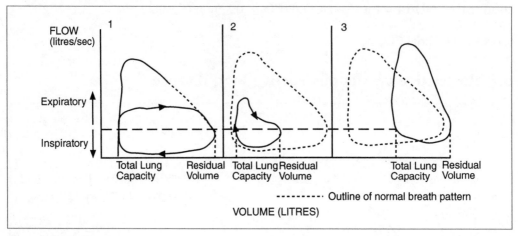

Flow volume loops

1. Tracheal/laryngeal obstruction
2. Obstructive lung disease
3. Restrictive lung disease

6.4 Gaseous exchange

- Occurs by simple diffusion
- Usually *not* a rate limiting step
- Measured using CO_2 uptake techniques
- Transfer coefficient = diffusing capacity of lungs for CO_2/accessible alveolar volume ($kCO_2 = DLCO_2/VA$)

6.5 Arterial blood gases

Partial pressures and pH measured by electrodes. Oxygen saturations and carbon monoxide measured via absorbance spectroscopy in a co-oximeter.

Normal values

pH	7.35 to 7.45	
Hydrogen ions	35 to 45	
$PaCO_2$	4.8 to 6.2 kPa	35 to 45 mmHg
PaO_2	13.3 kPa	100 mmHg
Bicarbonate	24 mmol	
BE	−1 to +1	

Base excess is the amount of acid or base required to restore 1 litre of blood to normal pH at $PaCO_2$ of 5.3 kPa and body temperature. In hypoperfusion in shock states the BE becomes negative and is a useful indicator.

Henderson-Hasselbach equation:

$$pH = 6.1 + \log_{10}\{[HCO^3]/(0.225 \times PaCO_2)\}$$

The kidneys excrete 80 meq acid per day
The lungs excrete 14,400 meq per day as CO_2

Interpretation

Look at acid and ventilation ($PaCO_2$) first then oxygenation.

1. **Is pH abnormal**
   pH <7.35 acidosis
   pH >7.45 alkalosis

2. **Look at $PaCO_2$**
   $PaCO_2$ – high in respiratory acidosis, low in respiratory alkalosis
   If $PaCO_2$ agrees with pH then respiratory acid or alkalosis, otherwise there is a metabolic problem

3. **Provisional diagnosis made, does BE agree**
   BE <−1 metabolic acidosis
   BE >+1 metabolic alkalosis

Compensation never over corrects. The lungs compensate quickly for metabolic problem and the kidneys compensate slowly for respiratory problems.

- Metabolic acidosis, negative BE with low $PaCO_2$ due to hyperventilation (e.g. shock, lactic acidosis, diabetic keto-acidosis, loss of intestinal fluid)
- Metabolic alkalosis, positive BE with normal to slightly raised $PaCO_2$ (e.g. low K+, loss of gastric acid via NG, hepatic failure, alkali use)
- Respiratory acidosis, high $PaCO_2$, bicarbonate and BE rise if chronic (e.g. respiratory failure, COAD chronic, restrictive disease, sleep apnoea)
- Respiratory alkalosis, low $PaCO_2$, bicarbonate and BE normal or low (e.g. hyperventilation, over ventilation, respiratory centre stimulation)
- Mixed metabolic and respiratory acidosis, high $PaCO_2$ and negative BE (e.g. cardiorespiratory failure)

Further information on metabolic acidosis can be determined from the anion gap.

- Serum values of electrolytes:
  (Sodium + Potassium) – (Chloride + Bicarb) normally equals a gap of 11–18 mmol/l
- Increased anion gap: lactic acidosis, ketoacidosis, salicylate, and uraemia
- Normal anion gap: bicarbonate replaced by chloride e.g. renal tubular acidosis, severe diarrhoea, uretero-sigmoidostomy

Lactic acidosis: Lactate >1
Type A: clear evidence of hypoxia or shock
Type B: ethanol, methanol, inborn errors

PaO_2 normal value 13.3
Less than atmospheric due to alveolar air equation giving an alveolar to arterial difference: $AaDO_2$.

This is normally about 10 but increases if shunt is present.

Saturations are either inferred on older machine from PaO_2 and derived from dissociation curve or measured directly with a co-oximeter.

6.6 Interpretation of a chest X-ray

On ICU are almost always AP views therefore heart size unreliable. They are also frequently supine films hence pneumothorax and effusions may not be apparent. CT scanning of the thorax can provide detailed information and ultrasound can help with isolation of effusions.

Remember

- Label
- Adequacy of film, exposure: thoracic vertebrae just visible
- Attached equipment (e.g. ECG leads, CVP/PA line, NG tube)

- Heart
- Mediastinum
- Endotracheal tube, tip level with lower edge clavicles
- Hilar regions
- Diaphragm
- Lungs, look for silhouette sign

Consolidation: air bronchogram, no volume change
Atelectasis: shift of fissures, decreased volume, compensatory hyperinflation

- Bones
- Soft tissues
- Special areas – apices, behind heart, look for pneumothorax
- Effusions – may appear at apex in supine patients (transudate: protein <30 g/l)

6.7 Respiratory function, surgery and trauma

Respiratory complications are a major cause of peri-op/trauma complications.

Risk factors

- Male
- Age
- Emergency surgery
- ↓ Anaesthetic score
- Obesity or abdominal distension (e.g. bowel obstruction)
- Length of procedure
- Surgery/trauma to chest or upper abdomen
- Pre-existing lung disease

Anaesthetic factors

- Reduced FRC resulting from supine position and raising of diaphragm
- V/Q mismatching: increased *shunt* – perfused but not ventilated; increased *dead space* – ventilated but not perfused
- Impaired host defences: impaired protective reflexes (e.g. gag and cough); dry anaesthetic gases hinder ciliary function

Post-operative factors

- Residual anaesthetic agents (muscle relaxants)
- Analgesia/sedatives (e.g. opiates)
- Pain restricting respiratory effort and adequate cough
- Lying supine

Trauma factors

- Cord lesions
- Analgesia
- Pain
- Pneumothorax
- Lung contusion

7. RESPIRATORY FAILURE

7.1 Definition

- PaO_2 <8 kPa or $PaCO_2$ >7 kPa
- Type I – low PaO_2 with normal or low $PaCO_2$
- Type II – low PaO_2 with high $PaCO_2$

Outline of management

- Exclude any airway problem and resuscitate as appropriate
- Oxygen. In type I failure CPAP can improve PaO_2 if high flow oxygen is inadequate
- Involve senior and ICU staff early for mechanical ventilatory support
- History (if possible) and examination
- Regular monitoring of ABGs
- Adjustment of inspired O_2 according to ABGs
- Bronchodilators (nebulized or IV), steroids and antibiotics as appropriate
- High level supervision – HDU or ICU*
- Repeated assessments

*Requirement of more than 40% O_2 to keep oxygen saturation >94% should be strongly considered for observation on HDU/ICU (a 'normal' oxygen mask, without a reservoir attached, can deliver at most approximately 40% O_2).

Physiotherapy

- Consider doxapram if respiratory effort is poor, but beware of exhaustion
- FRC: increased in upright and sitting positions
- Postural drainage
- Percussion to loosen secretions
- Bagging and suction
- Tracheostomy or mini-cricothyrotomy aid suction in non-ventilated patients

NB. As students, we all seem to remember being told that high concentrations of inspired O_2 can cause CO_2 retention and ultimately can stop a patient breathing in cases of hypoxic drive (low PaO_2 rather than raised $PaCO_2$ drives respiration). However, in reality this is unusual and the junior doctor should not be afraid to give a breathless/hypoxic patient high flow O_2. Respiratory depression in this situation does not occur immediately.

7.2 Alveolar–oxygen gradient

Measure of lung ventilation (or physiological shunt).

Alveolar gas equation
$PAO_2 = PIO_2 - (PACO_2 / RQ)$

where:

- PAO_2 is the alveolar PO_2
- PIO_2 is the inspired PO_2 (Atmos P – Saturated water vapour pressure) $\times$ FiO_2 where atmos p is 101 kPa and SVP water is 5 kPa
- $PACO_2$ is close to $PaCO_2$
- RQ is the Respiratory Quotient $CO_2/O_2 = 0.8$ for normal diet

From this we can calculate the alveolar partial pressure of oxygen (PAO_2).

In healthy lungs, $PAO_2 - PaO_2$ (measured from blood gases) is around 10 kPa. This gap is known as the $AaDO_2$. This explains why PaO_2 is approximately 10 less than FiO_2, as account must be taken of CO_2 and water vapour in the lung. In diseased lungs the $AaDO_2$ may be increased and is useful indicator of hypoxaemia. The A-a gradient is normal in hypo-ventilation related hypoxaemia, but decreased in VQ mismatch.

7.3 Intubation

Nasal intubation is preferred for paediatric ICU – there is an increased risk of haemorrhage in adults and risk of sepsis from sinus infection.

Endotracheal intubation:
Internal diameter 8–9 mm for males, 7–8 mm for females
Length 23 cm to teeth in males, 21 cm in females. Checked on CXR level with lower edge of clavicles.

Cuffs

- Create a seal
- Help prevent aspiration
- Can cause stenosis and tracheomalacia if high pressure
- Pressure should be monitored

Indications for intubation

- Unconscious patient who cannot maintain own airway (GCS <8)
- Impaired gag reflex
- To prevent rise in ICP (iatrogenic hyperventilation)
- Where there is a risk of upper airway obstruction

- Severe hypoxia or metabolic acidosis
- Mechanical ventilation
- To enable suction of secretions

Complications (DOPE)

- **D**isplacement (oesophagus or right main bronchus)
- **O**bstruction
- **P**neumothorax
- **E**quipment failure
- Trauma to mouth (chipped teeth) and upper airways – may cause later stenosis
- Aspiration and hypoxia during placement

Anaesthetic induction for intubation

Skilled operator trained in anaesthesia.
Preparation of equipment.
Prevention of pressor response on laryngoscopy with IV fentanyl or lignocaine especially if risk of raised ICP.
Cricoid pressure: application of pressure to the cricoid, the only complete ring cartilage in the airway, so that it impinges onto the body of C6. This will prevent passive regurgitation once induced.
Induction agent: if haemodynamically unstable there may be a precipitous drop in BP. Etomidate is reasonably cardio stable as is ketamine, which has the added value of bronchodilation.
Muscle relaxant: Suxamethonium has rapid onset (<1 min) characterized by fasciculations and is short acting. Side-effects include anaphylaxis, and hyperkalaemia especially following burns or in patients with paralysis when cardiac arrest can occur.

7.4 The surgical airway

Emergency surgical airway: cricothyroidotomy

Emergency when ET intubation not possible and impossible to ventilate by mask. An incision is made in the relatively avascular cricothyroid membrane and a cuffed tube approx 6 mm is inserted. This is a vital skill for all surgeons and can be placed very quickly.

Elective: surgical tracheostomy

Through 2nd and 3rd tracheal rings. High risk of stenosis if adjacent to first ring.

Indications

- Weaning off ET tube (less/no sedation, more comfortable)
- To enable suction of secretions
- Chronic/permanent ventilation
- Enables oral care and comfort

Complications

- Damage to surrounding structures
- Haemorrhage
- Displacement and false track
- Pneumothorax
- Infection
- Blockage
- Fistula
- Stenosis

Tracheostomy is not an emergency procedure as it cannot be performed as quickly and safely as cricothyroidotomy.

Percutaneous tracheostomy

This technique allows a full tracheostomy using placement of a 14G cannula into the trachea, insertion of a guide wire and serial dilation. This procedure can be performed in the ICU by non-surgical doctors thus avoiding transfer to theatre.

Advantages

- Avoids patient transfer
- Less incidence of haemorrhage and infection

Mini-tracheostomy

Small tracheostomy tube through cricothyroid membrane – to aid suctioning of secretions and physiotherapy. This is not suitable as a definitive airway as the tube is not cuffed.

7.5 Mechanical ventilation

Aims

- Elimination and control of CO_2
- Improve oxygenation – reduces 'work' of respiration and therefore O_2 consumed
- Enables high levels of inspired O_2 to be administered
- Can open collapsed alveoli

Complications of mechanical ventilation

- Airway (above)
- Barotrauma – pneumothorax, pneumomediastinum, pneumoperitoneum, surgical emphysema
- Cardiovascular – reduced venous return (high intrathoracic pressure)
- Increased pulmonary vascular resistance
- Gastric dilatation/ileus (Gastric tube must be inserted)
- Accidental disconnection or wrong setting of ventilator
- Na^+ and H_2O retention – increased ADH and atrial natriuretic peptide
- Atrophy of respiratory muscles if no spontaneous effort
- Infection/pneumonia

Physiotherapy

It is essential that secretions are cleared in ventilated patients who cannot cough especially with pneumonia. Chest physio with suctioning should be carried out frequently.

Intermittent Positive Pressure Ventilation (IPPV)

Ventilators on ICU have a choice of **mode** and **mandatory** or **spontaneous** features; all have pressure limitation cut off and sophisticated alarms.

Modes

Controlled mechanical ventilation (CMV)

- Sets rate for breaths and breath volume either by volume or pressure control
- Allows no spontaneous respirations e.g. as in anaesthetic ventilators

Intermittent Mandatory Ventilation (IMV)

- Delivers 'mandatory' minute volume but allows patient to take spontaneous breaths between mechanical breaths
- Can be synchronized with spontaneous breaths **(SIMV)** thus preventing stacking of breaths. This occurs when a mechanical breath is imposed after a spontaneous one. Sensors in the ventilator detect the patient's own breaths. This is the main mode used in ICU.

Mandatory type

This determines how breaths are delivered, either as a set volume or a set pressure.

Volume control

The tidal volume TV to be delivered is set on the ventilator. Normal settings are 10 ml per kg. This is the usual mandatory type, however if compliance is poor the inspired pressure will be very high with risk of barotrauma. Therefore not suitable in ARDS and asthma.

Pressure control

An inspiratory pressure is set on the ventilator and TV is dependent on compliance.
This type is used in ARDS. The inspiratory pressure is set to a value to achieve a satisfactory measured TV but peak pressures are usually limited to 34 cm H_2O to avoid barotrauma.

Spontaneous types

Pressure support

This adjunct supports spontaneous breaths with a set pressure to increase their tidal volumes. This allows very small breaths produced by the patient to be boosted to adequate volumes as an aid to weaning.

The sensitivity of breath detection can be altered via the trigger sensitivity and type.

The trigger for supported breaths is usually a drop in pressure, but flow triggering is more sensitive if required.

Assist control (trigger) ventilation
Uses patient's own respiratory rhythm to trigger delivery of a set tidal volume.

Positive End Expiratory Pressure (PEEP)

- Used *with* mechanical ventilation and improves oxygenation
- Expiratory pressure not allowed to fall below certain level (2.5 to 20 cm H_2O)
- Prevents alveolar collapse and recruits collapsed alveoli
- Increases lung volumes
- Reduces physiological shunting, but further reduces venous return and increases barotrauma

Continuous Positive Airways Pressure (CPAP)

- As PEEP but defined in a *spontaneously* breathing patient
- Requires ET tube or tightly fitting mask
- Same advantages and disadvantages as PEEP but also reduces respiratory effort
- Reduces cardiac work by reducing transmural tension

Weaning

- Patient must have recovered from original problem requiring ventilation
- Conscious level, metabolic state, cardiovascular function and state of mind to be considered including normal phosphate.
- SIMV mode aids weaning with Pressure Support (PS). As the patient starts taking spontaneous breaths the SIMV rate is reduced until all breaths are spontaneous and supported by PS. PS is then reduced until the patient self ventilates without support.
- The longer on a ventilator, the longer/more difficult the weaning.
  Prior to extubation the patient may be placed on a T Piece, which allows oxygenation without support. CPAP is sometimes helpful.

The most successful method of weaning is with spontaneous breaths from the patient supported by pressure support.

Extubation
Patient has to:

- Be able to breathe spontaneously indefinitely
- Have an effective cough reflex and be able to protect their airway
- Be conscious enough to co-operate
- Other factors include adequate TV without tachypnoea i.e. Resp rate / TV <100

  e.g. 12/0.7 = 17, 40/0.3 = 133

7.6 Acute respiratory distress syndrome (ARDS)

Respiratory component of SIRS or MODS (see later).

Brief pathogenesis

Lung injury causes an inflammatory response leading to damage to the alveolar-capillary membrane and microcirculatory changes. This causes an increased pulmonary vascular permeability leading to thickened alveolar membranes and leakage of fluid into interstitium and alveoli. This process may be the pulmonary manifestation of whole body capillary leak syndrome in MODS. This gives poorer *volumes, compliance* and *gaseous exchange* capabilities of lungs. There are three areas of the lung in this condition:

- Collapsed solid lung with consistency like liver
- Ventilated and perfused lung (termed baby lung as much smaller than normal)
- Potentially recruitable alveoli. This is where ventilatory techniques may be beneficial.

May resolve with or without pulmonary fibrosis.

Clinical features

There is a spectrum of Acute Lung Injury (ALI) up to severe which is termed ARDS.

Diagnostic features for ALI

- Pulmonary infiltrates on CXR
- PAWP <18 (hence infiltrates not due to cardiac pulmonary oedema)
- Hypoxaemia with ratio PaO_2/FiO_2 <40
- A known cause e.g. pancreatitis, aspiration, massive transfusion

ARDS is the above features but with severe hypoxaemia i.e. PaO_2/FiO_2 <27

Other features include respiratory distress and decreased compliance.

Causes of ALI

- **Direct**
  Chest trauma
  Aspiration
  Inhaled irritants (e.g. smoke)

- **Indirect**
  Sepsis
  Hypovolaemia
  Burns
  Pancreatitis
  Fat embolism
  Radiation
  DIC

Management

- Almost entirely supportive
- Treat underlying cause if possible
- Ventilation + PEEP
- Patient repositioning
- Careful fluid restriction/diuresis
- Corticosteroids in fibrosis stage
- Trial of blind antibiotics (controversial)

Ventilatory management

Optimisation of oxygenation by increasing mean airway pressure and increased FiO_2.

Increase mean airway pressure

- Increased peak inspired pressure limited to about 34 cm H_2O
- Increased PEEP
- Increased inspiratory time, even so far as reversing the I:E ratio to 2:1

Increase FiO_2

- Levels above 0.5 (50%) increase risk of oxygen toxicity hence the above measures are used to minimise the inspired oxygen and targets of PaO_2 of 8Kpa and saturations of 90% are acceptable.

Ventilation in ARDS

The usual method is pressure control ventilation, with PEEP and sometimes reverse ratio. To limit the peak pressures a low tidal volume can be allowed hence the $PaCO_2$ can be allowed to increase (permissive hypercapnoea). The tidal volume should also be restricted to around 6 ml/kg as excessive volumes cause shear stress damage to the alveoli.

In severely hypoxaemic patients Nitric Oxide maybe used to reduce the FiO_2 and improve oxygenation. The mainstay of therapy however is pressure support and PEEP to recruit collapsed alveoli and maintain them.

Ventilation in the prone position for periods of 4–8 hours may improve regional pulmonary VQ matching and improve oxygenation. This is due to non-homogeneous distribution of damage, which tends to be in dependent lung. Despite this benefit in some patients there are risks of dislodging the ETT, catheters and other tubes.

Fluid balance: this is difficult as over hydration is deleterious to injured lung but adequate cardiovascular performance is required. Judicious use of ventilation, fluids and inotropes is needed.

Outcome

- 50–60% mortality
- Those who recover may be left with diffuse interstitial fibrosis but mostly have good outcome

Nitric oxide (NO)

NO is a vasodilator that is formed naturally in almost all tissues (constitutive). It is also produced in excess in sepsis causing vascular dilatation.

When used clinically it is inhaled at a concentration of around 5–20 parts per million. Side-effects include pulmonary toxicity due to nitric acid formation when oxidised. It causes vasodilatation in ventilated lung only, improving V/Q match thus preventing systemic vasodilatation and reversal of pulmonary hypoxic vasoconstriction. The NO has a very high affinity for haemoglobin forming metheamoglobin, which deactivates NO and prevents systemic effects.

7.7 Specific respiratory infections in the ICU

Aspiration

- Current management dependent on what is aspirated into the lungs
- Particulate small airway obstruction
- Acid damage to alveolar membrane
- Possible infected material

Observe, oxygen, physiotherapy. Ventilation if necessary.
No antibiotics unless definitely infected material as promotes resistant organisms.
Do not use steroids.

Lung abscess

- Often caused by aspiration and hence anaerobic organisms
- Can be caused by: bronchial obstruction; pneumonia; infected pulmonary infarcts; haematogenous spread
- Treated by antibiotics, postural drainage and physio. <10% need surgical drainage.

Opportunistic pneumonia

- Relatively common on ICU
- May require bronchial lavage ± transbronchial biopsy to identify organism

Commonest infections are Gram-positive organisms but include Gram-negatives. After use of antibiotics candida may colonise and cause infection

Empyema

- Accumulation of pus in pleural cavity
- 50% caused by pneumonia, 25% post surgical infections
- Gram-ve inc Pseudomonas often found as well as Staphylococci
- Acutely low viscosity fluid accumulates, then becomes more turbid with increased WCC. At this point a fibrous peel develops on the lung surface limiting expansion. After 6 weeks this peel becomes organised with fibroblasts.
- Diagnosis from thoracentesis: pH <7, low glucose, LDH >1000 and Gram stain. CXR and CT scan.
- Treatment in acute phase with appropriate antibiotics, if thoracentesis shows progressive
- Empyema as above: chest drainage. Surgical drainage and decortication of the peel may be required.

7.8 Complications of thoracic operations

Patients at risk

- Elderly
- Smokers (IHD and COAD)

Immobility post-operatively (increases risk of DVT/PE).

Retained sputum

- Pain and opiate drugs post-operatively reduce respiratory effort and cough
- Ciliary function is reduced (smokers)
- Requires excellent pain control: intercostal nerve block or ablation (in theatre); epidural; PCA; NSAIDs (beware of ulcers)
- Deep breathing exercises to be encouraged
- Requires careful monitoring and aggressive chest physiotherapy, mini-tracheostomy to suction secretions

Pneumonectomy
Leaves an empty hemithorax that fills with fluid and gradually solidifies.

Complications

- Tension pneumothorax
- Haemothorax (can be massive)
- Pulmonary oedema
- Empyema – often *S. aureus* – requires drainage
- Bronchopulmonary fistula – patient starts coughing up fluid; requires moving patient onto side of operation, chest drain and surgical exploration unless small – rare but very serious

8. RENAL FAILURE

Renal failure is defined as failure of the kidneys to maintain the correct composition and volume of the body's internal environment.

Patients undergoing major surgery are at risk of developing renal failure, particularly in the post-operative period, where inadequate fluid rehydration is not uncommon.

Anuria is the absence of urine output. In most surgical patients, urinary retention is more likely to be due to a blocked or misplaced urinary catheter rather than to acute tubular necrosis.

Oliguria is defined as a urine output of less than 400 ml in 24 hours or less than 0.5 ml/kg/hr. This is a much more likely presentation of impending renal failure in surgical patients than anuria. It is not uncommonly seen after inadequate fluid replacement (see above).

Non-oliguric renal failure can also occur; this has a much lower morbidity.

8.1 Causes of renal failure

Pre-renal

Caused by underperfusion of the kidneys, the commonest type in ICU.

- Hypovolaemia: classified according to aetiology: loss of whole blood (haemorrhage); loss of plasma (burns); loss of crystalloid (dehydration, diarrhoea, vomiting).

NB. As far as possible one should replace like with like, i.e. blood after haemorrhage or water (given as 5% dextrose) in dehydration. However, in many hypovolaemic patients, the priority is initially to rapidly replace lost circulating volume. This is with either blood, colloid or isotonic crystalloid, such as 0.9% saline. The remaining fluid deficit can be made up more slowly, with whatever fluid most closely resembles the fluid losses.

The typical mechanism is that hypoxaemia and hypoperfusion reduces sodium absorption in the ascending loop of Henle, which is a high energy consuming process. Hence the Juxta Glomerular Apparatus detects increased filtrate sodium and therefore reduces renal blood flow to conserve blood volume hence reduced urine output. Appropriate treatment should reverse this process before ischaemic damage and acute tubular necrosis occurs.

Causes of renal failure

- Other causes of hypotension (e.g. drugs)
- Septic shock
- Anaphylactic shock
- Endocrine shock
- Low output cardiac failure
- Renovascular disease (e.g. renal artery stenosis)
- Raised intra-abdominal pressure (abdominal compartment syndrome)
- Renal artery emboli or trauma

Renal

Caused by intrinsic renal pathology.

- Acute tubular necrosis due to prolonged ischaemia or tubular toxins, including drugs (e.g. gentamicin)
- Glomerulonephritis or vasculitis (e.g. SLE, polyarteritis nodosa, Wegener's granulomatosis)
- Goodpasture's syndrome (antiglomerular basement membrane antibodies)
- Interstitial nephritis, drugs
- Vascular lesions, hypertension, emboli, renal vein thrombosis
- Infections, pyelonephritis

Post-renal

Caused by obstruction to the flow of urine along the urinary tract.

- **Pelvicalyceal**: (usually at pelvi-ureteric junction, e.g. bilateral PUJ obstruction)
- **Ureteric**: luminal/intramural extrinsic obstruction: retroperitoneal fibrosis, stone
- **Bladder/urethral outflow obstruction**: urinary retention, high pressure or atonic bladder, urethral stricture, blocked catheter, cervical prostatic neoplasm

NB. The most important causes that must not be missed (because they are so easily treatable) are pre-renal, especially hypovolaemia/dehydration, and post-renal (particularly prostate or catheter problems). Also inadequate rehydration of a post-obstructive diuresis commonly results in pre-renal failure.

Differentiating pre-renal and renal causes

This is initially on the basis of a history and examination. Where there is still a query as to the cause of renal failure, an analysis of the urine and serum biochemistry is performed. This is one of the simplest and most effective ways of differentiating pre-renal and intrinsic renal failure.

Urine analysis and serum biochemistry		
Measurement	**Pre-renal**	**Renal**
Urinary sodium	low, <20 mmol/l	high, >40 mmol/l
Urine:		
serum osmolarity ratio	>1.2	<1.2
serum creatinine ratio	high, >40	low, <20
Urine osmolality	>500	<350

Normal kidneys, in the presence of hypotension or hypovolaemia, will concentrate urine and conserve sodium (meaning that there will be less in the urine). If there is intrinsic renal pathology, the kidney will be unable to concentrate the urine or conserve sodium.

The fractional excretion of sodium is normally <1. In renal failure it is greater than 1 and can be used as a trend indicator.

Prevention of renal failure

- Prevention of hypotension or hypovolaemia
- Prevention of dehydration, especially in patients who continue to receive their 'normal' diuretic medication
- Early treatment of sepsis
- Care with potentially nephrotoxic drugs (e.g. NSAIDs, gentamicin)

8.2 Presentation and management

Acute renal failure usually presents as oliguria, or as progressively increasing urea and creatinine on serum biochemistry tests.

The important steps in the management of oliguria are

- Exclude obstruction (insert catheter or flush existing catheter, consider renal ultrasound)
- Correct hypovolaemia and hypotension (may need CVP +/– PA Cath and assessment of response of CVP to fluid boluses). When optimally filled inotropes or vasopressor may be required to provide adequate perfusion pressure.
  (Perfusion pressure may need to be increased in hypertensives)
  Fluid maintenance after resuscitation includes infusing urine output volume each hour plus insensible losses (about 1000 ml/24 hr) increased in pyrexia.
- Treat the cause or any contributing factors (e.g. stop NSAIDs and ACE inhibitors)
  Prostaglandin inhibition by NSAIDs causes renal vasoconstriction.

In addition, various treatments are often used to try to reverse/prevent renal failure.

Examples of such treatments are

- Frusemide, either as a bolus or as a continuous infusion. An infusion of 5–10 mg/hr is more effective than bolus therapy. The principle being a frusemide induced reduction of oxygen consumption by the nephron.
- Dopamine or Dopexamine causing stimulation of dopamine receptors, see section 2.10. Sodium loading with $NaHCO_3$ to reduce oxygen dependent sodium retention by the nephron.
  Mannitol increases urine output by osmotic diuresis. Does not prevent renal failure and some evidence of nephrotoxicity. Used successfully to reduce renal damage in jaundice and rhabdomyolysis. Beware that induced diuresis can cause hypovolaemia and reduce renal perfusion.

However, none of these treatments have been proven to prevent renal failure, and the other measures shown above are much more important.

In established renal failure, artificial support may be required. This is commonly achieved by haemodialysis.

Other aspects to consider in a patient with impending or established renal failure are

- Renal replacement therapy
- Hydration and fluid balance
- Optimization of serum biochemistry
- Nutrition
- Treatment of infection
- Review of drug therapy

8.3 Renal replacement therapy

Indications

- Hyperkalaemia (persistently >6.0 mmol/l)
- Metabolic acidosis (pH <7.2) with negative BE
- Pulmonary oedema/fluid overload without substantial diuresis
- The need to 'make room' for ongoing drug infusions and nutrition, and to aid clearance of drugs already given (e.g. sedatives)
- Complications of chronic uraemia (e.g. pericarditis/cardiac tamponade methods)
- High urea around 30–40 mmol/l
- Creatinine rising more than 100 mmol/l/day

Methods

CAVH	Continuous arterio-venous haemofiltration
CVVH	Continuous veno-venous haemofiltration
CVVHD	Continuous veno-venous haemo-diafiltration
HD	Haemodialysis

In **ICU**, both haemofiltration and haemo-diafiltration are commonly performed via a large bore dual lumen central venous cannula **CVVH**. As the flow of blood is both from and to the venous side of the circulation, a pump is required. The blood flow is in the region of 250 ml/min and alarms are incorporated to prevent air embolism. Anticoagulation is needed and heparin is usually used as an infusion or prostacyclin if thrombocytopaenia develops. Previously arterio-venous systems were used but a large bore catheter needs to be placed in an artery and filtration depends on arterial pressure. These techniques provide slow fluid shifts and maintain haemodynamic stability.

In **haemofiltration**, the blood is driven under pressure through a filter (a semi-permeable membrane). The 'ultrafiltrate' derived from the blood (which is biochemically abnormal) is disposed of, and is replaced with a replacement fluid. Small molecules such as sodium, urea, creatinine and bicarbonate pass through the filter with water (convection) but large molecules like proteins and cells do not. The usual volume of filtrate produced is 1 to 2 litres per hour and this volume is replaced with an electrolyte solution containing ions and buffer. The replacement fluid is buffered with lactate, acetate or freshly added bicarbonate. (Bicarbonate is unstable in solution and lactate is metabolised by the liver to bicarbonate.) The system provides a clearance equivalent approximate to 10 ml/min and if solute clearance is inadequate then augmentation with dialysis can be used (CVVHD).

In **haemodiafiltration (CVVHD)** the dialysate augments clearance by diffusion by running an electrolyte solution on the outside of the filter. The clearance increases to about 20 ml/min.

Fluid balance over 24 hours can be manipulated using these filters. If patient is oedematous then 2 litres negative may be appropriate and can be achieved by replacing 84 ml less per hour than is filtered.

In **haemodialysis (HD)** blood is pumped through the machine on one side of a semi-permeable membrane, similar to haemofiltration. However, in haemodialysis, a dialysis fluid is also pumped through the machine, on the other side of the semi-permeable membrane to the blood.

The biochemistry of the blood equilibrates with that of the dialysis fluid, by diffusion, although some ultrafiltration also occurs.

Haemodialysis tends to be more effective in terms of correcting acidosis and abnormal biochemistry in a short period of time. However, it is associated with more circulatory instability; continuous haemofiltration is often better tolerated in patients with pre-existing circulatory instability.

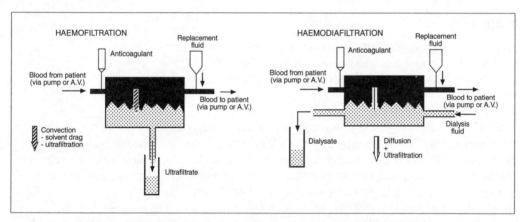

Haemofiltration   Haemodiafiltration

Continuous ambulatory peritoneal dialysis (CAPD) is becoming more common. Fluid is instilled into the peritoneum by a special catheter (e.g. Tenckhoff catheter). The peritoneum acts as the dialysis membrane. Increasingly, this method is chosen by patients as they can perform it at home but is unsuitable for patients post-laparotomy on ICU.

8.4 Optimization of serum biochemistry

The following biochemical abnormalities commonly occur:

- Progressive rise in urea and creatinine
- Hyperkalaemia
- Hyponatraemia (due to relative water overload)
- Acidosis
- Hypocalcaemia
- Hyperphosphataemia
- Hyperuricaemia

The abnormalities requiring most urgent correction are hyperkalaemia and acidosis.

Treatment

Hyperkalaemia

- 10 ml 10% calcium chloride IV (reduces risk of arrhythmia)
- 15 units IV insulin + 50 ml 50% dextrose
- Sodium bicarbonate infusion
- Salbutamol or other beta agonist

Neither insulin, beta agonist nor sodium bicarbonate reduces total body potassium. They increase intracellular potassium and so reduce the serum potassium. This reduces the risk of a fatal arrhythmia, but is only a short-term measure; haemofiltration/haemodialysis will be required in the medium-/long-term to prevent hyperkalaemia unless renal function improves.

- Calcium resonium – orally or PR (reduces total body potassium, but poorly tolerated orally, and works slowly)
- Stop potassium-containing infusions (which may include TPN or enteral feed), stop drugs such as potassium-sparing diuretics

Acidosis

- If artificially ventilated, increase the minute ventilation
- Sodium bicarbonate infusion (but this is controversial, may paradoxically increase intracellular acidosis, and is only a short-term measure)
- Artificial renal support

Nutrition

High-calorie diet needed, with adequate high-quality protein: maximum of 35 kcal/kg/day (approximately 2500 kcal) – 14 g nitrogen/day.

8.5 Treatment of infection

Infection and generalized sepsis may already be apparent as the cause or contributing factors in the development of renal failure. If the cause of renal failure (or other organ system failure) is due to sepsis, it is unlikely to improve until the source of the sepsis is eradicated (e.g. intra-abdominal collection).

In anuric patients the catheter should be removed and not replaced until urine output has recovered to prevent ascending urinary tract infection.

8.6 Review of drug therapy

All drug therapy given to patients in renal failure needs to be regularly and thoroughly reviewed.

- Drugs which may exacerbate renal failure or its complications (e.g. NSAIDs, ACE inhibitors, gentamicin and potassium-sparing diuretics) should be avoided
- Many drugs will need dose adjustment, to prevent overdosage as they or their active metabolites are excreted by the kidneys and this includes most antibiotics
- If possible, serum drug levels should be checked, and the drug doses adjusted accordingly

9. GASTROINTESTINAL FUNCTION AND NUTRITION

9.1 Gut function in the critically ill

The gastrointestinal tract plays an important role in the development of multiple organ failure and its outcome. The gut is considered to be the **motor** for sepsis and multi-organ failure. It is thought that the gastrointestinal mucosal function is impaired by many of the elements of critical illness, for example:

- Hypoxia
- Hypoperfusion, as part of circulatory failure
- An hypercatabolic state
- Inadequate oral nutrition

Once the gut mucosa has been damaged, it is thought that endotoxin and bacteria from the gut may pass through the gut mucosa and into the portal circulation. If the insult is large enough, or if there is concurrent hepatic dysfunction, the endotoxin and bacteria can pass into the systemic circulation, causing damage to various organ systems, either directly or through the systemic inflammatory response syndrome (SIRS). See section 11 on multiple organ failure.

On the basis of this theory, attempts have been made to carry out gut decontamination, to reduce the endotoxin/bacterial load on the systemic circulation. However, this procedure using non-absorbed antibiotics has been shown to have no effect on outcome in unselected intensive care patients, but may have a role in certain sub-sets of patients.

Gut tonometry

An early indicator of local gut hypoperfusion used mostly as a research tool. A modified NG tube with a semi-permeable balloon is inserted. A H2 blocker is used to eliminate local acidity. Saline is injected into the balloon and allowed to equilibriate and then withdrawn and analysed in a blood gas meter. An arterial blood gas is performed at the same time. A newer system uses gas in the balloon to automate this process and analyses CO_2 directly. The pHi is calculated by putting gut PCO_2 and serum bicarbonate into the Henderson-Hasselbach equation. Localised acidosis or an increased mucosal $PaCO_2$ indicates gut hypoperfusion.

Prophylaxis of stress ulceration

Gastric erosions in critical illness are probably due to regional hypo-perfusion rather than increased acidity. Prophylaxis includes:

- H2 receptor blocker – eradication of low pH allows bacterial overgrowth in the stomach which may promote nosocomial pneumonia (not proven).
- Sucralfate – protects gastric lining while preserving acid pH. This is highly effective but aluminium toxicity may occur in renal failure.
- Proton pump inhibitors – used when documented ulcer disease.
- Enteral feeding is the best prophylaxis.

9.2 Feeding and nutrition

Critical illness is usually associated with a hypermetabolic state.

In the absence of adequate nutrition, there is a severe hypercatabolic state, with extensive breakdown of body tissues, initially skeletal muscle, but followed by visceral protein breakdown leading to a worse clinical outcome. Even with adequate nutrition, some catabolism is inevitable; however, it can be minimized with good nutritional support.

Other benefits are

- Maintenance of immune function
- Fewer late complications relating to sepsis

Nutritional support should be instituted as soon as possible.

Enteral feeding is preferable to parenteral nutrition, on both theoretical grounds (maintenance of gut motor, secretory and mucosal function), and pragmatic (it is associated with improved outcome: reduction in sepsis associated with TPN). However, if no enteral route is available, then parenteral feeding should not be delayed.

9.3 Methods of feeding

Feeding methods

- **Enteral**
  Oral
  Not possible following bowel surgery,
    obstruction, perforation or ileus
  Nasogastric
  Gastric stasis and aspiration
    pneumonitis (Mendelson's syndrome)
    can be a problem
  Nasojejunal
  Often difficult to pass the tube and
    the procedure takes a long time, can be
    manipulated during laparotomy
  Percutaneous endoscopic gastrostomy
  (PEG) tube
  Gastric stasis can be a problem
  Jejunostomy
  In those patients who have had a laparotomy
  Risk of leak and infection
  Jejunal feed is often well tolerated and absorbed,
    when a similar volume of gastric feed may not be

- **Parenteral**
  Needs central venous access
  At risk of line-related sepsis
    and other complications can
    contribute to metabolic and
    electrolyte abnormalities
    (e.g. hyperglycaemia, hypo-
    or hypernatraemia)

9.4 'Immune-enhancing' feeding regimes

There has been much recent research activity on possible 'immune-enhancing' nutritional supplementation; current evidence seems to show improvement in outcome of critical illness.

Examples of feeding regimes

- Glutamine (50% of gut mucosal cell energy is from glutamine use). Important for gluconeogenesis, fundamental for purine, pyridamine and nucleotide synthesis. Antioxidant metabolism and immune function (T-Helper and monocyte). Becomes depleted in critical illness, scientific evidence for glutamine to be given in all parenteral feeds.
- Arginine
- Omega 3 polyunsaturated fatty acids: anti-inflammatory
- Nucleotides

10. NEUROLOGICAL ASPECTS OF CRITICAL CARE

10.1 Sedation, analgesia and muscle relaxation

Sedation

- Relieve anxiety
- Help synchronisation with the ventilator
- Encourage natural sleep
- Permit unpleasant procedures

Drugs

- Bolus dosing. Prevents oversedation but inconvenient.
- Infusion. Risk of oversedation, can be discontinued each day until rousable then restarted as necessary.
- Benzodiazepines (e.g. Midazolam): reduce anxiety and amnesic. Can accumulate with infusions. Inexpensive.
- Propofol: rapid elimination, does not accumulate but expensive, however avoiding increased length of stay due to oversedation may offset cost. May cause hypotension.

Analgesia

- Reduces stress response due to pain
- Respiratory depression helps ventilator synchronisation
- Epidural analgesia post surgery gives excellent analgesia avoiding IV administration

Drugs

- Opioids are the mainstay administered by infusion.
- Morphine: analgesia and anxiolysis, apnoea may occur, gastrointestinal stasis.
- Inexpensive but may accumulate. Metabolite morphine-6–glucuronide accumulates in renal failure and is more potent than morphine.
- Alfentanil: cleared by hepatic clearance, accumulation less likely but variable metabolism in the critically ill. Expensive.

Regulation

- Ramsay score 1–6 points. 1 – anxious, 6 – unresponsive, 2–4 appropriate normally.
- Sedation may not be required if a tracheostomy is used
- To assess pain, visual analogue scales or pain scores can be used

Neuromuscular blockade

- Used infrequently in modern practice. Sedation must be ensured before use as it is unpleasant to be paralysed if awake.
- Used with unnatural ventilation modes such as inverse ratio and in raised ICP to prevent coughing

Drugs

- Bolus or infusion
- Atracurium: metabolised by temperature and pH hence ideal in renal and hepatic failure (Hoffman elimination). Can cause histamine release.
- Rocuronium: rapid onset, metabolised by the liver
- Monitoring. Can be assessed with peripheral nerve stimulator.

10.2 Intracranial pressure (ICP), monitoring and control

ICP is normally approximately 10 mmHg. It is considered critical above 24 mmHg.

Within the cranium are

- Brain tissue
- Blood
- CSF

Any increase in one causes a compensatory reduction in one or more of the others until compliance is lost and ICP rapidly rises.

Causes of raised ICP

Intracranial bleeding
Cerebral oedema; head injury, liver failure, changes in osmolality
Secondary brain injury; hypoxaemia, shock,
Hypercapnia (CO_2 induced cerebral vasodilatation)

Raised ICP decreases cerebral perfusion pressure CPP

$$CPP = MAP - ICP$$

CPP below 70 mmHg may lead to inadequate cerebral oxygenation.

It is vital that CPP is maintained by ensuring an adequate MAP if ICP is raised. Hypotonic fluids such as dextrose are harmful due to osmotic changes in the brain but isotonic fluids to optimise the BP should not be withheld. Vasopressors may be required to ensure an adequate CPP.

ICP monitoring

- **Pressure transducer** inserted through the skull
- **Fibre-optic subdural transducer** – easy to place.
- **Ventriculostomy** – more accurate, higher complications, but able to withdraw CSF if acute rise in ICP.

Cerebral blood flow monitoring

- Jugular venous saturation
- A catheter is placed retrogradely into the jugular vein with the tip lying at the base of the skull. Samples of blood or a fibre optic oximeter tip measure the global oxygen saturation of blood draining from the brain. A low saturation implies poor perfusion and a higher saturation suggests increased blood flow.

Taken in conjunction with ICP monitoring it can be helpful in determining therapy for raised ICP. If high cerebral blood flow then hyperventilation to a lower $PaCO_2$ around 3.5 to 4 will reduce vessel diameter and hence ICP. If there is poor perfusion then hyperventilation is harmful as perfusion is decreased to critical levels. Diuretics should be considered instead.

Other therapies in reducing ICP include:

- Nursing slightly head up
- Avoiding cervical collars when ventilated
- Avoiding tight tube ties round the neck and jugular CVP lines
- Ventilating to $PaCO_2$ around 4.0 kPa. Over ventilation leads to rebound increase in ICP.
- Mannitol causes transient decrease in ICP by osmosis and improved rheology, but transient with rebound increase. (D/w neurosurgeon first in head injuries)
- Keep sedated if ventilated, consider paralysis and care with suctioning

10.3 Brain stem death

Irreversible cessation of brain stem function.
In the UK diagnosed by specific tests as follows:

Preconditions

- Apnoeic coma requiring ventilation
- Known cause of irreversible brain damage e.g. head injury, cerebral haemorrhage

Exclusions

- Hypothermia. Temperature below 35°C.
- No depressant drugs e.g. sedation, opiates, muscle relaxants
- No metabolic derangements e.g. Na, glucose, hepatic encephalopathy

NB. Na at time of diagnosis is taken as otherwise it may be difficult to normalise the value in diabetes insipidus.

Tests
These look for activity in the cranial nerves (CN).

- **Pupil responses**: CN 2. No direct or indirect reaction to light.
- **Corneal reflex**: CN 5 & 7. Direct stimulation with cotton wool.

- **Pain reflex** in facial distribution, motor. CN 5 & 7. Reflexes below the neck are ignored as they may be spinal reflexes.
- **Caloric test**. Instillation of cold water into auditory canal, looking for nystagmus towards the stimulation. CN 8, 3 & 6. Check canal is not blocked with wax first.
- **Gag reflex**. CN 9 & 10.
- **Apnoea test**. Pre-oxygenate with 100% oxygen then disconnect from the ventilator. Insufflate oxygen into trachea via catheter at 4 L/min. Observe for any sign of respiration for 10 mins until $PaCO_2$ is above 6.65 kPa. May need to stop test if sats drop or becomes bradycardic and unstable.

If the patient shows no response to the above tests then brain death can be diagnosed after two sets have been performed. Legal time of death is after the first set.

The tests are performed by two doctors, both 5 years post registration, one of which must be a consultant, and neither should be members of a transplant team. There is no set time between the two sets but at least 6 hours should have elapsed between the onset of coma and the first set.

Organ donation

The possibility of donation must be discussed with the relatives, usually after the first set of tests. If they agree to donation then the local transplant co-ordinator is contacted who arranges viral and histocompatibility testing. They will come to the hospital and talk in detail with the relatives and liaise with the transplant surgeons.

11. MULTI-SYSTEM FAILURE

Multiple organ system failure (MOF) is an important cause of death in intensive care. It refers to the process whereby more than one organ system has deranged function and requires support. Patients do not often die from single organ failure but from MOF following the initial insult.

- The degree of dysfunction can be difficult to quantify, (e.g. dysfunction of the gastrointestinal tract), or easily quantifiable (e.g. renal dysfunction, quantified by the degree of oliguria, serum biochemistry and acid-base status).
- When assessing the degree of dysfunction, account must be taken of the support being provided for the organ system (e.g. for respiratory failure the concentration of inspired oxygen and ventilatory support must be considered when assessing arterial PaO_2).
- MOF is a process that develops over a period of time, and can be in response to an initial severe stimulus (e.g. major burns, sepsis, multiple trauma, major surgery or following several seemingly minor insults).

The development of MOF depends more on the body's response to a given stimulus rather than the stimulus itself. This may explain why different patients, with seemingly similar pathology or injuries, differ in their tendency to develop MOF.

11.1 Pathophysiology

Any localized injury stimulates an inflammatory response. This response involves recruitment of inflammatory cells (such as macrophages and neutrophils) to the area, release of inflammatory mediators (e.g. cytokines, IL-1, 6, 8, TNF-alpha), and changes in vascular permeability.

- These localized inflammatory responses are responsible for minimizing further damage (e.g. from infection) and optimising conditions for healing.
- Under certain conditions (e.g. major trauma), the extent of the inflammatory activity throughout the body is activated in an apparently uncontrolled manner, with an imbalance between inflammatory and anti-inflammatory responses.
- The widespread activity of this systemic inflammation (Systemic Inflammatory Response Syndrome (SIRS)) and activation of a mediator network is such that it damages organs throughout the body, initiating MOF.

Important components of the inflammatory response

Oxygen free radicals
Occur after initial hypoxic injury and subsequent reperfusion i.e. reperfusion injury. Mechanism involves the formation of xanthine oxidase during ischaemia from xanthine dehydrogenase which converts adenosine to hypoxanthine. When oxygen becomes available the hypoxanthine is metabolised to uric acid via the enzyme xanthine oxidase and free radicals are formed in the process. Cause direct endothelial damage and increased permeability.

Cytokines

- Peptides released by various cell types which are involved in the immune response
- Produced by macrophages

TNF Central mediator in sepsis, produces deleterious effects similar to effects of infection, pivotal role in Host response

IL-1 Synergistic with TNF, initiator of Host response, stimulates Helper T cells,

IL-6/8 Reparative processes, production of acute phase proteins

Macrophages

- Phagocytosis of debris and bacteria
- Act as antigen presenting cells to T-lymphocytes
- Release inflammatory mediators, endothelial cells and fibroblasts

Neutrophils

- Migrate to inflamed tissue from the blood
- Release mediators
- Release proteolytic and hydrolytic enzymes, which cause vasodilatation, increased permeability, myocardial depression and activation of clotting mechanisms.

Inducible Intercellular Adhesion Molecules (ICAMs)

- Mediation of adhesion and migration of neutrophils through endothelium
- Induced by Lipopolysaccharides (LPS) and cytokines

Platelet Activating Factor (PAF)

- Released by neutrophils and monocytes
- Cause hypotension, increased permeability and platelet aggregation

Arachidonic acid metabolites

- Essential fatty acid. Metabolised by cyclooxygenase to form prostaglandins and Thromboxane, and lipoxygenase to form leukotrienes.

Vascular endothelium

- Increased permeability, allowing both inflammatory cells and acute phase proteins from the blood to reach the injured (inflamed) area
- Complex organ in its own right involved in vascular tone, permeability, coagulation, phagocytosis and metabolism of vascular mediators.
- Nitric oxide, induced form stimulated by TNF and endotoxin via nitric oxide synthase. Causes sustained vasodilatation.
- Endothelin-1, powerful vasoconstrictor, increased in trauma and cardiogenic shock.

Complement cascade

Occurs in early septic shock via the alternative pathway. Attracts and activates neutrophils.

Vasodilatation

- Allowing increased recruitment of inflammatory cells from the blood

In the systemic inflammatory response syndrome, it is these changes in the vascular endothelium which, when widespread, cause circulatory failure and hypotension, contributing to MOF.

11.2 Definitions

Systemic inflammatory response syndrome

Harmful excessive reaction of acute phase response. Defined by two or more of the following:

- Tachycardia >90 bpm
- Respiratory rate >20 breaths per minute or $PaCO_2$<4.3 kPa
- Temperature >38°C or <36°C
- White cell count >12 or <4 x 10^3/mm^3 or >10% band forms

- **Sepsis**: body's response to infection which includes two or more of the above
- **Severe sepsis**: sepsis with evidence of organ dysfunction or hypoperfusion

- **Septic shock**: severe sepsis with hypotension (<90) despite fluid resuscitation
- **Septicaemia**: clinical signs and symptoms associated with multiplying bacteria in bloodstream
- **Endotoxin**: toxin that remains within cell wall of bacteria. Heat stable. Lipid A conserved amongst different organisms are responsible for effect of triggering mediator network.
- **Exotoxin**: toxin actively secreted by bacteria, specific effects according to organism
- **Carriage:** two consecutive surveillance samples of throat and rectum positive for micro-organisms
- **Colonisation:** Presence of micro-organisms in normally sterile organ without host response e.g. blood, bladder, bronchi and CSF
- **Infection:** microbiologically proven clinical condition with host response
- **Bacteraemia**: bacteria in bloodstream but not necessarily symptomatic or requiring treatment

Definitions of organ system failure

Cardiovascular failure (one or more of the following)

- HR <54 or symptomatic bradycardia
- MAP <49 mmHg or (>70 mmHg requiring inotropic support)
- Occurrence of VT or VF
- Serum pH <7.24 with normal pCO_2

Respiratory failure

- RR <5 or >49
- $PaCO_2$ >6.65 kPa
- $AaDO_2$ >46.55
- Ventilator dependent on day 4 ICU

Renal failure

- Urine output <479 ml 24 hr, or <159 ml 8 hr
- Urea >36
- Creatinine >310
- Dependent on haemofiltration

Haematological failure

- White cell count <1
- Platelets <20
- HCT <0.2
- DIC

Neurological failure

- GCS <6 in the absence of sedation

Gastrointestinal failure

- Ileus >3 days
- Diarrhoea >4 days
- GI bleeding
- Inability to tolerate enteral feed in absence of primary gut pathology

Skin failure

- Decubitus ulcers

Endocrine

- Hypoadrenalism or abnormal thyroid function tests

Outcome from MOF

In two organ failure mortality is in the region of 50% and increases to 66% on 4th day.

In three organ failure mortality around 80% on first day increasing to 96% if does not resolve. Survival from four organ failure is unlikely.

Pre-existing medical condition and age must be taken into account.

Treatment and prevention

The prognosis of established multi-organ failure is extremely poor. (Where three or more systems are in failure for more than three days, the prognosis is dismal.)

The emphasis must therefore be on identifying at-risk patients early, and intervening quickly to prevent MOF.

In order to optimise the chances of recovery, the initial insult (e.g. intra-abdominal sepsis) must be treated if possible. Early nutritional support, particularly via the gut (enteral feeding) is increasingly being recognized as important in improving outcome.

Various anti-inflammatory treatments have been attempted, affecting different parts of the inflammatory response (e.g. anti-endotoxin antibodies, IL-1 antibodies), but in clinical trials none seem to have any effect on outcome. This is due to the complex and multiple pathways involved and some beneficial effects of mediators such as TNF.

11.3 Predisposing factors to sepsis in ICU

Impaired barriers

- Gag reflex – reduced level of consciousness, drugs
- Cough reflex – drugs, pain
- Ciliary function – high-inspired O_2, dry O_2, intubation
- Gut mucosal barrier – ischaemia, change in gut flora (antibiotics)

- Urinary catheters predispose to UTI
- Intravenous/arterial lines breach skin barrier

Impaired defences

- Cell-mediated immunity
- Humoral immunity
- Reticulo-endothelial system
- Caused by trauma, shock, post-op, sepsis, age, malnutrition, malignancy, splenectomy (humoral) and immunosuppressive drugs

Gram-positive are commonest cause of infection e.g. Staphylococci and have taken over from Gram-negatives such as Pseudomonas, *E. coli* and proteus. Organisms such as Acinetobacter are a particular problem on ICUs after use of broad spectrum antibiotics or immunosuppression as are fungal infections e.g. Candida and Aspergillus.

Local antibiotic policy on ICU should be formulated by collaboration with the Microbiologist so that appropriate antibiotics for local organisms are used as well as based on culture and sensitivity. Typical policies follow patterns such as:

- Cephalosporin plus metronidazole +/- gentamicin (renal toxicity).

If unsuccessful moving up to broad spectrum anti-pseudomonals such as

- Piperacillin plus Tazobactam
- Ciprofloxacin
- Ceftazidime
- Or Imipenem/Meropenem

Guided by culture and sensitivity of sputum, blood, wound and urine samples, but quite often this is not available hence broad spectrum agents are used.

For MRSA – Teicoplanin, or Vancomycin (beware toxicity).
For fungal infections – Fluconazole followed by Amphotericin if resistant or Aspergillus.

Infection on ICU

Community acquired: tend to be sensitive organisms. Nosocomial: resistant species, Gram-positive commoner, but Pseudomonas and other Gram-negatives still occur. EPIC (European Prevalence of Infection in ICU) study shown 21% infections acquired within ICU.

11.4 Septic shock

Classically high cardiac output, low systemic resistance, maldistribution of blood flow and increased vascular permeability. Suppression of contractility but tachycardia increases CO. Vasodilatation from NO production. Effects induced by inflammatory responses but not always infection e.g. pancreatitis.

Features

- Pyrexia
- Tachycardia
- Warm skin/flushed or cold/mottled
- Hypotensive, low CVP
- Acidotic (lactic acidosis)

NB. NSAIDs and corticosteroids can mask pyrexia. Corticosteroids may also mask peritonitis.

Management

Treat the cause and support organ function.

- High flow oxygen
- History (if available) and examination
- Urine, sputum, drainage (if appropriate) and blood cultures before antibiotics
- Broad-spectrum antibiotics whilst awaiting results
- CXR and relevant basic bloods
- Change catheter, IV/arterial lines (new sites if possible) unless newly inserted
- Send tips of removed lines for culture
- CVP (or PA catheter) and urinary catheters for monitoring shock/fluid balance
- Haemodynamic support – optimise intravascular volume
- Increase perfusion pressure with noradrenaline
- Monitor pH as a guide to optimal tissue perfusion
- Early enteral feeding or TPN if not possible
- Remember, prevention is better than cure

Complications

- Stress ulcers
- Pulmonary hypertension
- Hypercatabolic state and hyperglycaemia
- Metabolic acidosis
- DIC
- MODS/MOF

Outcome

Approximately 50% mortality.

12. PRINCIPLES OF INTENSIVE CARE (ICU)

12.1 Admission to ICU

- Can be elective, emergency or prophylactic
- For potentially reversible condition, not futile
- For specialized/high level of monitoring
- For mechanical support of organs (ventilation, dialysis)
- Failure of more than one system

The High Dependency Unit (HDU) is appropriate for patients who require more input than a general ward can give, have single organ failure but do not require ICU care or ventilation. Outreach services may provide early access to skilled advice and allow earlier initiation of critical care. Referral should be specialty consultant to ICU consultant.

Reasons for poor outcome in the critically ill

- Inadequate ward care
- Late referral to ICU
- Cardiac arrest (80% are predictable prior to arrest)

Improvement in survival

- Earlier critical care intervention
- Better critical care training of Medical and Nursing staff in critical care principles
- Systems to identify physiological deterioration earlier
- ICU staff expanding role onto wards and Emergency rooms

Early warning systems
To recognise ill patients on the ward early and institute critical care.

- Can be based on a physiological score including parameters:
  - Airway compromise
  - Respiratory rate and effort
  - Heart rate
  - Blood pressure
  - Urine output
  - Glasgow Coma Score
  - And anything that makes ward staff suspicious

12.2 Discharge from ICU

- To an HDU can occur earlier than to a general ward
- Is decided by senior ICU staff
- Care is handed over to specialty team

12.3 ICU Transfers

Required for

- Clinical escalation of care e.g. neurosurgical
- Lack of bed availability
- Patient must have been fully assessed, resuscitated and be stable
- Direct Dr-to-Dr referral and discussion by telephone by both ICU and specialty teams
- Appropriate monitoring should be in place
  Invasive BP as non-invasive unreliable in transit
  ECG, Pulse Oximeter, $EtCO_2$, CVP

- Escort by experienced doctor (senior anaesthetist) and trained nurse
- Any equipment or drugs that may possibly be required should be to hand; include all Radiology, Lab results and copy of notes.
- A good handover on arrival is essential

12.4 Location of ICUs and definitions of critical care

ICU beds in the UK comprise 1% of total beds. An ICU should have a minimum of 4 beds to be efficient and have up to 8 to 12 beds. Bed occupancy should be around 70% but is often much higher due to insufficient capacity.

Should ideally be near and on the same floor as

- A&E
- Theatres
- Radiology
- Blood bank

Critical care provision is classified into 4 levels.

Level 0   Normal ward
Level 1   Enhanced care, approx. 3 to 1 nurse ratio, monitored.
Level 2   High Dependency, 2 to 1 nurse ratio, single organ failure (not ventilated).
Level 3   Intensive Care, 1 to 1 nurse ratio. MOF, ventilation.

Medical staffing

- ICU Director. Should have specialty training in ICM (CCST in the future), base specialty from Anaesthetics, Medicine, Surgery or A&E. More than 80% consultants from Anaesthetics.
- ICU consultants covering all daytime sessions and on-call rota.
- Trainee: 24 hour dedicated cover, SHO, SpR, Fellows from above specialities.

It is recommended that trainees in acute specialties should have at least 3 months training in ICU.

Nurse staffing

About seven whole time equivalents per ICU bed. Increased degree of nursing autonomy with role in fluid therapy, weaning and ventilation, and inotrope titration.

Costs
Approximately £1000 to £1800 per bed per day. Non-survivors consume greater costs.

12.5 Scoring systems

These enable comparison between units and evaluation of new/existing treatments by case mix adjustment for differences in the severity of illness of patients. Average mortality in ICU is 25–30%.

SMR: Standardised Mortality Ratio. Calculated on unit for diagnostic groups and can be compared with national standards e.g. ICNARC or RIYAD.

Acute Physiology, Age and Chronic Health Evaluation (APACHE I, II and III). It has three point-scoring components:

- Acute physiology based on GCS, blood results, haemodynamic and urine output variables
- Age
- Chronic health

Simplified Acute Physiology Score (SAPS) reduces the APACHE scoring system to 14 variables.

Other scoring systems

- Injury Severity Score (ISS): correlates severity of injury in 3 anatomical areas, scoring up to 5 and squaring the result. Max score in 75. Used for audit
- Revised Trauma Score (RTS); TRISS = ratio of RTS and ISS
- Mortality Prediction Model or Mortality Probability Model (MPM)
- Standardized Mortality Ratio (SMR) = ratio of estimated deaths (MPM) and actual deaths
- Therapeutic Intervention Scoring System (TISS): used to measure nursing workload; points are attributed to different therapeutic interventions received by patients
- Quality of life data (e.g. QALYs)

NB. No scoring system can predict with certainty outcomes in individual patients and should not be used to influence clinical decision-making.

13. SUGGESTED FURTHER READING

Textbooks

Clinical Intensive Care, Hillman and Bishop, 1996, Cambridge
Handbook of Drugs in Intensive Care, Paw and Park, 2000, Greenwich M M
Handbook of ICU Therapy, McConachie, 1999, Greenwich Medical Media
Intensive Care Manual, T E OH, 1997, Butterworth Heinemann
Intensive Care: A Concise Textbook, Hinds and Watson, 1996, Saunders
Imaging in Anaesthesia and Critical Care, Hobbs and Mahajan, 2000, Churchill Livingstone
Key Topics in Critical Care, Craft Nolan and Parr, 1999, Bios
Textbook of Intensive Care, Goldhill and Withington, 1997, Chapman and Hall
The ICU Book, Marino, 1998, Williams and Wilkins

Reference books

Anaesthesia and Intensive Care A to Z, Yentis, Hirsch and Smith, 2000, BH
Oxford Textbook of Critical Care, Webb, Shapiro, Singer and Suter, 1999

Study Aids

Critical Care Cases, Armstrong and Salmon, 1997, Oxford

Courses

Care of the Critically Ill Surgical Patient, CCrISP, Royal College of Surgeons of England
Textbook for the course:
Anderson Care of the Critically Ill Surgical Patient, Arnold. 1999
Fundamentals of Critical Care Support, FCCS, Society Critical Care Medicine.
An American course run under licence in the UK.
Advanced Life Support Course. ALS. Resuscitation Council UK.

Chapter 5

Neoplasia

CONTENTS

Neoplasia

1. PRINCIPLES OF ONCOLOGY

1.1 Epidemiology and cancer registries

The study of disease frequency in populations.

Prevalence: proportion of population with a condition at a given time.
Incidence: proportion of population developing a condition in a given time.
Risk factor: an agent or characteristic predisposing to the development of a condition.
Relative risk: strength of association between risk factor and condition.
Disease-free survival: an outcome measure in oncology for the time period from diagnosis to detection of recurrence.
Life table: a calculation predicting the cumulative probability of surviving a given number of years e.g. five year survival rate.
Survival curve: plot of probability of survival against time, e.g. Kaplan-Meier curve.
Cancer registries: registries set up to monitor the incidence and mortality of various cancers in the population, and determine any changes in these parameters.

e.g. information from death certificates is collated by the national cancer registry in England and Wales and followed up by case note analysis, post mortem diagnoses etc. Statistical information from cancer registries should be viewed with caution due to potential errors from differences in accuracy of data collection, geographical variations in diagnosis rates and post mortem rates etc.

1.2 Disorders of growth

Hyperplasia

This is an increase in the number of cells. The cells mature to normal size and shape. It can occur in response to inflammation, increased workload, excess endocrine drive, or increased metabolic demand, for example:

331

- Benign prostatic hyperplasia
- Renal hyperplasia (in response to contralateral dysfunction)

Hypertrophy

This is an increase in cell size but not in number. It occurs in response to a demand for increased function, for example:

- Increased skeletal muscle volume in athletes
- Increased cardiac muscle volume in hypertension
- Pregnant uterus

NB. Both hyperplasia and hypertrophy can occur simultaneously.

Metaplasia

This is the reversible replacement of one differentiated cell type with another. It is an adaptive response and the replacement cells are of the same tissue type. It can be due to chronic irritation or altered cell function. There is greater susceptibility to neoplastic transformation (via dysplasia) but it is not inevitable (e.g. squamous epithelium changing to gastric type in the distal oesophagus – Barrett's oesophagus).

Dysplasia

This is disordered cellular development characterised by increased mitosis and pleomorphism. This is frequently pre-neoplastic and it may follow metaplasia.

Hamartoma

This is the overgrowth of mature cells which are usually found within the tissue but with disordered architecture (e.g. haemangioma).

Teratoma

This is a growth of cells originating from more than one germ cell line. Teratomas contain a variety of tissues in a variable state of differentiation. They arise in the gonads or the midline of the body (e.g. mediastinum, retro peritoneum, base of skull). They can behave in a benign or malignant manner.

Neoplasia

Abnormal mass of tissue, the growth of which is uncoordinated and exceeds that of the normal tissues and persists in the same manner after the cessation of the stimuli which evoked the change.

The cell cycle

Phases of neoplasia

- **G1:** pre-synthetic
- **S:** DNA synthesis
- **G2:** pre-mitotic
- **M:** mitotic
- **GO:** quiescent (resting phase)

Labile cells

These are cells which are constantly renewed (e.g. stratified squamous epithelium of the skin).

Stable cells

These cells are usually quiescent but can be stimulated to divide (e.g. hepatocytes).

Permanent cells

These cells do not undergo mitosis in post-natal life (e.g. neurones, skeletal muscle tissues, glomeruli).

1.3 Naming, grading and staging

- **Benign neoplasms**
  Expansile, usually slow growing
  Don't metastasise
  Low mitotic rate, little pleomorphism
  Normal chromosome numbers
  Necrosis and haemorrhage unusual

- **Malignant neoplasms**
  Infiltrative, irregular or fast growth rate
  May metastasise
  Pleomorphic, frequent mitotic figures
  Abnormal chromosome numbers
  Necrosis and haemorrhage may occur

Naming

Neoplasms are named according to whether they arise from **epithelium** or **stroma**.

Epithelial neoplasms

Adenoma: benign epithelial neoplasm forming a glandular pattern or arising from a gland but not necessarily forming a glandular pattern.

Papilloma: benign epithelial neoplasm protruding from a surface which produces finger-like fronds made up of connective tissue processes covered by epithelial cells

Cystadenoma: benign epithelial neoplasm arising from duct or gland epithelium with secretion and distension of the lumen due to lack of drainage

Carcinoma: a malignant epithelial neoplasm

Mesenchymal neoplasms

These are named according to cell type:

- **-oma**: if benign (e.g. lipoma)
- **-sarcoma**: if malignant (e.g. osteosarcoma)

Naming of neoplasms

Cell of origin	Benign	Malignant
Epithelium		
Squamous	Squamous cell papilloma	Squamous cell carcinoma
Transitional	Transitional cell papilloma	Transitional cell carcinoma
Columnar	Adenoma or papilloma or cystadenoma	Adenocarcinoma Cystadenocarcinoma
Stromal		
Blood vessel	Haemangioma	Haemangiosarcoma
Lymph vessel	Lymphangioma	Lymphangiosarcoma
Fibrous tissue	Fibroma	Fibrosarcoma
Smooth muscle	Leiomyoma	Leiomyosarcoma
Striated muscle	Rhabdomyoma	Rhabdomyosarcoma
Cartilage	Chondroma	Chondrosarcoma
Bone	Osteoma	Osteosarcoma
Complex cell origin		
Lymphoid		Lymphoma
Haemopoietic cells		Leukaemia
Plasma cells		Multiple myeloma
Embryonic tissue		Blastoma (e.g. nephroblastoma, hepatoblastoma, retinoblastoma)
Specialised		
Breast	Fibroadenoma	Ductal or lobular carcinoma
Melanocytes	Naevus	Malignant melanoma
Mesothelium	Benign mesothelioma	Malignant mesothelioma
Salivary gland	Pleomorphic adenoma	Carcinoma arising in a pleomorphic adenoma

NB. These are just a few examples.

Tumour grading

This is an assessment of the degree of differentiation of a tumour and corresponds to the aggressive behaviour of the tumour. Tumours are graded as:

- Well differentiated
- Moderately differentiated
- Poorly/undifferentiated/anaplastic

(but many different grading systems exist for different tumours).

Differentiation refers to the degree to which neoplastic cells resemble their tissue of origin. Features of poor differentiation are:

- Increased nuclear pleomorphism
- Atypical mitoses
- Hyperchromatic nuclei
- Increased nuclear:cytoplasmic size ratio
- Giant cells may be present

Tumour grading is important for prediction of behaviour and prognosis.

Tumour staging

This refers to the size and spread of the neoplasm as assessed by clinician, pathologist or radiologist. Used for decisions on management and prognosis.

Examples   Dukes' classification for colorectal carcinoma
Clarke's classification for malignant melanoma
TNM (tumour, node, metastasis) system

The TNM classification was first developed by the American Joint Committee on Cancer Staging and End Result Reporting and has now been modified for systems for most solid tumours.

e.g. breast, colon, thyroid

T = primary tumour	T_0	no primary tumour
	T_{is}	in situ primary tumour
	T_x	unknown primary
	T_{1-4}	sizes of primary tumour
N = nodal metastasis	N_0	no nodes
	N_1	few node(s)
	N_{2-3}	relates to number, fixity, or distant lymph node group involvement
M = distant metastasis	M_0	no metastasis
	M_1	distant metastasis present

1.4 Carcinogenesis

This arises from genetic mutation or damage to a single cell (monoclonal cell theory), or from a defect inherited in the germ cell line. Knudson's two-hit hypothesis of 1974 states that both normal alleles of Rb gene on chromosome 13q14 had to be lost before retinoblastoma developed.

Therefore, this implies that tumours are monoclonal. There are four classes of genes that can be affected to produce a neoplasm:

- **Growth-promoting proto-oncogenes**: up-regulated by mutation to oncogene
- **Growth-inhibiting cancer suppressor genes (anti-oncogenes)**: down-regulated by mutation
- **Genes regulating programmed cell death (apoptosis)**: down-regulated by mutation
- **DNA repair genes**: excise mutated gene segments; are down-regulated in neoplasia

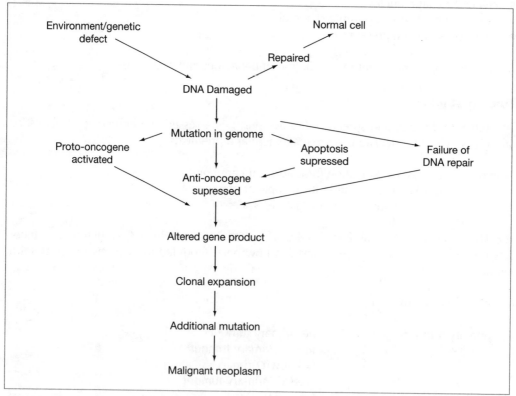

Overview of carcinogenesis

Gene	Associated malignancy
Proto-oncogenes	*Oncogenes*
Nuclear regulatory proteins	
myc Burkitt's lymphoma	
N-myc	Neuroblastoma
L-myc	Small cell carcinoma of lung
Signal transduction	
ras Lung, colon, pancreas, leukaemia	
abl Chronic myeloid leukaemia	
(c-abl – Philadelphia chromosome)	Acute lymphoblastic leukaemia
Growth factors	
sis Astrocytoma	
hst-1 Osteosarcoma	
int-2 Gastric cancer	
Bladder cancer	
Breast cancer	
Growth factor inhibitors	
Erb B1	Gliomas
Erb B2	Breast, ovary, stomach
ret Medullary carcinoma of thyroid	
Tumour suppressor genes	
E-cadherin	Stomach carcinoma
APC	Familial adenomatous polyposis coli
	Colon
	Stomach, pancreas
DCC	Stomach, colon, pancreas
NF1	Neurofibromatosis, sarcomas & schwannomas
NF2	Meningiomas, schwannomas
	Neurofibromatosis type II
	Acoustic neuromas
p53	Approximately 50% of human cancers
	Osteosarcoma
	Breast
	Glioma
	Li-Fraumeni syndrome
Rb	Retinoblastoma
	Osteosarcoma
WT-1	Wilms' tumour
DNA repair genes	
Msh-2	Hereditary non-polyposis colon cancer
Genes regulating apoptosis	
bcl-2	B-cell lymphoma

1.5 Carcinogens

These can be divided into:

- Chemical
- Physical
- Oncogenic viruses, bacteria, protozoa

Carcinogens (historical and contemporary)

Carcinogen	Associated carcinoma	
Chemical		
B-naphthamine	Bladder	(e.g. dye workers)
Benzopyrene	Lung	(painters, printers
Aflatoxin	Hepatocellular	(peanut farmers)
Asbestos	Mesothelioma	(builders, shippers)
Chromium	)	
Arsenic	) Lung carcinoma	(miners, smelters)
Nickel	)	
Vinyl chloride monomers	Angiosarcoma of liver	
Diethyl stilbestrol	Adenocarcinoma of the vagina	
Benzol/Benzene	Blood and lymphatic cancers	
Nitrates	Gastric cancer	
Physical		
UV light	Melanoma (esp UVB)	
	Squamous cell carcinoma	
	Basal cell carcinoma	
Ionising radiation	Leukaemia (blood)	(radium workers)
	Bone	
	Breast	
	Thyroid	
	Skin, tongue, tonsil	
Viruses, bacteria and protozoa		
Human immunodeficiency virus	Leukaemias, lymphomas, Kaposi sarcoma	
Hepatitis B & C	Hepatocellular carcinoma	
Epstein–Barr virus	Nasopharyngeal carcinoma, B-cell	
	Burkitt's lymphoma, Hodgkin's lymphoma	
Human papilloma virus (16 & 18)	Cervical cancer	
Helicobacter pylori	Gastric cancer	
Schistosoma	Squamous cell carcinoma of the bladder	

1.6 Natural history of a typical malignant tumour

Neoplastic transformation of a cell
Clonal expansion
Local invasion
Distant spread

Formation of tumour depends on the following:

Speed of tumour cell growth

- **Doubling time of tumour cells**: cells can be pushed into the cell cycle more easily
- **Growth fraction**: this is the proportion of cells within the tumour cell population that are in the replicative pools; cells continue to leave the replicative pools; most cells are not in the replicative pool at the time of detection; growth fraction is 20% even in rapidly growing tumours.
- **Cell loss and production**: growth depends on balance between production and loss

Clinical application

- **Latent period**: accumulation of cells is slow therefore it can take several years for a single cell to proliferate into a clinically detectable mass.
- **Chemotherapy**: chemotherapeutics are most effective on cycling cells; tumours with a high growth fraction are more susceptible to antinuclear agents; debulking tumours or radiation pushes more cells into the cell cycle.

Tumour angiogenesis

- Formation of new blood vessels
- Required when tumour is more than 1–2 mm in diameter
- Angiogenic factors are secreted by tumour cells and macrophages: fibroblast growth factor; vascular endothelial growth factor; tumour necrosis factor α (from macrophages); transforming growth factor α.

Factors inhibiting angiogenesis

- Angiostatin
- Thrombostatin
- Transforming growth factor β

Tumour progression

Some tumours become more aggressive with time. This produces a heterogeneous group of cells despite their monoclonal origin.

1.7 Invasion and metastasis

Invasion can be:

- Direct e.g. direct invasion of bladder from adenocarcinoma of the sigmoid colon
- Transcoelomic e.g. ovary
- Lymphatic e.g. axillary nodes from Ca breast
- Haematogenous e.g. bone metastases from follicular carcinoma of the thyroid

Mechanisms of invasion

Loss of cell-to-cell adhesion

- E-cadherin is the major cell adhesion molecule in epithelia; these are down-regulated in several carcinomas
- Integrins bind epithelial cells to the basement membrane; loss of integrins is associated with increased metastatic potential.

Migration through the interstitium and invasion of vessels

- Increased motility of cells: hepatocyte growth factor
- Cell adhesion to basement membrane: in normal epithelial cells laminin receptors are expressed on one side of the cell and bind to laminin on the basement membrane; tumour cells have increased numbers of laminin receptors on all sides
- Protease secretion: these break down the extracellular matrix (e.g. metallo-proteinases (also stimulate angiogenesis))

Dissemination in the circulation

- Malignant cells avoid detection by decreased expression of MHC-1
- They also shed ICAM-I molecules which interact with cytotoxic T-cell receptors stopping their destruction

Extravasation

- Cells attach to the vessel wall and migrate through it (e.g. increased expression of integrin VLA-4 in melanoma); reduced expression of *nm23* gene is associated with increased metastases of breast cancer, but its mechanism of action is unknown.

Establishment of metastasis

- This is poorly understood
- Requires blood supply, i.e. angiogenesis occurs

Common patterns of metastasis

Site of metastasis	Possible primary source
Liver	GI
	Pancreas
	Lung
	Breast
	GU
	Malignant melanoma
Skeletal	Lung
	Breast
	Prostate (osteosclerotic)
	Kidney
	Thyroid
Brain	Lung
	Malignant melanoma
Adrenal	Lung
	Breast
Trans-coelomic	Stomach
	Colon
	Ovary
Lung	Kidney
	Breast
	Colorectal
	Ovary

1.8 Tumour markers

These are substances in the blood whose presence may be useful in monitoring of specific cancers. Includes

- Enzymes
- Hormones
- Oncofetal antigens

Useful in diagnosis, staging, treatment and detection of recurrence.

PSA (prostatic specific antigen)

- A prostatic epithelial protein
- Elevated if >4 ng/dL (in general)
- Used in conjunction with digital rectal examination, transrectal sonography and needle biopsy for 'screening', diagnosis and monitoring of treatment of prostatic cancer
- It is also elevated in benign prostatic hyperplasia, prostatitis, prostatic infarction, urinary retention, instrumentation and even ejaculation
- Thought *not* to rise significantly following rectal examination
- PSA velocity measures rate of change of PSA with time (>0.75 ng/dL/year suggests malignancy)
- PSA density compares PSA value with volume of prostate (>0.15 suggests malignancy)
- Age-related PSA (older patients have a higher 'normal' cut-off)
- Free-total PSA ratio (<25% suggests malignancy)

CEA (carcinoembryonic antigen)

- An oncofetal antigen, normally expressed in embryonic gut, liver, pancreas
- Elevated in colorectal carcinoma in 60–90% of cases
- May also be elevated in ovarian and breast carcinoma
- Also occasionally elevated in cirrhosis, alcoholic hepatitis, inflammatory bowel disease, pancreatitis
- Not specific or sensitive enough to be used as a screening tool
- Used to monitor efficacy of therapy and detection of recurrence

Alpha-fetoprotein

- An embryonic antigen
- Elevated in carcinoma of liver (also in cirrhosis, chronic hepatitis, normal pregnancy, fetal neural tube defects)
- Also elevated in non-seminomatous germ cell tumours of the testes (NSGCT)

b-hCG (human chorionic gonadotrophin)

- A hormone
- Elevated in pregnancy
- Elevated in choriocarcinoma, NSGCT and in 7% of seminomas where syncytiotrophoblastic elements are present

CA 125

- For non-mucinous ovarian cancers
- A high concentration is more likely to be associated with malignancy
- Can be used to monitor therapy
- Can be raised in other conditions (e.g. pancreatitis, endometriosis, breast and pancreatic carcinomas)

CA 15–3

- A glycoprotein, occasionally elevated in breast carcinoma

CA 19–9

- A glycoprotein sometimes elevated in pancreatic and advanced colorectal carcinoma

Thyroglobulin

- Elevated in some thyroid carcinomas

Calcitonin

- Elevated in medullary thyroid carcinoma

ACTH/ADH

- Elevated in some small cell lung carcinomas

2. CLINICAL FEATURES OF COMMON CANCERS

2.1 Gastric

Epidemiology

- Peak incidence is 55–65 years
- Male to Female ratio is 2:1
- Occurs more commonly in the lower social classes
- High incidence in Japan (but decreases in second-generation Japanese migrants)
- Represents 90% of gastric cancers
- Second commonest cause of cancer deaths world-wide.
- Annual mortality 7000

Risk factors

Interstitial type

- Diet
  - Nitrates (smoked food and fish)
  - High salt intake
  - Low vitamin intake (A, C, E)
  - Low fruit and vegetable intake
- *Helicobacter pylori*
- Pernicious anaemia
- After sub-total distal gastrectomy
- Family history

- Chronic gastritis
- Ulcers, polyps

Diffuse type

- Blood group A

Morphology

Location

- Pylorus and antrum: 50–60%
- Cardia: 25%
- Body and fundus: remainder

Macroscopic

- Exophytic: tumour mass extends into lumen
- Flat: no obvious tumour mass within the mucosa
- Excavated
- Linitis plastica (leather bottle stomach): extensive infiltration of large area or entire stomach

Microscopic (Lauren classification)

- Intestinal type: malignant cells forming neoplastic intestinal glands resembling those of colonic adenocarcinoma
- Diffuse type: malignant cells are gastric type mucous cells which permeate the mucosa as scattered 'signet-ring' cells or small clusters in an infiltrative pattern; occur in younger patients.

Spread

- Local and regional lymph nodes
- Supraclavicular node (Virchow's node, Troisier's sign – *left*)
- Transcoelomic (e.g. ovaries – Krukenberg tumour)
- Liver

Clinical features of gastric cancer

- Anorexia
- Weight loss
- Vomiting
- Increasing satiety
- Indigestion
- Dyspepsia
- Anaemia
- Succussion splash
- Perforation
- Hepatomegaly
- Troisier's sign
- Ascites
- Jaundice

- They can be present within perforated or bleeding ulcers
- Most patients present late

Diagnosis

- Upper GI endoscopy: biopsy or brush cytology of suspicious areas
- US + CT/laparoscopy: used for assessing disease advancement, i.e. lymph node involvement and liver metastases

Staging

Nodes
    Supra/infra pyloric
    R+L cardiac
    Greater or lesser curves
    Those at origin and along arterial supply
N_1 – all nodes are within 3 cm of primary;
N_2 – all nodes mentioned above which are >3 cm from primary.

Treatment

Radical gastrectomy with Roux-en-Y loop (gastrectomy with radical lymph node dissection).

Complications of gastrectomy (occur in >20%):

- Diarrhoea
- Biliary reflux
- Anaemia – B12 and Fe deficiency
- Malnutrition
- Dumping syndrome

Dumping syndrome

Lack of pylorus
↓
No controlled release of digesting load into small bowel
↓
Large osmotic load
↓
Fluid absorbed into bowel lumen (diarrhoea)
↓
Hypovolaemia
↓
Collapse
↓
Absorption of large quantities of glucose into bloodstream
↓
Large amount of insulin secreted
↓
Post-prandial (approx 2 h) hypoglycaemia

Prognosis

- Most are detected at an advanced stage in the UK
- In UK, five-year survival is 5–10%

Gastric lymphoma

- Accounts for 4% of gastric malignancies
- Occurs at 50–60 years of age. It is the most common site for GI lymphoma.

Clinical features

- Anaemia
- Abdominal pain
- Perforation
- Haemorrhage

Arise from B cells.

Treatment
Surgical resection, chemotherapy.

Carcinoid tumour

Accounts for 3% of gastric malignancies
Tumour of gut neuroendocrine cells.
May be asymptomatic.
May secrete gastrin, ACTH, insulin, 5–HT (carcinoid syndrome – if liver metastases present).

Treatment
Resection.

2.2 Oesophagus

Epidemiology and aetiology

Most patients are middle aged or elderly with a male to female ratio of 2.5:1.

Squamous cell carcinomas may arise from any part of the oesophagus.

Alcohol and tobacco are the main risk factors.

World-wide variations such as Northern China, Kazakhstan, areas of southern Africa and Iran have much higher incidences (>35/100,000 whereas Europe and USA 2–8/100,000).

Other lesser risk factors include: diet, achalasia, coeliac disease, caustic stricture and hereditary tylosis.

Adenocarcinoma is now the most common (65%) and incidence is rising faster than any other solid organ cancer (5% per year).

Adenocarcinomas occur mainly in the lower third of the oesophagus, and oesophagogastric junction.

Believed to arise from areas of dysplasia in Barrett's oesophagus

Barrett's oesophagus

Barrett's oesophagus was first described in 1950 and is the replacement of the normal squamous epithelium of the lower third of the oesophagus with columnar epithelium (metaplasia). It can progress to dysplasia and adenocarcinoma.

It is due to GORD and about 10% of patients with GORD develop Barrett's. Of these 1% develop adenocarcinoma per year. There is a 30 fold increased risk of developing a malignancy. Bile reflux is thought to be an important contributing factor.

Management consists of life-long acid suppression, but there is limited evidence to show that there is any regression of the metaplasia. At present there is controversy about the benefits of endoscopic surveillance of patients with Barrett's. However, it is known that the 5–year survival after resection of adenocarcinomas detected by surveillance is greater than 95%.

Clinical features
Progressive dysphagia, initially solids, but progressing to fluids.

Weight loss and wasting are common.

Uncommon presentations include cervical node, left recurrent laryngeal nerve palsy and overspill respiratory complications.

Patients with early disease often have no clinical signs.

Diagnosis
Endoscopy is the investigation of choice, as biopsies can be taken. Many are diagnosed at routine endoscopy for reflux type symptoms.

Staging
Once the diagnosis has been made the stage and spread of the cancer is assessed initially by CT of the thorax and abdomen. If this does not show inoperable or metastatic disease, endoscopic ultrasound is used to stage tumour depth, and less effectively, local lymph node spread. There is little benefit of further investigation after CT if the tumour is inoperable.

Tumour (T)	Nodes (N)	Metastasis (M)	Stage
is	0	0	0
1	0	0	1
2–3	0	0	2a
1–2	1	0	2b
3–4	1	0	3
Any	Any	1	4

Treatment

Surgery

- Only 40% of tumours are resectable, the operative mortality is 5%
- There are a number of procedures including:
  - Ivor-Lewis two-stage and McKeown three-stage (with thoracotomy)
  - Ong Transhiatal (without thoracotomy)
  - Thoraco-abdominal oesophago-gastrectomy with jejunal reconstruction
- Post-operative nutrition is given via a feeding jejunostomy, which is sited at the time of operation

Chemotherapy

- Adenocarcinomas of the oesophagus are not radiosensitive
- MRC multicentre trial has shown that neoadjuvant chemotherapy with 5FU and cisplatin prior to surgery confers a survival benefit over surgery alone

Palliation

- Stenting may be performed either radiologically or endoscopically. Self expanding covered metal stents have now mainly replaced the traditional rigid tubes. Middle and lower third tumours are more successfully stented than upper third.
- Exophytic tumours are most suitable to endoscopic laser therapy, where effective recanalisation of the lumen is produced, with good swallowing
- Radiotherapy can be used to reduce pain and dysphagia, but is of limited use in larger tumours

Outcome

Less than 40% of patients are suitable for surgery and 70% of these have lymph node involvement. Patients with stage 1 disease have a 5 year survival of >80%. However for stage 2b and 3 the 5–year survival is 10%. With palliation alone, the median survival is only 4 months.

2.3 Pancreas

Epidemiology and aetiology

- Pancreatic carcinoma is a common (10/100,000) highly malignant tumour of the acinar cells of the exocrine pancreas. The incidence is rising and also increases with age. The male to female ratio is 2:1.
- The main risk factor is smoking, however diabetes and high dietary fat intakes are also implicated
- 60% are in the head of the gland and there is frequent obstruction of CBD. There is rapid spread to draining lymph nodes.
- Usually adenocarcinoma

Clinical features

- Classically there is painless jaundice, however 50% of patients experience epigastric pain. Back pain is a sign of poorer prognosis as it suggests invasion into the prevertebral structures.
- If there is obstruction of the pancreatic duct then patients may present with pancreatitis
- May invade the duodenum leading to symptoms of gastric outlet obstruction
- Anorexia and weight loss is present in 90% of patients
- 75% already have metastasis at presentation

Diagnosis

- Ultrasound and duplex ultrasound have a sensitivity of 85% and can also help in the assessment of vascular involvement
- Spiral CT has over 95% sensitivity for detection of tumour. However the distinction between carcinoma and chronic pancreatitis can be difficult.
- Biopsies can be performed either by US or CT guidance
- ERCP to obtain cytological samples by brushings
- Laparoscopy can pick up many small peritoneal and liver metastases missed by US or CT scanning. Laparoscopic ultrasound can help to ascertain suitability of resection.

Treatment

Curative surgery

- Resection is only hope of cure – but only 15% are resectable (tumours <2cm without liver or lymphatic spread)
- Whipple's procedure is performed for tumours in the head, and distal pancreatectomy with splenectomy for those in the tail

Whipple's procedure consists of:
Cholecystectomy and choledochojejunostomy
End to side pancreaticojejunostomy
Gastrojejunostomy

Palliation

- Surgical palliation is in the form of biliary bypass, (loop cholecystojejunostomy or choledochojejunostomy) and duodenal bypass by an antecolic gastrojejunostomy
- Stenting can be performed endoscopically in 95% of patients, and has a low mortality. They are useful in relieving obstructive jaundice.
- Plastic stents do require regular changing as they become blocked after 3–4 months, or they can migrate
- Adequate analgesia, as pancreatic carcinoma is notoriously painful

Outcome

The mean survival after diagnosis is just 6 months without resection.
Whipple's procedure has an operative mortality of 5%, and the overall 5–year survival is just 5% following resection. Tumours of the ampulla that present earlier have a 15% 5–year mortality.

2.4 Colorectal

Epidemiology

- Peak incidence 60–70 years
- More common in developed countries
- 1–3% associated with FAP
- Ulcerative colitis
- Second most common cancer death in the UK in males and the third in females
- Equal incidence in males and females

Risk factors

- Diet: low roughage diet; high carbohydrate intake; high fat intake; low vitamin A, C, E intake, high meat intake
- Family history
- Familial adenomatous polyposis coli (Chr 5q21)
- Gardner's syndrome
- Hereditary non-polyposis colorectal carcinoma
- Genes: K-ras (Chr 12p12), p53 (Chr 17)
- Ulcerative colitis

Morphology

- 98% adenocarcinomas
- May produce mucin (poorer prognosis)

Distribution

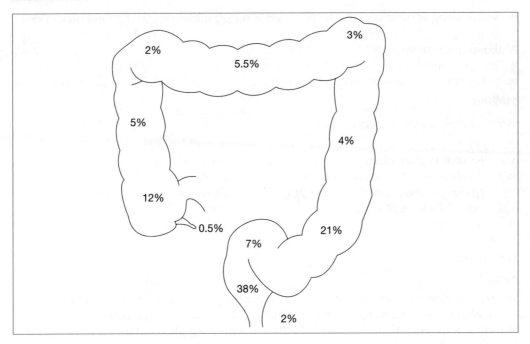

Distribution of colorectal carcinoma

Clinical features

- Altered bowel habit
- Per rectum bleeding/mucus
- Abdominal distension/obstruction
- Weight loss
- Iron deficiency anaemia
- Tenesmus
- Back pain and sciatica
- Perforation
- Fistula formation

Thirty per cent of people present as an emergency. Twenty per cent of people have metastases at the time of presentation.

Diagnosis

- Colonoscopy
- Barium enema and rigid sigmoidoscopy
- Chest and liver must be imaged to exclude metastasis, US or CXR
- CT and MRI scans of the pelvis can be used for staging

Spread

- Nodes along vessels: superior rectal; inferior rectal; middle rectal; internal iliac nodes (rare)
- Blood: liver; pulmonary
- Transperitoneal

Staging

Modified Duke's classification

		5–year survival
A	Limited to muscularis	90–100%
B	Involves serosa, or extra-rectal tissue	75%
C1	Nodes positive, apical node negative	50–75%
C2	Apical node positive	25%
D	Metastases	0%

Treatment

Colon

Surgery – remove primary and local and regional lymph nodes (with blood supply):
Caecum/ascending colon: right hemicolectomy with end-to-end anastomosis
Hepatic flexure: resection extended to halfway down descending colon
Transverse colon: excise right and transverse colons, splenic flexure, greater omentum, end-to-end anastomosis
Carcinoma of splenic proximal descending colon: excise transverse colon, flexures and halves of the ascending and descending colon; end-to-end anastomosis
Sigmoid colon: descending colon to upper third of rectum, anastomosis

Rectum

Those tumours which are less than 15 cm from the anal verge on rigid sigmoidoscopy: Abdomino-perineal (AP) resection or anterior resection (if 1 cm distal clearance can be achieved with total mesorectal excision)
Emergency surgery: for obstruction or perforation; remove carcinoma – Hartmann's procedure or primary anastomosis – subtotal colectomy with ileosigmoid or ileorectal anastomosis

Oncological therapies

Chemotherapy: Duke's A tumours do not require chemotherapy. As yet no firm evidence for chemotherapy in Duke's B, at present either taken on an individual basis or part of a multi-centre trial. For Duke's C tumours 5–fluorouracil (5FU) ± folinic acid. The UK QUASAR trial however did not show any benefit conferred by the addition of folinic acid or levamisole for Duke's C tumours. The second arm of QUASAR looks at the 'uncertain indications' for chemotherapy. (QUASAR stands for Quick and Simple and Reliable).

Pre-operative radiotherapy: can downstage tumour. Trials have shown that there is a decrease in local recurrence, but there is only one trial (Swedish rectal cancer trial) that shows that this confers a survival benefit. There is an MRC trial (CR07) to address this question further.

Post-operative radiotherapy: is offered to patients with a high risk of recurrence. Trials have shown reduced recurrence, but no survival benefits. Unresectable tumours have high dose radiotherapy with or without chemotherapy. This neoadjuvant chemotherapy can downstage a tumour and allows a potentially curative operation to be performed.

Liver metastases

50% of patients with colorectal cancer develop hepatic metastasis.
The median survival is one year without hepatic resection.
Ultrasound or CT scan can detect liver metastases. Serial tumour marker levels can monitor progress (e.g. CEA).

Hepatic resection is the only chance of cure, but only 10% of patients with metastases are suitable for resection.

Criteria for resection are:

- Single lobe involvement
- Less than three lesions
- No IVC invasion
- At least 20% of the liver spared

2.5 Lung

Epidemiology

- Most common cancer death in men and women in UK
- 228.5/100,000 deaths in men
- 63/100,000 deaths in women

Risk factors

- Cigarette smoking
- Asbestos exposure
- Radon exposure
- Male sex

Histological classification

Squamous cell carcinoma

- 50% of lung cancers
- Most found in larger bronchi
- Metastasise to hilar, mediastinal or supraclavicular lymph nodes
- Spread to brain and bone

Adenocarcinoma

- 5–15% of lung cancer
- Often lesions are located peripherally
- Metastasise to distant sites more often than squamous cell
- Spread to liver, brain, bone, adrenals

Large cell carcinoma

Two types:
- Giant cell tumour (aggressive)
- Clear cell carcinomas (less common benign behaviour)

Small cell carcinomas (oat cell carcinomas)

- 20% of lung cancers
- Often disseminated at time of presentation
- Often presents with systemic symptoms because 15% of patients have paraneoplastic syndromes
- Staged according to whether disease is limited, i.e. confined to one ipsilateral hemithorax, ipsilateral or contralateral mediastinal or supraclavicular node involvement, ipsilateral pleural effusion, extensive (beyond)

Staging

TNM classification		
T_x	:	occult cancer
T_{IS}	:	carcinoma *in situ*
T_1	:	<3 cm diameter, completely surrounded by lung parenchyma
T_2	:	>3 cm, invasion of pleura, invasion of main bronchus; >2 cm from carina, atelectasis extending to hilar region
T_3	:	extrapulmonary extension of primary tumour with limited involvement of parietal or mediastinal pleura, fat or pericardium
T_4	:	extensive extension involving the mediastinal structures, great vessels or vertebral bodies
Nodes		
N_0	:	no regional nodes
N_1	:	intrapulmonary lymph nodes
N_2	:	ipsilateral mediastinal or hilar nodes
N_3	:	contralateral mediastinal or hilar nodes; scalene/supraclavicular nodes on either side
Metastases		
M_0	:	no metastases/extrathoracic lymph node involvement
M_1	:	metastases

STAGE GROUPING

Stage	TNM	Prognosis
Stage 0	T_{IS}	
Stage I	$T_1 N_0 M_0, T_2 N_0 M_0$	60–85% five-year survival
Stage II	$T_1 N_1 M_0, T_2 N_1 M_0$	
Stage IIIa	$T_1 N_2 M_0, T_2 N_2 M_0, T_3 N_2 M_0$ $T_3 N_0 M_0, T_3 N_1 M_0$	40% one-year survival
Stage IIIb	$T_4 N_0 M_0, T_4 N_1 M_0, T_4 N_2 M_0$ $T_1 N_3 M_0, T_2 N_3 M_0, T_3 N_3 M_0$ $T_4 N_3 M_0$	10% five-year survival
Stage IV	M_1	15% one-year survival

Clinical features

- Cough ± haemoptysis
- Weight loss
- Dyspnoea
- Chest pain
- Lymphadenopathy
- Hoarseness
- Loss of power in arm
- Pancoast tumour (NB. Horner's syndrome)
- Bone pain
- Finger clubbing

Diagnosis

- CXR: masses, effusion, osteolytic lesions, raised hemidiaphragm
- CT
- Sputum cytology with bronchoscopy
- Percutaneous transthoracic needle biopsy: peripheral and some hilar and mediastinal lesions
- Mediastinoscopy: for lymph node sampling, for pre-op staging

Pre-op assessment

ECG

Stage:
CT
Bronchoscopy
PFTs

Management

Small cell lung cancer

Combination chemotherapy (etoposide and cisplatin, cyclophosphamide, doxorubicin and vincristine)

Five-year survival: limited disease 10–20%, extensive disease 1–3%

Non-small cell disease

Aim for complete resection

Lobectomy (mortality 2%)

Pneumonectomy (mortality 5–6%) indicated when lobectomy will not completely remove the tumour, or spread to lobar or hilar lymph nodes

Segmentectomy for small peripheral lesions (<2 cm)

Complications of surgery

- Atelectasis
- Pneumonia
- Bronchopleural fistula
- Empyema
- Haemothorax
- Cardiac dysrhythmia
- PE/MI

Therapeutic options

- Radiotherapy – palliative
- Laser therapy
- Endobronchial prosthetic stent devices for very advanced disease

Surgery indicated in T_1, T_2 and some T_3 tumours with N_1 and N_2 nodes. Not in N_3, M_1, disease.

2.6 Thyroid

Thyroid – benign

Follicular adenomas

Diagnosis can only be made histologically NOT by cytology (FNAC).

Hypothyroidism makes malignancy very unlikely.

Treatment

Lobectomy, if adenocarcinoma is shown histologically then completion thyroidectomy is indicated.

Thyroid – malignant

Epidemiology

- 4 per 100,000
- <1% of cancer deaths
- Most common in middle age
- Women affected more than men in middle age (F:M = 3:1)
- At extremes of age there is equal sex incidence

Risk factors

- Family history (medullary)
- Radiotherapy in childhood with radioactive iodine (papillary)
- Iodine deficiency goitre
- Autoimmune thyroiditis (lymphomas)

Clinical features

- Thyroid swelling
- Enlarged cervical nodes
- Hoarse voice – recurrent laryngeal nerve palsy

Diagnosis

- Ultrasound and FNAC

Pathology

- Papillary   75–85%
- Follicular   10–20%
- Anaplastic   5%
- Medullary   5%
- Lymphoma   <5%

Histological classification

Papillary carcinoma
- Tumour of follicular cells
- Can be solitary or multifocal
- Ground glass or 'Orphan Annie' (clear) nuclei
- Lymph node involvement in 1/3 of cases

Follicular carcinoma
- Tumour of follicular cells
- Hurthle cells (abundant cytoplasm)
- Equal sex incidence
- More malignant than papillary carcinoma
- Spreads to bone, lung, liver

Anaplastic carcinoma
- Older patients
- More women
- Rapidly growing
- 20% survival after 1 year

Medullary carcinoma
- C-cell tumour
- Familial (MEN) or sporadic
- Spindle-shaped cells
- Solitary or multiple
- May have amyloid deposits

Management

Papillary: total thyroidectomy; thyroxine to suppress TSH; secondaries – node picking; 90% ten-year survival
Follicular: surgical – total thyroidectomy and thyroxine therapy as above
Anaplastic: palliative debulking surgery; palliative radiotherapy
Medullary: look for phaeochromocytoma/MEN; surgery – total thyroidectomy; six-year survival = 50%

Complications of thyroidectomy

- Haemorrhage
- Recurrent laryngeal nerve palsy – 0.2%; indirect laryngoscopy prior to surgery
- Superior laryngeal nerve palsy – loss of pitch
- Hypoparathyroidism
- Hypothyroidism and hypocalcaemia
- Thyrotoxic crisis

2.7 Multiple Endocrine Neoplasia (MEN)

Familial autosomal dominant disorder. Disorder of amine precursor uptake and decarboxy-lation cells (APUD cells).

MEN Type I – Werner's syndrome
Tumours of:

- Pituitary adenoma 65%
- Pancreatic islets 80%
- Hyperplasia of parathyroid 90%
- Adrenal cortex

It is inherited in an autosomal dominant pattern with complete penetrance, however it may occur sporadically.

MEN Type II

Genetic screening is now used in the diagnosis of MEN II and is due to mutations of the ret oncogene.

MEN IIa – Sipple's syndrome
Tumours of:

- Medullary thyroid carcinoma
- Phaeochromocytoma (in 20–50%, half will be bilateral)
- Parathyroid adenoma hyperplasia

MEN Type IIb
Tumours of:

- Parathyroid
- Medullary thyroid carcinoma
- Phaeochromocytoma
- Multiple mucosal neuromas
- Marfanoid habitus

2.8 Lymphoma

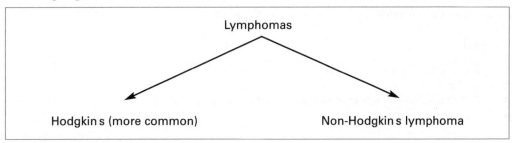

Hodgkin's lymphoma (Hodgkin's disease)

- Males
- Young adults

Clinical features

- Painless progressive lymph node enlargement (cervical/supraclavicular)
- Malaise, fever, weight loss, pruritus
- SVC obstruction
- Bone pain (secondaries)
- Splenomegaly, hepatomegaly

Pathology

- Must have Reed–Sternberg (RS) cells
- Rubbery nodes
- Spreads to bone and liver

Rye classification

1. Lymphocyte predominant 15% Worsening
2. Nodular sclerosing 40% prognosis
3. Mixed cellularity 30%
4. Lymphocyte depleted 15% ↓

Staging

Based on Ann Arbour classification:

- A Absence of systemic symptoms, i.e. weight loss, fever, anaemia
- B Presence of above symptoms

Stage:

I Confined to one lymph node site
II In more than one lymph node site but all on one side of diaphragm
III Nodes above and below diaphragm
IV Spread beyond lymphatic system (e.g. liver and bone)

Diagnosis

- Node excision biopsy
- CXR: mediastinal nodes
- IVU: retroperitoneal nodes compress renal calyces
- CT scan

Staging laparotomy is now rarely used due to improved imaging techniques.

Treatment

- Stage I: radiotherapy
- Stages II–IV: combination chemotherapy

80% cure rate in good prognostic groups (i.e. lymphocyte predominant Stage I).

2.9 Prostate

Epidemiology

- Increasing incidence with age
- Introduction of PSA has detected many more tumours and at earlier stages
- Most common in Black Americans
- Second most common cause of cancer in males in the UK (most common in the USA)

Risk factors

Not known for certain, but:

- **Hormonal**: androgens (does not occur in males castrated before puberty)
- **Genetic:** increased incidence in those with a first-degree relative who has had the disease
- **Environmental**: low incidence in Japan, high incidence in Scandinavia; offspring of immigrants have an intermediate incidence of the disease

Morphology

Macroscopic appearance:

- 70% occur in periphery of gland (peripheral zone)
- Firm, grey ill-defined lesions
- Usually are hypoechoic lesions on ultrasound

Microscopic – almost all are adenocarcinoma.

Spread

Locally

- Seminal vesicles
- Urinary bladder (can cause bilateral ureteric obstruction)
- Pelvic lymph nodes
- Rarely spreads to rectum (due to Denonvilliers fascia)

Distant

- Bony metastases (usually axial skeleton)
- Produce osteosclerotic lesions
- Lung metastases not infrequent

Clinical presentation

- An incidental finding of an elevated PSA (a Kallikrein-like protein)
- Bladder outflow obstruction
- Haematuria
- Lower limb swelling due to pelvic lymph node involvement or DVT
- Bone pain or pathological fractures
- Anaemia
- Renal failure

May present late with symptoms of advanced disease.

Diagnosis

- Per rectum: craggy, loss of midline sulcus, hard nodule
- Biopsy: almost all are performed using transrectal ultrasound-guided biopsies under antibiotic cover; biopsies taken of suspicious areas + six random biopsies
- PSA: >4 ng/ml is elevated level; >10 ng/ml is suggestive of cancer – used in conjunction with the above; however, also elevated in benign prostatic hyperplasia and other conditions (see Section 1.8, PSA); PSA velocity, PSA density and free-total PSA ratio are helpful (NB. May be detected at time of TURP).
- Radio-isotope bone scan
- CXR
- IVU/US: effect of tumour on upper tract
- TRUS assesses extent of local tumour and seminal vesicle involvement
- Histology following routine TURP (T1a, T1b)

Staging

> **TNM classification:**
>
> | | |
> |---|---|
> | T_1 | not palpable nor visible |
> | T_{1a} | <5% prostatic chips following TURP |
> | T_{1b} | >5% prostatic chips following TURP |
> | T_2 | confined within prostate |
> | T_{2a} | one lobe |
> | T_{2b} | both lobes |
> | T_3 | through prostatic capsule |
> | T_{3a} | extracapsular |
> | T_{3b} | seminal vesicles |
> | T_4 | fixed or invades adjacent structures |
> | N_1 | regional lymph node(s) |
> | M_{1a} | non-regional lymph node(s) |
> | M_{1b} | bone |
> | M_{1c} | other site(s) |

NB. Prostatic intra-epithelial neoplasia (PIN) may be found; it is high or low grade. Low grade is of little clinical significance, high grade is associated with the finding of cancer in subsequent biopsies in up to 50% of patients.

Treatment

Organ-confined disease T_1/T_2:

- Radical prostatectomy (if life expectancy >10 years)
- External beam radiotherapy or brachytherapy (implantation of radioactive seeds into prostate)
- Watch and wait (T_1, well-differentiated tumours, older patients)
- Locally advanced/metastatic disease T_3/T_4:

- Hormonal therapy (in asymptomatic patients complications may be more severe if treatment delayed; survival **may** be reduced)
- Radiotherapy (locally – palliative, treatment of symptomatic bone metastases)

Hormonal treatment of prostate cancer

The aim is the suppression of androgens:

- 80% of prostate cancers are androgen dependent
- Anti-androgenic antagonists (e.g. cyproterone acetate (steroidal), flutamide (non steroidal), megestrol acetate)
- Luteinizing hormone-releasing hormone agonists: initially stimulate the release of gonadotrophins before causing inhibition by negative feedback (e.g. goserelin), therefore must cover 'tumour flare' with an anti-androgen. Continuous levels act to inhibit pituitary and down-regulate LH receptors on testis.
- Androgen suppression can be achieved by bilateral subcapsular orchidectomy but some patients find this unacceptable.

Criteria for radical prostatectomy

- Histological confirmation
- Localised (i.e. T_1 or T_2)
- Patient has at least a ten-year life expectancy
- No surgical or medical contraindications
- Partin's tables predict positive margins following radical prostatectomy
- Patient accepts risks of impotence and incontinence

Complications of treatment

- Radical prostatectomy: impotence 50–70%; urinary incontinence 2–10%
- Anti-androgens: GI upsets; gynaecomastia; weight changes; hot flushes
- Radiotherapy: prostatitis; possible decreased cure rate; bladder wall fibrosis; impotence

2.10 Bladder

Superficial Transitional Cell Carcinoma

Risk Factors
Smoking

Symptoms
Painless haematuria

Diagnosis
Cystoscopy, biopsy and cystoscopic resection.

STAGING

Stage

P_{is}	*in situ*
P_a	Papillary, non-invasive (incidence 70%)
P_1	Lamina propria invasion
P_2	Into superficial muscle
P_{3a}	Deep muscle invasion
P_{3b}	Into perivesical tissue
P_{4a}	Prostate invasion
P_{4b}	Extravesical (pelvic wall)

Treatment

- Transurethral resection
- Intravesical chemotherapy
- Laser
- BCG immunotherapy

Invasive Transitional Cell Carcinoma

- Radical cystectomy
- Radiotherapy however preserves bladder and potency
- No evidence for neoadjuvant chemotherapy
- Adjuvant chemotherapy has response rates up to 70%

5 YEAR SURVIVAL RATES FOR INVASIVE TCC

Stage	Surgery %	Radiotherapy %
T_1	85–95	35
T_2	75	40
T_3	44	26
T_4	16	12

Methods of urinary diversion include

- Ileal conduit
- Valved rectal pouch
- Continent cutaneous diversions – requires intermittent self catheterisation
- Continent orthotopic reservoir (bowel segment anastomosed between ureter and urethra)

Squamous Cell Carcinoma

Very common in areas of the world endemic with schistosomiasis, but accounts for less than 5% of bladder tumours in the UK.

2.11 Kidney

Renal cell tumours arise from the proximal tubule and are also known as

- Clear Cell Carcinoma
- Grawitz tumour
- Hypernephroma

They spread via the venous system leading to pulmonary metastasis.

Staging

- US and CT scan (check for renal vein and IVC spread)
- Robson staging
  - Confined within the kidney
  - Gerota's fascia intact
  - Renal vein
  - To other organs

Treatment

- Radical nephrectomy
- No role for chemo or radiotherapy

2.12 Testicle

- Usually seminoma or teratoma
- Present late
- Woody insensate testicle
- 20–30 year olds
- May complain of backache
- α-FP (teratomas) and β-hCG (seminomas and teratomas)
- Ultrasound
- Open biopsy and frozen section before orchidectomy
- Avoid needle biopsy to avoid seeding

Treatment

- Orchidectomy (groin incision)
- Seminomas – radiosensitive
- Teratomas – chemotherapy

2.13 Skin

Benign skin tumours

Naevi – benign tumour of melanocytes.

The following are types of benign pigmented naevi:

- **Lentigo**: within basal layer of epidermis
- **Junctional naevus**: in basal layer of epidermis and project into the dermis
- **Dermal naevus**: entirely within the dermis
- **Compound naevus**: features of junctional and dermal naevus
- **Blue naevus**: arrested migration within the dermis, overlying normal dermis

They are usually compound or junctional.

Treatment
Excision indicated if:

- Malignant change suspected
- Cosmetic
- Nuisance

Malignant skin tumours

- Malignant melanoma
- Basal cell carcinoma
- Squamous cell carcinoma

Malignant melanoma
Can arise *de novo* or in pre-existing benign naevus (60%). Features suggesting malignant change in a naevus are:

- Change in size or shape
- Change in colour
- Bleeding
- Ulceration
- Crusting
- Itching
- Satellite spots

Risk factors

- Fair skin and redheads
- Celtic origin
- UV light
- Family history
- Albinism
- Xeroderma pigmentosum

Epidemiology

- Fair skins near the equator
- Increasing incidence
- Accounts for almost all skin cancer deaths
- Most common in Australia
- Women and men affected (women: legs, men: trunk)
- 10% are autosomally inherited with incomplete penetrance

Pathology

Group of melanocytes that are malignant. There are five clinical types:

- **Lentigo maligna 7%**: sun damage, face and hands
- **Superficial spreading 65%**: most common
- **Nodular 27%**: younger age group, poor prognosis
- **Acral lentiginous 1%**: Blacks and Asians, hands and soles of feet
- **Amelanotic**: poor prognosis, present with lymph node involvement

Initially there is a radial then a vertical growth phase.

Diagnosis

- Excision biopsy (2 mm clearance margin)
- Differential diagnosis: basal carcinoma; seborrhoeic wart; haemangioma; naevus

Spread

Local: satellite lesions
Regional: lymph nodes
Blood: lung, liver, brain, skin

Staging – Breslow's thickness		
Tumour thickness	Risk of metastasis	5 year survival
<0.75 mm	Low	95–99%
0.76–1.49 mm	Moderate	80–90%
1.5–3.99 mm	High	60–75%
>4.0 mm	High	<50%

Clinical staging

- I: no regional spread
- II: satellite lesions, lymph node spread, 'in-transit' i.e. in between.
- III: distant spread

Treatment of malignant melanoma

Resection margins

- Over time the resection margins have reduced, as studies (such as WHO Melanoma Group 1990) have shown no survival benefit with extended margins.

- Generally accepted margins based on clinical appearance are:
  - Impalpable lesions   1cm
  - Palpable lesions   2cm
  - Nodular lesions   3cm

Treatment

- Excision of the primary ± regional lymph node dissection
- Isolated limb perfusion – for recurrence of limb disease – now rarely used

Basal cell carcinoma

- Commonest malignant skin condition
- Malignant tumour of epidermal cells
- Almost never metastasise
- Most commonly occur on face
- Associated with UV light exposure
- Also known as rodent ulcer
- Can be nodular, cystic or ulcerated
- Slow growing
- Can invade deeper tissues

Treatment

- Cryosurgery : smaller lesions
- Surgery: excision (0.5 cm margins), primary closure or skin grafts
- Radiotherapy: fractionation; elderly – extensive lesions

Squamous cell carcinoma

- Five-year survival 90%
- Malignant tumour of epidermal keratinocytes
- UV light exposure
- Can occur in pre-existing skin lesions (such as in ulcers – Marjolin's ulcer)
- More common in males
- Occurs on back of hands, forearms, face (i.e. areas exposed to sun)

Treatment

- Surgery: 1–2 cm clearance; excision biopsy, (± lymph node dissection)
- Radiotherapy: for head and neck tumours; older patients (less satisfactory scar); with surgery if in doubt about clearance

2.14 Liver

Epidemiology

- Hepatocellular carcinoma is uncommon in the West, where secondaries are much more common
- Common in East Africa and SE Asia
- Male:Female = 4:1
- In Europe the age of presentation is 80 years, whereas in Africa and Asia it is 40 years

Pathology

- Cirrhosis
- Viral Hepatitis (B and C)
- Alcohol
- Anabolic steroids
- Mycotoxins e.g. aflatoxin
- Primary liver diseases

Presentation

- There is a massive liver swelling usually in an already cirrhotic liver, usually with rapid deterioration. Jaundice usually occurs late.
- Investigation by Ultrasound and CT scanning
- Disease progress can be monitored by α-fetoprotein

Treatment

- Only 25% of tumours are amenable to surgery
- Resection
- Transplantation

Palliation

- Chemotherapy
- Cryotherapy
- Embolisation
- Thermotherapy
- Devascularisation

2.15 Salivary glands

- Benign
- Pleomorphic adenoma
- Adenolymphoma (Warthin's tumour)
- Intermediate
- Mucoepidermoid
- Acinic
- Oncocytoma
- Malignant
- Adenoid cystic carcinoma
- Adenocarcinoma
- Squamous cell carcinoma

Parotid tumours

- 80% of all salivary tumours are found within the parotid
- 15% of these are malignant
- Divided into the deep and superficial lobes by the facial nerve
- Facial nerve palsy is highly suggestive of malignancy
- Diagnosis by FNA and CT
- Surgery is carried out with VII nerve sparing
- Radical surgery for malignant disease includes VII sacrifice

Frey's syndrome

- Gustatory sweating
- Occurs 6–9 months post surgery
- Due to cross regeneration of secretomotor fibres to cutaneous fibres

2.16 Brain

Tumours may arise from any of the structures within the brain

- Gliomas arise from glial cells – the supportive structure of the brain
  - Astrocytomas
  - Oligodendromas
  - Ependymoma
  - Medulloblastoma
- Meningiomas arise from the arachnoid cells
- Cerebral metastases
  - Most commonly from bronchus and breast
  - Usually multiple
  - Cause extensive oedema
- Schwannoma (Acoustic Neuroma)
  - Usually arise from VIII nerve
  - Consider in all patients with unilateral sensorineural deafness

2.17 Bone

Cell of origin	Malignant	Benign
Bone	Osteosarcoma	Osteoma Osteoid osteoma Osteoblastoma
Cartilage	Chondrosarcoma	Chondroma Osteochondroma (commonest)
Synovium	Synovial sarcoma	
Fibrous tissue	Fibrosarcoma	Fibroma
Marrow	Ewing's sarcoma myeloma	Eosinophilic granuloma
Unknown	Malignant Giant cell tumour	Giant cell tumour

Presentation

- Pain
- Swelling
- Tenderness

Investigation

- Plain radiography
- CT
- Nuclear bone scan
- Biopsy

3. PRINCIPLES OF CANCER TREATMENT

Active treatment modalities include:

- Surgery
- Radiotherapy
- Chemotherapy
- Hormonal manipulation
- Monoclonal antibodies
- Novel approaches

Palliative care, including close attention to adequate pain control, is also a fundamental pillar of management.

3.1 Chemotherapy

Drugs used to treat cancer which inhibit the mechanisms of cell proliferation. They are therefore toxic to normally proliferating cells, i.e. bone marrow, GI epithelium, hair follicles. They can be:

- Cycle-specific: effective throughout the cell cycle
- Phase-specific: effective during part of the cell cycle

Alkylating agents

- Work by forming covalent bonds with nucleic acids, proteins, nucleotides and amino acids. This inactivates enzymes involved in DNA production and protein synthesis.

	Disease	**Side-effects**
Mustargen	Hodgkin's disease	Very toxic so rarely used
	Non-Hodgkin's lymphoma	Vomiting
	CML, CLL	Bone marrow depression
Cyclophosphamide	Many cancers including:	Bone marrow depression
	Lymphoma	Nausea & vomiting (mild unless high
	Breast	dose)
	Lung	Haemorrhagic cystitis (high doses)
	Ovary	Pulmonary interstitial fibrosis
Chlorambucil	CLL	Bone marrow suppression
	NHL (low grade)	Nausea, vomiting, diarrhoea
	Ovary	Jaundice, pulmonary fibrosis
Melphalan	Multiple myeloma	Bone marrow depression
		Nausea and vomiting
		Diarrhoea
		Rash
		Pulmonary fibrosis

Non-Classical Alkylating Agents

Cause cross-linkage of DNA strands.

	Disease	Side-effects
Cisplatin (C-DDP) (toxic to cycling & resting cells)	Testis Ovary Head and neck Bladder Lung Oesophagus Stomach	Renal failure Electrolyte disturbance (hypomagnesaemia) Peripheral neuropathy Ototoxicity Bone marrow depression
Carboplatin	Ovary Lung Seminoma	Less toxic analogue, but more bone marrow suppression

Anti-Metabolites

Interfere with purine or pyrimidine synthesis and hence interfere with DNA synthesis.

	Disease	Side-effects
Methotrexate (S-phase specific)	ALL Breast cancer Lung	Bone marrow depression GI symptoms Stomatitis Renal failure Hepatic failure
5–Fluorouracil (5FU) (toxic to resting & cycling cells)	Colon Breast Stomach Oesophagus Pancreas	Bone marrow depression GI symptoms Alopecia Rash Palmar-plantar syndrome and cardiotoxicity with high dose infusional treatments
Gemcitabine	Pancreas Lung	Nausea Flu-like symptoms Oedema

Antibiotics

These intercalate between base pairs and prevent RNA production. Several groups with differing actions.

Anthracycline antibiotics
Complex actions (not fully understood)

- Intercalate into DNA strands
- Bind membranes
- Produce free radicals
- Chelate metals – producing cytotoxic compounds
- Alkylation

	Disease	Side-effects
Doxorubicin	Acute leukaemias	Bone marrow depression
	Lymphomas	Nausea and vomiting
	Breast cancer	Alopecia
	Small cell lung cancer	Cardiac-dose dependent congestive
	Sarcomas	cardiac failure
	Bladder	
	Ovary	
	Wilms' tumour	
	Neuroblastoma	
Epirubicin	Breast	Doxorubicin analogue with less cardiac toxicity

Non-anthracycline antibiotics

Act by intercalation, free radical production and/or alkylation

	Disease	Side-effects
Mitozantrone	Breast cancer	Bone marrow depression
		Congestive cardiac failure
		Alopecia
		Nausea and vomiting
Bleomycin	Lymphomas	Bone marrow sparing
	Testicular cancers	Pneumonitis and pulmonary fibrosis
	Head and neck cancers	Rash
		Fever
Mitomycin C	Breast	Bone marrow depression
	Bladder (intravesical)	Renal failure (haemolytic-uraemic
	Pancreatic	syndrome with tamoxifen)
	Gastric	Stomatitis, rash, alopecia
		Nausea and vomiting

Vinca Alkaloids

Inhibit mitosis by preventing spindle formation. M-phase specific.
INTRATHECAL ADMINISTRATION IS FATAL

	Disease	Side-effects
Vincristine	Acute leukaemias Lymphomas Neuroblastoma Wilms' tumour Rhabdomyosarcoma	Highly vesicant Neuropathy Bronchospasm
Vinblastine	Testis Hodgkin's lymphoma Non-Hodgkin's lymphoma Choriocarcinoma	Highly vesicant Bone marrow depression Bronchospasm Abdominal pain and ileus (mimics acute abdomen) Peripheral neuropathy
Vinorelbine	Breast Lung	Highly vesicant Bone marrow depression Abdominal pain and constipation Local phlebitis

Taxanes

Inhibit mitosis through stabilisation of microtubules.

	Disease	Side-effects
Docetaxel	Breast Ovary	Allergic reaction Severe neutropaenia Alopecia Peripheral oedema Myalgia Peripheral neuropathy
Paclitaxel	Ovary Breast Lung	Anaphylaxis Severe neutropaenia Sudden total alopecia Myalgia Peripheral neuropathy

Topoisomerase inhibitors

Inhibit topoisomerase I, an enzyme involved in DNA replication.

	Disease	**Side-effects**
Irinotecan	Colorectal	Cholinergic syndrome
		Profuse diarrhoea (may be life threatening)

Monoclonal antibodies

The first two monoclonal antibodies in clinical use are rituximab (Mab Thera) and trastuzumab (Herceptin).

Rituximab is a monoclonal antibody that causes lysis of B lymphocytes and is licensed for treatment of relapsed low grade lymphoma. It is being used earlier in the course of disease in clinical trials.

Trastuzumab can used in metastatic breast cancer, if the tumour over-expresses human epidermal growth factor receptor 2 (HER 2). About 16–18% of patients are likely to be strongly HER2 positive

Infusion related side-effects are common with both: chills, fever, hypersensitivity reactions.

Both can exacerbate chemotherapy related cardiotoxicity.

3.2 Radiotherapy

This is the therapeutic use of ionizing radiation for the treatment of malignant conditions.

Mechanism of action:

- Kills cells by causing high-energy interactions between molecules
- Multiple 'sublethal' doses given at intervals
- This allows normal tissues to recover (takes at least 4 hours), whilst malignant tissues take longer – allows targeting of malignant cells
- Cell is most sensitive during M phase
- Killing cells leads to stimulation of other cells to divide, i.e. enter the M phase:
  1. **Repair**: normal cells take 4 hours to recover (6+ hours for CNS), malignant cells take longer
  2. **Repopulation**: more cells are stimulated to divide due to death of others, after about 3–4 weeks of standard fractionated treatment
  3. **Redistribution**: pushes cells into the M phase – more radiosensitive
  4. **Reoxygenation**: oxygen is a radiation sensitizer; cell death facilitates reoxygenation – increases cytotoxicity

Types of radiation

- **Particulate**
  Electrons
  Protons
  Neutrons
  a particles
  pi mesons

- **Electromagnetic**
  X-rays
  Gamma rays

- Source can be implanted into tissue to be treated (e.g. brachytherapy for prostate cancer)
- Can be given systemically (e.g. Iodine 131 – thyroid cancer)
- Fractionation: describes the number of individual treatments and their time course

Method of action

- Molecular action
- Packets of energy
- Interact with molecules in tissues
- DNA damage via release of kinetic energy (oxygen-dependent process)
- Chromosomal abnormalities: prevents mitosis
- May trigger apoptosis in some cells

This has two effects:

- Cells may not appear abnormal until they attempt to divide
- Slow-growing tumours may not respond or respond slowly to radiotherapy

Depends on:

- Radiosensitivity of tumour – sensitive: seminoma, Hodgkin's lymphoma, resistant: melanoma
- Tolerance of normal tissue: surrounding tissue may be very sensitive to treatment (e.g. nervous tissue, small bowel), which limits the amount of radiotherapy that can be delivered

For radical treatments aim for maximum possible dose in the smallest volume which will encompass all of the tumour and likely occult spread.

Primary treatment

- Sensitive tumours
- Better cosmetic/functional result
- Inoperable or high mortality/morbidity with surgery
- Patient not fit for surgery

Adjuvant radiotherapy

- Post-operative
- Can be given at site of disease or at site of potential metastatic spread

Neo-adjuvant radiotherapy

- Pre-operatively, can downstage tumours (e.g. rectal tumour) and can reduce risk of seeding at operation.

Palliation

- Aiming for symptom relief, from either primary or metastatic disease e.g. relief of bone pain, bleeding, dyspnoea, cord compression, superior vena caval obstruction
- Short courses of treatment, with simple set-ups, to minimise toxicity
- Single fractions often used for bone pain

Complications of radiotherapy

- Oesophagitis
- Ulceration
- Bleeding
- Premature menopause
- Oligospermia
- Stricture formation
- Delayed wound healing
- Lymphoedema
- Acute leukaemia
- Hypothyroidism/renal failure – after many years treatment

3.3 Hormonal manipulation

Prostate

- Subcapsular orchidectomy (bilateral)
- Antiandrogens
- LHRH analogues
- Stilboestrol (oestrogen)

Breast

- Tamoxifen: pre- and post-menopausal women if ER and/or PR positive
- Aromatase inhibitors: prevent oestrogen production from peripheral fat – no effect on ovarian oestrogens, so post menopausal only. Recent evidence of superior survival in advanced disease compared with tamoxifen for 3rd generation aromatase inhibitors e.g. anastrazole.
- Progestogens: now tend to be used 3rd line, as aromatase inhibitors superior.
- LHRH analogues:**monthly** goserelin in pre-menopausal women (3 monthly preparation does not reliably suppress menstruation in all)

Thyroid

- Thyroxine (see Section 2.6 Thyroid neoplasms): to suppress TSH secretion. Liothyronine used.

3.4 Immune modulation

Renal cancer

- Radioresistant
- Chemoresistant
- Some success with IL-2 and α-interferon

Bladder cancer

- BCG vaccine used intravesically. Used in treatment of cis and high-grade (non-invasive) tumours. May be used long-term as 'maintenance therapy'.

3.5 Novel approaches

- Anti-angiogenesis agents currently being developed
- On-going trials of gene-therapy with glioblastoma

3.6 Cryotherapy

- Probe inserted into tumour
- Freezing temperature causes 'ice ball'
- Mainly used in palliation

3.7 Palliative care

Analgesics in terminal care

- by mouth (where possible)
- by the clock (prn = **p**ain **r**elief **n**egligible!)
- by the analgesic ladder

Analgesic ladder

- step 1   simple analgesics   paracetamol/NSAID
- step 2   compound analgesics   co-proxamol/co-codamol etc
- step 3   opiate   oral morphine remains drug of choice

- Little to choose between various analgesics at step 2
- For bone pain add NSAID to level 2/3 drugs
- Co-proxamol 2 qds = morphine 6–8 mg 4 hourly

Starting dose of morphine should be 10mg 4 hourly, unless elderly, hepato-renal impairment etc.

- **Non-opioids** (e.g. aspirin/NSAIDs/paracetamol) can control bone pain; can be given rectally
- **Opioids**: Oral (e.g. morphine); increase dose by 50% if 1st dose is ineffective; MST – twice daily; modified release; to calculate dose, start on oral four-hourly dose and divide total in two daily doses + morphine for breakthrough pain.
  May need anti-emetic for first 2 or 3 days
  Should have aperient prescribed routinely
  Transdermal fentanyl or alternative oral drugs e.g. Oxynorm useful if tolerance poor

Parenteral analgesia

For patients who cannot take things by mouth.

Subcutaneous administration has been shown to be as effective an intramuscular in terminal care.

Diamorphine is drug of choice.

May need anti-emetic in pump if not previously on opiate.

- Diamorphine: SC dose = one-quarter to one-third of oral dose of morphine.
- SC infusion preferable to IV infusion
  Less potentiation
  Easier management
  Can discharge to home/hospice with SC pump

Potential problems with pumps

- Miscalculations with rate and delivery of setting of pump
- Mechanical failure of pumps
- Reaction at injection site (IV/SC)

Treatment of specific symptoms

- **Pain**

Colic	loperamide 2–4 mg q.d.s tyoscine
Gastric distension	domperidone
Muscle spasm	relaxant (e.g. diazepam, baclofen)
Nerve pain-compression	dexamethasone
Nerve irritation	amitriptyline, carbamazepine, TENS
	nerve blocks
Liver pain	dexamethasone
(capsular stretching)	

- **Respiratory**

Dyspnoea	morphine, diazepam, dexamethasone
Excess respiratory secretions	hyoscine
Cough	morphine (short acting better than MST)

- **GI**

Hiccoughs	antacid, metoclopramide, chlorpromazine
Anorexia	prednisolone, dexamethasone, Megace
Constipation	lactulose, co-danthrusate
Nausea & vomiting	haloperidol (due to morphine)

- **Skin/mucus membranes**

Pruritus	antihistamine
Dry mouth	artificial saliva, oral candidiasis treatments

- **Neurological**

Headache	dexamethasone if raised ICP
	oxygen if hypoxia
Confusion/sedation	consider drugs/hypercalcaemia/brain mets
Confusion/agitation	haloperidol, chlorpromazine
Convulsions	phenytoin, carbamezapine, diazepam rectal

4. THE BREAST

4.1 Anatomy of the breast

Embryology

- Modified apocrine sweat gland
- Ectoderm: epithelial lining of ducts and acini
- Mesenchyme: supporting tissue
- Downward growth of the ectoderm into the underlying mesenchyme at 4 weeks gestation
- Thickened mammary ridges (ectoderm) called the milk line grow bilaterally from axilla to groin
- Branching epithelial cords as 15–20 buds become lactiferous ducts
- Breast bud: mammary tissue growth beneath areola at age 10
- Nipple development at 12 years

Gross anatomy

Position

- Vertical: base 2nd to 6th ICS
- Horizontal: sternum to anterior axillary line
  2/3 on pectoralis major muscle
  1/3 serratus anterior muscle
  (axillary tail of Spence = extension of upper outer quadrant of breast to 3rd rib in axilla, found in 95% female breasts)
- Fascia: superficial fascia – two layers
  Condensation of fibrous tissue forms suspensory
  Ligaments of Cooper, divides breast into lobes
  and acts as supportive framework

Blood supply

- Arterial
  Axillary artery branches:
    thoracoacromial
    subscapular
    lateral thoracic – main contribution
  Internal mammary artery branches:
  Mainly second perforating branch
  (need to preserve in subcutaneous mastectomy)

- Venous
  Drainage via intercostal, internal mammary and axillary veins

Nerve supply

Sensory: cutaneous branches of intercostal nerves T4 to T6 (especially nipple). Sympathetic nerves to breast parenchyma (blood vessels and glands).

Lymphatic drainage

75% to axillary nodes; three main groups:

- **Level 1**: lateral to pectoralis minor
- **Level 2**: posterior to pectoralis minor
- **Level 3**: medial to pectoralis minor

(See below for more details.)

25% to internal mammary nodes: 2nd to 4th ICS.

Surgical anatomy of the axilla

Space between upper arm and thorax. Bordered anteriorly and posteriorly by axillary folds.

- **Anterior wall**: pectoralis major and minor, subclavius and clavipectoral fascia
- **Medial wall:** upper serratus anterior, lower limit 4th rib
- **Lateral wall**: anterior and posterior walls converging humeral bicipital groove
- **Posterior wall**: subscapularis, teres major, tendon of latissimus dorsi
- **Apex**: bordered by clavicle, first rib, scapula – links axilla to post triangle
- **Floor**: axillary fascia from serratus anterior to deep fascia of the arm

Contents of axilla

Neurovascular bundle (from neck to upper limb):

- Axillary artery
- Axillary vein
- Brachial plexus
- Lymph nodes

Brachial plexus cords embrace second part of axillary artery under pectoralis minor. Axillary vein lies medial to axillary artery and nerves. Lymph nodes lie in fibrofatty areolar tissue of axilla.

Axillary artery

Continuation of 3rd part of subclavian artery. Starts at outer border of 1st rib. Invested in fascia: the axillary sheath. Becomes brachial artery at lower border of teres major.

Three part division by pectoralis minor; second part embraced by brachial plexus cords under cover of pectoralis minor.

Branches

- 1st part – 1 branch: superior thoracic artery – supplies both pectorals.
- 2nd part – 2 branches: lateral thoracic artery – supplies both pectorals and breast; thoracoacromial artery – supplies clavicle, deltoid, pectorals and acromion.
- 3rd part – 3 branches: subscapular artery – gives off thoracodorsal to supply latissimus dorsi; anterior circumflex humeral artery – supplies biceps and shoulder joint; posterior circumflex humeral artery – supplies deltoid, triceps and shoulder joint.

Axillary vein

Formed by basilic vein and venae comitantes. Starts lower border of posterior axilla. Situated medial to the artery. Becomes subclavian vein at outer border of 1st rib. Tributaries of 2nd and 3rd part same as the artery. Cephalic vein drains into 1st part. No axillary sheath around vein.

Brachial plexus

(See Chapter 3, *Trauma*, Section 4.4.)

Lymph nodes of axilla

There are many scattered nodes in axillary fibro-fatty tissue. The average number of nodes is 35, but there can be up to 50. They are grouped into:

- **Anterior or pectoral group**:
  Position – medial wall with lateral thoracic artery, lower border pectoralis minor
  Drainage – anterior upper trunk and breast
- **Posterior or subscapular group**:
  Position – posterior part medial wall with subscapular artery
  Drainage – posterior upper trunk and axillary tail
- **Lateral group**:
  Position – medial side of axillary vein
  Drainage – upper limb
- **Central group**:
  Position – fat of axilla
  Drainage – above nodes
- **Apical group**:
  Position – apex of axilla
  Drainage – all above nodes; apical nodes drain into supraclavicular nodes which ultimately drain into the thoracic duct or the right lymphatic trunk

Latissimus dorsi

Origin (O)	Spinous processes and supraspinous ligaments T7 to T12 Lumbar and sacral vertebrae, inferior angle of scapula, 8th to 12th ribs, lumbar fascia, posterior 3rd iliac crest
Insertion (I)	Spirals around teres major then into humeral intertubercular groove

Nerve supply (NS)   Thoracodorsal nerve (C6, 7, 8)
                                Risk of injury in axillary operations

Blood supply (Bld)   Thoracodorsal artery

Action   Arm extension, adduction and medial rotation
                                Resp accessory – deep inspiration and forced expiration

NB. White tendon forms lower posterior axillary wall.

Serratus anterior

O   Digitations from 1st to 8th ribs and anterior intercostal membrane
                                Lower 1/2 interdigitate with external oblique

I   Inner medial border of scapula

NS   Long thoracic nerve (of Bell) (C5, 6, 7)

Bld   Branch of thoracodorsal artery and intercostal branches

Action   Lateral rotation and protraction of scapula

NB. Forms medial wall of axilla; covered with a strong fascia; paralysis causes winged scapula.

Pectoralis major

O   Medial half of clavicle, anterior sternum, 1st to 6th costal cartilages, anterior upper rectus sheath

I   Lateral lip of intertubercular sulcus of humerus

NS   Medial and lateral pectoral nerves (clavicular fibres C5, 6 and sternocostal part 6, 7, 8, T1)

Bld   Deltoid and pectoral branches of thoracoacromial artery
                                Superior and lateral thoracic artery, perforating branches of internal thoracic artery

Action   Assists adduction and medial rotation of the humerus
                                Swings extended arms forward and medially
                                Active in deep inspiration

NB. Thick, fan-shaped muscle; overlies pectoralis minor.

Pectoralis minor

O   3rd to 5th (or 2nd to 4th) ribs, external intercostal fascia

I   Medial border and upper surface of coracoid process of scapula

NS   Medial and lateral pectoral nerves (C5, 6, 7, 8, T1)

Bld   Deltoid and pectoral branches of thoracoacromial artery
                                Superior and lateral thoracic artery

Action   Assists serratus anterior in drawing scapula forward
                                Rotates scapula depressing the point of shoulder
                                Active in forced inspiration

NB. Thin, triangular muscle; lies deep to pectoralis major.

4.2 Congenital and developmental disorders

- **Athelia**: absence of a nipple (rare)
- **Polythelia**: supernumerary nipples irregularly placed over the breast
- **Amastia**: absence of a breast (rare)
- **Polymastia**: presence of accessory breast
- **Amazia**: absence of a breast with the nipple present = hypoplasia of the breast; 90% have absent or hypoplastic pectoral muscles; Poland syndrome = above anomaly with hand deformity but 90% of pectoral muscle defects have normal breasts; breast asymmetry can be normal (L>R).

Supernumerary (accessory) breasts or nipples

Persistence of extramammary breast ridge in 1–5% of people.

Abnormal breast enlargement

- **Female**
  Prepubertal breast enlargement in absence of other sexual development is normal, if other sexual development signs are present then investigate to exclude endocrine tumours
  Virginal or juvenile hypertrophy: adolescent overgrowth of the breast is a normal variant
  Rx – reduction mammoplasty
  Hormonal treatment using Danazol

- **Male**
  Gynaecomastia = growth of male breast tissue at any age and to any extent
  Bilateral in 25%
  Mostly benign and reversible
  Physiological causes:
  neonatal
  pubertal hormone imbalance
  old age
  Other causes:
  hypogonadism
  neoplasms
  systemic disease: hepatic disease
  renal failure
  hyperthyroidism
  drug-induced*

*Drugs include: cimetidine, spironolactone, ketoconazole, digitalis, oestrogens, androgens, anabolic steroids, HCG, methyldopa, TCA, phenothiazines, metoclopramide, busulphan, vincristine, nitrosureas.

4.3 Aberrations of normal development and involution (ANDI)

The majority of benign breast conditions can be classified into the concept of aberrations of normal development and involution (ANDI). Many benign breast conditions can be thought of as disorders rather than disease. In the early reproductive years this is well illustrated by the progression from normal development (lobule formation), to benign change (fibroadenoma – hypertrophy of one lobule) to benign disease (giant/multiple fibroadenoma).

Fibroadenoma

- Aberration of development rather than benign neoplasm
- Develops from a single lobule
- Shows hormonal dependence: lactating during pregnancy; involuting in perimenopausal period
- Present most commonly 15–25 years

Ex: well-circumscribed, smooth, firm, mobile lumps (breast mouse). May be multiple and bilateral. Some increase in size; majority do not and may disappear.

Ix: clinical diagnosis inaccurate in 50%, therefore need FNA, NCB or excision biopsy. Mammography in >35 years shows a well-rounded opacity. Ultrasonography in all age groups.

Rx: reassurance; removal if large (>2cm) and on request.

Giant fibroadenoma and phylloides tumour

- Giant fibroadenoma = fibroadenoma >5 cm in diameter
- More common in African countries
- Not synonymous with Phylloides tumour
- Phylloides tumour is uncommon; most over 3 cm in diameter

Ix: mammogram and USS. Need NCB (giant fibroadenoma indistinguishable by FNAC).

Rx: complete excision – risk of recurrence: giant fibroadenoma age 10–20 years; Phylloides tumour median age 50 years.

Disorders of breast involution

Cystic disease

- Impalpable microcysts considered normal
- Palpable macrocysts in 7% of women in the West
- Common age 38–53 years
- Cause unknown

Hx: breast lump

Ex: discrete, smooth, maybe fluctuant

Ix: Aspirate fluid – send for cytology only if bloodstained; cystic carcinoma (rare); USS all ages, mammography if >35

Rx: aspiration; if persistent then excision

Sclerosing lesions

- Due to aberrations of involution, includes sclerosing adenosis, papillomatosis or duct adenoma
- Diagnostic problem, mimic cancer
- Radial scars – present via screening – potential underlying breast cancer – FNA is inaccurate all should be excised following wire localisation

Hx: breast pain or lump, screen detected (radial scars)

Ix and Rx: mammography and excision biopsy

Epithelial hyperplasia

- Epithelial cell increase in the terminal duct lobular unit
- Can be mild or moderate; common in premenopausal women
- If atypia is present in addition to hyperplasia there is an increased risk of breast cancer
- Hyperplastic cells are either ductal or lobular
- Atypical ductal or lobular cells – $\times$ 4–5 greater risk of breast cancer

Hx: breast lump or incidental finding on biopsy

Ix: FNA or NCB; mammography

Rx: Excision biopsy; need follow-up with screening – increased risk of cancer in both breasts

On histology it is difficult to differentiate between atypical ductal hyperplasia with severe atypia and low grade DCIS as these conditions represent two overlapping stages on the continuum between benign and malignant breast disease. It is important to remember that LCIS is conventionally thought of as a marker of increased risk of breast cancer and that DCIS is a pre-invasive form of the disease.

4.4 Breast pain and inflammatory lesions

Mastalgia = breast pain

There are two types:

- Cyclical
- Non-cyclical

Causes: hormonally-based; not psychological.

Cyclical mastalgia

- Any age up to menopause
- Mostly young women (mean age 34 years)
- 3–7 days pre-menstrual cycle
- Improving at menstruation
- Usually lateral part of breast affected

Ex: clinical examination

Rx: reassure, only 15% require treatment; advice including weight loss, dietary change, supportive/sleep bra; Evening primrose oil – effective in 70%; NSAIDS; danazol

Non-cyclical mastalgia

- Older women (mean age 43 years)
- Less common than cyclical mastalgia

Ex: again, clinical; exclude costochondritis (Tietze's syndrome) or periductal mastitis

Ix: women >40 mammography

Rx: well-supporting bra, NSAIDs

Inflammatory lesions of the breast

Breast abscess: lactating; non-lactating

Lactating

Mastitis neonatorum

- First few weeks of life
- Infected enlarged breast bud

Cause: *S. aureus* and *E. coli*

Rx: antibiotics, I&D

Lactating breast abscess

- This is a puerperal mastitis

Cause: *S. aureus, S. epidermidis*, streptococci. Common in the first two months after breast feeding.

Hx: breast pain, swelling and tenderness

Ix: tender, erythema, may be fluctuant; not usually axillary lymphadenopathy

Rx: flucloxacillin or augmentin; aspiration or I&D; advise to continue breastfeeding if mastitis only – if an abscess develops stop; if persistent inflammation consider inflammatory carcinoma which can mimic breast abscess – core Bx

Non-lactating

Periareolar

- Complication of periductal mastitis
- More common than lactating breast abscess
- Average age 35 years
- 90% cases are smokers

Hx: nipple discharge and retraction, central breast pain

Ix: FNA and cytology to exclude inflammatory breast carcinoma

Rx: antibiotics, aspirate or I&D; complication: mammary duct fistula

Peripheral

- Less common than above
- Associated with DM, RA, steroid therapy, trauma, granulomatous mastitis (rare)

Cause: *S. aureus,* occasionally TB

Ix and Rx: as above

Periductal mastitis

- Periductal inflammation but no enlargement

Cause: bacterial involvement, cigarette smoking – autoimmune basis

Hx: breast pain, periareolar inflammation, nipple discharge

Ex: tender mass, periareolar, nipple discharge and retraction or inversion

Rx: antibiotics (e.g. augmentin)

Complications: non-lactating breast abscess, mammary fistula.

Duct ectasia

- Duct dilatation without marked inflammation
- Affects older women

Hx: nipple discharge or retraction

Rx: microdochectomy, total duct excision

Mammary duct fistula

- Communication between periareolar skin and a duct
- Complication mainly of periductal mastitis or rarely of granulomatous mastitis
- Common age 35 years

Ex: nipple retraction

Rx: excision and antibiotics cover

Fat necrosis

- Traumatic fat necrosis but in 50% no history of trauma

Ex: skin dimpling and retraction, mimics breast cancer

Ix: mammography, focal calcification and scarring; USS – oil cyst – may mimic breast cancer, excision or biopsy

Benign neoplasms

Duct papilloma

- Single or multiple
- Very common
- Usually small and symptom free
- If duct involvement: bloodstained nipple discharge

Ix: mammography, ductography

Rx: microdochectomy

Lipoma

- Soft, lobulated, radiolucent lesion
- Exclude pseudolipoma (soft mass felt around breast cancer)
- If >35 years need mammogram and FNA cytology
- Hamartoma

Discrete lesions with pseudocapsule – benign – similar to hamartomas elsewhere.

Multiple hamartomas (slightly different pathological features) seen in Cowden's syndrome where there is a high risk of breast cancer.

4.5 Nipple discharge and retraction; miscellaneous lesions

Discharge

Single duct or multi-duct discharge should be ascertained from the history. Multiduct discharge is not usually pathological except in the case of hormone producing endocrine tumours. Single duct discharge requires further investigation.

- Most common cause – physiological
- Other causes
  - Galactorrhoea
  - Periductal mastitis/duct ectasia (slit-like nipple inversion)
  - Duct papilloma
  - Epithelial hyperplasia
  - Breast cancer – single duct discharge; either serous or bloodstained; 5% due to DCIS
- Bloodstained discharge is feature of duct carcinoma but not pathognomonic of breast cancer

Ix: Haemo-stix testing, cytology, mammography, USS, ductography, ductoscopy

Rx: microdochectomy, excision

Ductoscopy is a new technique – ductal pathology including DCIS can be seen and washings taken for cytology – where ducts are normal, a washout may prevent further discharge.

Nipple discharges		
Colour	**Nature**	**Cause**
White	milk	lactating breast
Yellow	exudate	abscess
Green	cellular debris	duct ectasia
Red	blood	ductal papilloma or carcinoma

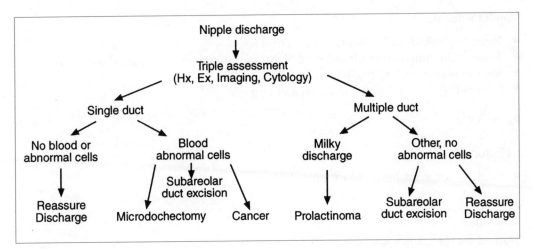

Nipple discharge

Retraction

- Congenital or acquired
- Higher incidence of periductal mastitis infections
- Acquired causes: periductal mastitis, duct ectasia, TB, previous biopsy, malignancy
- Simple breast involution in elderly

Ix: Triple assessment

1. Clinical
2. Radiological
3. Pathological

If negative, no treatment is required.

Miscellaneous lesions of the breast

Haematoma

- Post-traumatic (e.g. from car seat belts)
- Spontaneous on anticoagulants

Complication: fat necrosis

Rx: aspiration, supporting bra

Mondor's disease

- Thrombophlebitis of a subcutaneous vein
- Tender skin dimpling; indurated cord about 3 mm in diameter of variable lengths
- Seen in both male and female
- Occurs in breast, anterior chest wall and arm

Rx: NSAIDs

Galactocoele

- Cystic lesion containing breast milk

Rx: aspiration

Blocked Montgomery's tubercle

- Blocked blind – ending ducts in the areola

Hx: periareolar lump

Rx: local excision

4.6 Breast carcinoma: aetiology and clinical features

Breast carcinoma

- Risk factors
  Age
  Hyperplasia with atypia (x5 risk)

- Other putative risk factors
  Dietary
  HRT
  OCP
  Smoking
  Ionizing radiation

Aetiology

Incidence of breast cancer correlates well with lifetime oestrogen exposure. Genetic factors are modified by environmental factors – particularly diet and reproductive history. BRCA-1 and -2 genes are implicated in 2% of breast cancer cases. It is estimated 10–15% of cases may have one or more genetic predispositions to the disease.

It is more common in nulliparous women in developed countries, those with early menarche and late menopause and in those with obesity. It is less common in multiparous women with first pregnancy at an early age, in underdeveloped countries, and in those with artificial early menopause by ovarian ablation or irradiation. The incidence is increasing: latest figures for the US (lifetime risk) 1:7 and UK 1:9.

Epidemiological features of breast carcinoma

- Linear increase with age
- Continuing rise with age in high-incidence countries

Genetic factors

- 5–10% familial predisposition
- 2% all breast cancers associated with BRCA-1 gene (17Q)
- BRCA-2 gene (13Q) also implicated
- Li–Fraumeni syndrome
- Loss of heterozygosity of p53 on 17Q

Possible risk if following relatives affected

- Mother × 1.8
- Mother *and* sister × 5.6
- Sister × 2.5
- Mother *and* sister developed breast cancer <40 years × 9.0

Clinical features

- Painless breast lump: most common feature
- Pain or skin ulceration: less common
- Nipple discharge: serosanguinous and bloodstained

Examination

Most breast cancers present as a discrete lump with few special features, the sensitivity for detecting breast cancer by clinical examination alone is 50%.

Advanced breast cancers have more obvious clinical features:

- Hard, irregular lump fixed to tissue, skin or muscle
- Nipple retraction, skin tethering and fixity
- Nodal masses, skin ulceration, oedema and satellite nodules in advanced breast carcinoma (ABC)
- Infiltration of skin of chest, back and neck: cancer en cuirasse
- Localized dermal oedema: peau d'orange
- Automastectomy
- Weight loss, ascites, jaundice, central nervous system symptoms, pathological fractures associated with metastatic disease

NB. T_{1a} lesion (5 mm or less) impalpable, found by mammography; T_{1b} lesion (6–10 mm) possibly palpable.

4.7 Staging, pathology and diagnosis of breast carcinoma

Staging

There are three major clinical systems:

- UICC
- Manchester
- Columbia

By reference to primary tumour, regional nodal areas and systemic disease.

The **UICC** system is the most comprehensive and universal:

- T_0: subclinical
- T_1: 2 cm or less
- T_2: >2 cm but <5 cm
- T_3: >5 cm
- T_4: any size with chest wall or skin extension
- N_0: no node metastasis
- N_1: ipsilateral axillary (mobile)
- N_2: ipsilateral axillary (fixed)
- N_3: ipsilateral internal mammary nodes
- M_0: no distant metastases
- M_1: distant metastases

Breast cancer staging systems

TNM	Manchester	Columbia
T_0–T_1 N_0–N_1	Stage1	Stage A
$T_2 N_{1b}$	Stage 2	Stage B
T_3–T_4 N_2–N_3	Stage 3	Stage C
M_1	Stage 4	Stage D

Pathology

WHO classification: Epithelial cell or connective tissue origin.

Epithelial tumours

- **Non-invasive**: DCIS – ductal carcinoma *in situ*; LCIS – lobular carcinoma *in situ*
- **Invasive**: ductal carcinoma 80–90%; lobular 1–10%; mucinous 5%; medullary 1–5%; atypical medullary; papillary, adenoid cystic rare; tubular, Paget's disease 2%; apocrine 1%.
- **DCIS**: pre-malignant condition; 25–50% risk of breast cancer at 10–15 years; risk of metastasis and nodal invasion 1%. When DCIS recurs – 50% will be invasive tumours.

Paget's disease of the nipple

- Nipple skin infiltrated with large pale cells, then nipple erosion
- Associated with invasive or intraductal carcinoma

Features distinguishing eczema from Paget's disease

Paget's disease will start at the nipple with some evidence of destruction. Eczema may predominantly affect the areola.

	Eczema	**Paget's disease**
Cause	Atopy	Ductal carcinoma involving epidermis
Bilateral	Yes	No
Vesicular	Yes	No
Pruritus	Yes	No

Pathological prognostic factors

- Positive nodes – cancerous invasion of regional nodes
  >5 positive nodes – survival <20%
  Sampling lower axillary nodes or axillary clearance
- Tumour grade – cytological and structural pattern of tumour
  Bloom and Richardson grading system: Grade 1 (well-differentiated) to Grade 3 (poorly differentiated); based on tubule formation, nuclear pleomorphism and mitotic activity
- Tumour size – the bigger the tumour the worse the prognosis
- Vascular invasion in primary tumour and multicentricity – poor prognosis
- Oestrogen receptor protein in primary tumour based on histochemical (H) score out of 300: ER +ve – Estrogen receptor positive, H Score >50; ER -ve – Estrogen receptor negative, H score <50

Tumour marker

- CA 15–3 mucin marker (two monoclonal antibodies)
- Increased in 55–100% advanced breast cancer
- Increased in 10–46% early breast cancer
- Poor prognosis if increased levels pre-therapy
- Poor prognosis and recurrence if increased post-therapy

Fine needle aspiration and needle core biopsy. There are two recognized methods of needle sampling:

- FNA: fine needle aspiration
- NCB: needle core biopsy

Pre-operative diagnostic sensitivity of >95%

Needle sample gradings

- **FNAC (cytology)**
  C1 inadequate
  C2 benign
  C3 equivocal
  C4 suspicious
  C5 malignant
- **NCBH (histology)**
  B1 normal
  B2 benign breast tissue
  B3 equivocal
  B4 suspicious
  B5 malignant

Nottingham Prognostic Index (NPI)

Predicts survival for breast cancer. Depends on three pathological prognostic factors:

- Tumour size (max diameter in cm)
- Tumour grade (1 – well-differentiated to 3 – poorly differentiated)
- Lymph node involvement (stage 1: no lymph node, stage 2: 1–3 nodes, stage 3: >4 nodes or high lymph node)

Nottingham Prognostic Index (NPI)

NPI = size x 0.2 + stage + grade

Example:

- Prognosis is excellent if NPI <3.4 –15-year survival is 90%
- Prognosis is poor if NPI >5.4 – 15-year survival is 8%

Diagnosis: this is best achieved by attention to detail.

Triple assessment:

1. Clinical examination
2. Radiological – mammography (>35yr) or ultrasound (<35yr)
3. Pathological – cytology or histology (biopsy)

Multi-disciplinary clinical team working to clearly defined clinical protocols. Diagnostic breast team includes the surgeon, radiologist, pathologist and breast care nurse.

4.8 Management of breast cancer

The primary aim of surgery in the management of early breast cancer is to adequately stage disease to facilitate appropriate adjuvant therapy, and to prevent local recurrence. A secondary aim is to provide good cosmesis.

Radiotherapy reduces the risk of local recurrence after breast conserving surgery to a level similar to that seen after mastectomy. It is also used after mastectomy in poor prognostic groups to reduce local recurrence, but may also have a survival benefit (controversial).

The aim of adjuvant therapy (endocrine and chemotherapy) is to improve mortality and disease free survival.

In advanced disease the aim of surgery is to improve symptoms of local disease. Systemic therapy is used to prolong survival and prevent disease progression. Neo-adjuvant therapy (chemotherapy before surgery) is used to downstage inoperable disease to operable disease (control of local symptoms). It can also be used to reduce the size of large tumours to make breast conserving surgery possible instead of mastectomy. It does not prolong survival.

Treatment options

There is no single best method of treatment of breast cancer – each case has to be taken on its own merits and decisions made as part of a multidisciplinary approach, which must include the patient herself.

Surgery

- Many breast conserving operations (WLE, quadrantectomy or segmentectomy)
- Little data to distinguish between them
- Aim is to remove the tumour and obtain clear resection margins
- Less than 5 mm is inadequate, and less than 1 mm incomplete
- Incomplete excision requires further wide local excision or mastectomy. If margins are still inadequate after the second wide local excision, statistics show that complete excision can only be achieved by mastectomy
- Whole breast radiotherapy is required after breast conserving surgery to ensure low local recurrence rates. It is not a substitute for inadequate margins
- Local recurrence rates of up to 5% at 5 years are acceptable

- Mastectomy removes 90% of the breast tissue
- Adequate skin flaps are required for cover
- Radiotherapy is given post-operatively if the risk of local recurrence is thought to be high (>15%), the poor prognostic factors associated with this include large tumour, Grade 3, positive lymph nodes or vascular invasion
- Reconstruction may be immediate or delayed
- Many options for reconstruction and they should be discussed with the patient
- Immediate skin sparing mastectomy and reconstruction with Becker prosthesis or free/pedicled flaps
- Delayed reconstruction with tissue expansion or free/pedicled flap

Management of the axilla

The status of the nodes of the axilla is one of the main prognostic indicators and determines the need for further adjuvant treatment. The only way to assess the nodes accurately is histologically.

- The axilla can be sampled or cleared.
- Sampling provides diagnostic information, but may miss positive nodes as only four are removed (so called skip nodes).
- The axilla can be cleared to three levels.
- Level II clearance – all nodes up to medial border of pectoralis minor being removed, is accepted as the best balance between adequate staging and morbidity (lymphoedema)
- Sentinel node technique attempts to identify the first draining lymph node
- Combination of technetium and a blue dye.
- Histological examination
- Radiotherapy may be used to treat the axilla if positive nodes are found on sampling – alternatively a surgical clearance to level II can be performed
- The axilla is cleared or irradiated to prevent loco-regional recurrence – no reduction in mortality is achieved
- Both surgery and radiotherapy can cause lymphoedema, however if both are given the rate is much increased

Systemic treatment

Can be given as primary therapy prior to loco-regional treatment or as adjuvant therapy following treatment.

Hormonal therapy

- Usually given as a post-operative adjuvant or treatment of systemic disease
- Tamoxifen can be used as primary treatment in the elderly

- **1st line**

Tamoxifen – Selective Estrogen Receptor Modulator (SERM) peripheral oestrogen antagonist
Reduce circulating oestradiol
Others – **faslodex** = pure anti-oestrogen

- **2nd line**

Aromatase inhibitors – blocks oestrogen via the aromatase pathway:
Licensed for first-line treatment in post-menopausal women:
Anastrazole (Arimidex) blocks oestrogen pathway but not oestradiol
Formestane (Lenetran) only blocks oestrogen
Aminoglutethimide (Orimeten) also blocks production of other steroids therefore need
steroid replacement therapy
Letrozole (Femara) only blocks oestrogen

LHRH antagonist – prevents oestrogen production by the ovaries: used in pre-menopausal
women
Goserelin (Zoladex)

- **3rd line**

Progesterone, megestrol (Megace)
Medroxyprogesterone (Provera)

Chemotherapy

- Many chemotherapeutic agents are effective
- Cyclophosphamide
- Methotrexate
- 5–fluorouracil
- Doxorubicin
- Epirubicin
- Vincristine
- Taxols – useful in advanced disease, adjuvant value being evaluated
- Response rates of about 50%
- Significant side-effects (bone marrow depression, nausea, vomiting, diarrhoea and
  alopecia)
- Corticosteroids and ondansetron have helped

Adjuvant therapy

Tamoxifen reduces the death rate at 10 years by 5.6% for node negative women and 10.9%
for node positive women. This is increased in women over the age of 50. ER –ve patients
gain a small benefit with tamoxifen if they have nodal involvement.

Adjuvant chemotherapy reduces mortality in the medium term. The absolute survival benefit
at 10 years is 6–8%. Chemotherapy reduces the annual risk of death by 30% for at least 10
years. Absolute reduction in death rate depends on the chance of dying. A 30% reduction
in the relative risk of odds of dying reduces a 10% mortality (low risk group) at 10 years by
3% and a 60% mortality (higher risk group) by 20%.

It is accepted that for most patients this benefit results from a delay in the onset of recurrence rather than a long-term cure. Premenopausal women benefit most from chemotherapy and those with positive nodes show the greatest benefit of all. All premenopausal node positive women should be offered chemotherapy. It should also be considered and discussed with fit postmenopausal women with poorly differentiated tumours and positive nodes and node negative premenopausal women with other poor prognostic features.

There is now evidence to suggest that Zoladex by itself or in combination with tamoxifen is as effective as adjuvant chemotherapy in young women with poor prognosis ER+ disease (ZEBRA trial).

Follow up

Clinical follow up of breast cancer patients has not been shown to have any benefit in terms of mortality but has been shown to provide psychological support. In addition it provides a convenient focal point for mammographic follow up and a point of contact for patients with concerns or new symptoms.

- Early detection and treatment of local recurrence
- Detection of local recurrence – a marker of adequacy of original surgery and quality of histological reporting
- Assess contralateral breast
- Detect psychiatric morbidity
- Provide a prosthesis
- Early detection and treatment of metastatic disease
- Audit

Annual follow up is sufficient once treatment is complete.

Advanced disease

Advanced disease can be conveniently thought of as any breast cancer beyond stage 1 or 2 (see above).

Patients may present with

- Advanced disease (suggestive of aggressive tumour behaviour or neglect)
- Local recurrence or disseminated disease (blood or lymphatics)
- Lymphatic dissemination
- Supraclavicular fossa, internal mammary nodes, intra-thoracic and intra-abdominal nodes
- Blood borne dissemination
- Lungs
- Liver
- Brain
- Bone (esp ER +ve tumours)

Treatment

- Treatment of advanced breast cancer is complex
- A good response to treatment of a patient with advanced breast cancer can be defined as prolongation of survival with good quality of life
- Treatment of lesions that pose a threat to life or function should be identified, monitored and treated.

Palliation

- Must treat all aspects of the patients disease including emotional and psychological
- Surgery can be used to treat unpleasant local disease and may require chest wall reconstruction to achieve this
- Analgesia
- Radiotherapy for symptomatic bony metastasis
- Antiemetics

Recurrence

Late recurrences are well documented and no woman can ever be assured that she is cured; however studies have shown that early diagnosis and treatment reduce the number of deaths (HIP and Swedish studies).

Recurrences are classified into:

- **Local recurrence**: local involvement of the breast or chest wall. Single spot, multiple spot or field recurrence.
- **Regional recurrence**: regional spread to axilla, brachial plexus and supraclavicular nodes, lymphoedema.
- **Distant metastases**: metastases to bone, lungs and liver and brain. Hypercalcaemia, pleural effusion, jaundice.

Palliative treatment for associated symptoms

- Blood transfusion for anaemia
- Bisphosphonates or radiotherapy for bone pain
- Orthopaedic fixation for pathological fractures
- Bisphosphonates for hypercalcaemia
- Chest drainage and pleurodesis for pleural effusion
- Adequate analgesia
- Social and psychological support

DCIS

DCIS is a proliferation of malignant cells within the duct system that has not yet breached the basement membrane and as such is not capable of metastasising. Positive lymph nodes are found in 1% of cases of pure DCIS and this is thought to be due to small invasive tumours missed by histological sectioning.

DCIS is significant because up to a third of these lesions will go on to become invasive cancers – this may be higher in high grade DCIS. Clearance of disease is also important, as recurrent disease will be invasive in 50% of cases. It is accepted that low grade DCIS is associated with low grade invasive tumours and high grade DCIS with high grade invasive tumours.

DCIS makes up 3–4% of symptomatic and 25% of screen detected cancers.

Treatment of DCIS

- Ductal Carcinoma *in situ* has a good prognosis and can be cured by total mastectomy (5 year survival 98%)
- Localised DCIS (<4cm)
  Wide local excision with clear margins
  Consider radiotherapy
  Consider tamoxifen
- Widespread DCIS(>4cm)
  Mastectomy
  Consider tamoxifen

Breast Cancer prevention

The NSABP P1 trial of tamoxifen chemoprevention showed a 50% reduction in the risk of invasive ER+ breast cancer across all sub-groups. The relative risk of developing endometrial cancer was 2.53. There was also a slight increase in thromboembolic events in women over 50. Risk reduction can be achieved by life style changes; these include avoiding postmenopausal weight gain, regular exercise in adult life and a low fat, vitamin C rich diet.

Management of women at high risk

Are usually managed within the Family History Clinic at a Specialist Breast Unit. The clinic provides

- Regular screening
- Referral to genetics centre for High Risk women
- Bilateral prophylactic mastectomy with/out reconstruction when indicated (BRCA carriers)
- One study has shown prophylactic oophorectomy reduces the risk of breast cancer by 70% and is one strategy available for high risk women from breast/ovarian families (avoids mastectomy)

5. SCREENING, AUDIT AND ECONOMICS

5.1 Screening

In order to reduce mortality from various cancers, screening programmes have been set up to try to detect cancer at an early curable stage. Examples of current population-based screening programmes for women in the UK include cervical and breast cancer.

Screening test prerequisites (WHO – Wilson and Junger, 1968)

- Sensitive, i.e. detects most cases, few false negatives
- Specific, i.e. detects only certain disease, few false positives
- Safe
- Acceptable test with high compliance
- Inexpensive
- Disease must be important; natural history must be understood
- Facilities for treatment available
- Benefits outweigh adverse effects
- There must be a detectable latent or pre-clinical phase
- Screening must result in reduced mortality and morbidity
- Results must be audited and criteria must be met

Requirements of a screening programme

- Accurate register of people to be screened, i.e. those at risk
- Available resources

Advantages and disadvantages of a screening programme

- **Advantages**
  Increased survival
  Reduced radical therapy
  Reduced costs in treatment
  Reassurance

- **Disadvantages**
  Increased morbidity with unaffected
    prognosis
  Excessive therapy of doubtful cases
  Increased anxiety
  Lack of co-operation of target
    population
  Costs involved in the screening process
  Dangers of screening
  Ineffective screening tests
    (low sensitivity and specificity)
  False reassurance

NHS screening programme for breast cancer

- Set up in 1987 following recommendation by the Forrest report
- All 50–64-year-old women are invited for three-yearly screening
- First mammogram has two views, thereafter single oblique view mammogram taken
- Abnormal mammograms are recalled to specialist breast units for further assessment and treatment
- Trials have shown reduction in mortality following randomized trials of mammography
- Approximately one-quarter of cancers detected are not palpable clinically

New recommendation for breast screening

- All 49–64-year-old women to be invited for three-yearly screening
- Double view mammograms taken on first round visit
- Single view on subsequent visit
- Self-referral after age 65
- Single radiological reading

Cervical cancer screening programme

- Begins three years following commencement of sexual activity
- False negative rate is 10%
- Very labour intensive
- Compliance about 80%
- Lower compliance in lower social classes

Colorectal cancer

- For family history of FAPC and other high-risk populations, not general population
- Ideal test is colonoscopy, but low compliance and costly
- FOB: low sensitivity, low specificity

Carcinoma of the stomach

- Only in Japan
- Incidence is declining

5.2 Audit

Definition: *Interdisciplinary process by which clinical staff collectively review, evaluate and improve their practice with the common aim of improving standards.*

Functions:

- Encourage improvement in clinical procedure
- Educate all members of the team
- Raise overall quality of clinical care
- Compare with current best practice
- Provides peer comparison

Requirements of College

- Audits in each surgical discipline
- Everyone attends (all disciplines)
- One consultant is responsible for the audit programme
- Must be undertaken regularly
- Records are kept

Data

From medical notes, notes audit is required regularly. Data should investigate:

- Access patients have to care (e.g. waiting time, cancellations)
- Process (e.g. investigations)
- Outcome (e.g. deaths, complications)
- Organization of hospital, resources
- Financial implications

Should be consultant-led (has to be in attendance)

Minutes of meeting must include:

- Who attends
- Topics discussed
- Conclusions and recommendations
- Date for reviewing the topic
- Action to be taken on unresolved topics

Evidence of regular audit meetings is mandatory for educational approval of training posts.

National Confidential Enquiry into Peri-operative Deaths

- Aim is to improve standards of surgical practice
- Can recommend actions for specific clinical situations
- Independent of DOH

Medical audit

- Doctors looking at what they do

Clinical audit

- Interdisciplinary

Audit of structure, process or outcome

- **Structure**: 'Availability and organization of resources required for the delivery of a service' (e.g. resources can include staff, equipment, accommodation)
- **Process**: 'The way the patient is received and managed by the service from time of referral to discharge'
- **Outcome**: 'Results of clinical intention'

Constructing an audit

- Standard: best practice
- Indicator: thing to be measured
- Target: what would be the desired result
- Monitoring method: method of data collection, who is collecting and frequency

The audit cycle

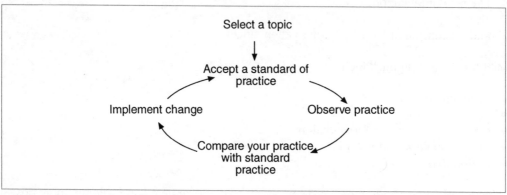

Audit cycle

5.3 Economic aspects of surgical care

QUALY – Quality Adjusted Life Year

Clinical 'profit': the gain expected from a clinical decision once the patient has paid the price of pain, disability and financial loss whilst under treatment.

Laboratory tests

Sensitivity: number with the condition who had a positive result/total number tested with the condition.

Specificity: number tested who had negative result/number tested who did have the condition.

When selecting a test consider:

- Sensitivity and specificity
- Cost
- Probability of diagnosis
- Cost per day in hospital whilst awaiting test

Cost of complications

Infections

- Prolonged hospital stay
- Antibiotics
- Cost of investigations

Post-operative bleeding

- Prolonged hospital stay
- Re-operation
- Investigations
- Replacement blood
- ICU bed

6. SUGGESTED FURTHER READING

Concise notes in oncology, Mokbel, K, 1999, Petroc Press, Newbury.
Pathology: Basic and systemic, Woolf, N, 1998, WB. Saunders + Co, London.

Index

411